Chemistry of Materials for Energy and Environmental Sustainability

Chemistry of Materials for Energy and Environmental Sustainability

Guest Editor
Qingguo Shao

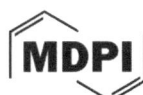

Basel • Beijing • Wuhan • Barcelona • Belgrade • Novi Sad • Cluj • Manchester

Guest Editor
Qingguo Shao
School of Intelligent Manufacturing
and Control Engineering
Shandong Institute of Petroleum
and Chemical Technology
Dongying
China

Editorial Office
MDPI AG
Grosspeteranlage 5
4052 Basel, Switzerland

This is a reprint of the Special Issue, published open access by the journal *Molecules* (ISSN 1420-3049), freely accessible at: www.mdpi.com/journal/molecules/special_issues/773D78MXR4.

For citation purposes, cite each article independently as indicated on the article page online and using the guide below:

Lastname, A.A.; Lastname, B.B. Article Title. *Journal Name* **Year**, *Volume Number*, Page Range.

ISBN 978-3-7258-3088-6 (Hbk)
ISBN 978-3-7258-3087-9 (PDF)
https://doi.org/10.3390/books978-3-7258-3087-9

Cover image courtesy of Qingguo Shao

© 2025 by the authors. Articles in this book are Open Access and distributed under the Creative Commons Attribution (CC BY) license. The book as a whole is distributed by MDPI under the terms and conditions of the Creative Commons Attribution-NonCommercial-NoDerivs (CC BY-NC-ND) license (https://creativecommons.org/licenses/by-nc-nd/4.0/).

Contents

About the Editor vii

Preface ix

Qinguo Shao
Chemistry of Materials for Energy and Environmental Sustainability
Reprinted from: *Molecules* **2024**, *29*, 5929, https://doi.org/10.3390/molecules29245929 1

Yu Liu, Yan Li, Zhuohao Liu, Tao Feng, Huichuan Lin and Gang Li et al.
Uniform P-Doped MnMoO$_4$ Nanosheets for Enhanced Asymmetric Supercapacitors Performance
Reprinted from: *Molecules* **2024**, *29*, 1988, https://doi.org/10.3390/molecules29091988 6

Talgat M. Inerbaev, Aisulu U. Abuova, Zhadyra Ye. Zakiyeva, Fatima U. Abuova, Yuri A. Mastrikov and Maksim Sokolov et al.
Effect of Rh Doping on Optical Absorption and Oxygen Evolution Reaction Activity on BaTiO$_3$ (001) Surfaces
Reprinted from: *Molecules* **2024**, *29*, 2707, https://doi.org/10.3390/molecules29112707 21

Kaijie Ni, Yanlong Chen, Ruiqi Xu, Yuming Zhao and Ming Guo
Mapping Photogenerated Electron–Hole Behavior of Graphene Oxide: Insight into a New Mechanism of Photosensitive Pollutant Degradation
Reprinted from: *Molecules* **2024**, *29*, 3765, https://doi.org/10.3390/molecules29163765 36

Wenjing Chen, Hong Yin, Ivan Cole, Shadi Houshyar and Lijing Wang
Carbon Dots Derived from Non-Biomass Waste: Methods, Applications, and Future Perspectives
Reprinted from: *Molecules* **2024**, *29*, 2441, https://doi.org/10.3390/molecules29112441 53

Bharti Gaur, Jyoti Mittal, Syed Ansar Ali Shah, Alok Mittal and Richard T. Baker
Sequestration of an Azo Dye by a Potential Biosorbent: Characterization of Biosorbent, Adsorption Isotherm and Adsorption Kinetic Studies
Reprinted from: *Molecules* **2024**, *29*, 2387, https://doi.org/10.3390/molecules29102387 74

Shasha Liu, Mei Sun, Can Wu, Kaixuan Zhu, Ying Hu and Meng Shan et al.
Fabrication of Loose Nanofiltration Membrane by Crosslinking TEMPO-Oxidized Cellulose Nanofibers for Effective Dye/Salt Separation
Reprinted from: *Molecules* **2024**, *29*, 2246, https://doi.org/10.3390/molecules29102246 90

Guoshun Liu, Xuhui Liu, Xingdong Ma, Xiaoqi Tang, Xiaobin Zhang and Jianxia Dong et al.
High-Performance Dual-Ion Battery Based on Silicon–Graphene Composite Anode and Expanded Graphite Cathode
Reprinted from: *Molecules* **2023**, *28*, 4280, https://doi.org/10.3390/molecules28114280 101

Geethanjali Kuppadakkath, Sreejith Sudhakaran Jayabhavan and Krishna K. Damodaran
Supramolecular Gels Based on C_3-Symmetric Amides: Application in Anion-Sensing and Removal of Dyes from Water
Reprinted from: *Molecules* **2024**, *29*, 2149, https://doi.org/10.3390/molecules29092149 113

Guangtao Fu and Xinfa Dong
Enhanced Stability of Dimethyl Ether Carbonylation through Pyrazole Tartrate on Tartaric Acid-Complexed Cobalt–Iron-Modified Hydrogen-Type Mordenite
Reprinted from: *Molecules* **2024**, *29*, 1510, https://doi.org/10.3390/molecules29071510 129

Haixia Xie, Lei Li, Jiawei Zhang, Yihao Zhang, Yong Pan and Jie Xu et al.
[BMP]$^+$[BF$_4$]$^-$-Modified CsPbI$_{1.2}$Br$_{1.8}$ Solar Cells with Improved Efficiency and Suppressed Photoinduced Phase Segregation
Reprinted from: *Molecules* **2024**, *29*, 1476, https://doi.org/10.3390/molecules29071476 . . . . . . **142**

Zhiwen Yang, Longjiang Li and Yalan Wang
Mechanism of Phosphate Desorption from Activated Red Mud Particle Adsorbents
Reprinted from: *Molecules* **2024**, *29*, 974, https://doi.org/10.3390/molecules29050974 . . . . . . **153**

Meng Wang, Tingting Huang, Meng Shan, Mei Sun, Shasha Liu and Hai Tang
Zwitterionic Tröger's Base Microfiltration Membrane Prepared via Vapor-Induced Phase Separation with Improved Demulsification and Antifouling Performance
Reprinted from: *Molecules* **2024**, *29*, 1001, https://doi.org/10.3390/molecules29051001 . . . . . . **171**

About the Editor

Qingguo Shao

Qingguo Shao received his Ph.D. in Materials Science and Engineering from the University of Tsukuba (Japan) in 2015. Then, he conducted postdoctoral studies at the National Institute for Materials Science (Japan) from 2015 to 2016 and the City University of Hong Kong (CityU) from 2016 to 2018. After that, he joined the China University of Petroleum (East China) as an Associate Professor. In 2024, he moved to the Shandong Institute of Petroleum and Chemical Technology. His research interests focus on the design and synthesis of novel nanomaterials for energy storage and conversion. He has published more than 40 peer reviewed academic papers in *Adv. Mater., Adv. Funct. Mater., J. Mater. Sci. Technol., Energy Storage Mater., J. Mater. Chem. A., Nano Research*, etc. His papers have been cited over 3000 times.

Preface

Today's industry trends are moving towards energy conservation, environmental protection, and planetary sustainability in the development of new products. Many efforts have been devoted to developing various renewable energy resources, such as wind, solar, and tidal energy sources. Due to the intermittent and uncontrollable characteristics of these energy resources, energy storage devices are required to deal with such problems. Advanced electrode materials are the key components of electrochemical energy systems. However, traditional electrode materials can no longer meet the needs of electrochemical materials in the fields of energy and environmental protection in the future. This reprint introduces the recent research progress made in the chemistry of materials for energy and environmental sustainability and comprises over 150,000 words. The topics included cover rational designed composite electrode materials for energy storage, effective additives for promoting solar cells, powerful adsorbents for hazardous dyes in water, versatile membranes for oil–water separation, etc. I hope that interested researchers and practitioners will be inspired by this content and find it valuable to their own research.

February 1, 2025.

Qingguo Shao
Guest Editor

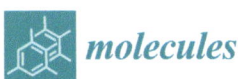

Editorial

Chemistry of Materials for Energy and Environmental Sustainability

Qinguo Shao [1,2,3]

[1] School of Intelligent Manufacturing and Control Engineering, Shandong Institute of Petroleum and Chemical Technology, Dongying 257061, China; qgshao@upc.edu.cn
[2] Dongying Key Laboratory of Mechanical Surface Engineering and Corrosion Protection, Shandong Institute of Petroleum and Chemical Technology, Dongying 257061, China
[3] Shandong Provincial Engineering Research Center for Green Manufacturing and Intelligent Control, Shandong Institute of Petroleum and Chemical Technology, Dongying 257061, China

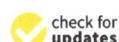

Citation: Shao, Q. Chemistry of Materials for Energy and Environmental Sustainability. *Molecules* **2024**, *29*, 5929. https://doi.org/10.3390/molecules29245929

Received: 12 December 2024
Accepted: 13 December 2024
Published: 16 December 2024

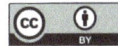

Copyright: © 2024 by the author. Licensee MDPI, Basel, Switzerland. This article is an open access article distributed under the terms and conditions of the Creative Commons Attribution (CC BY) license (https://creativecommons.org/licenses/by/4.0/).

In contemporary society, energy serves as the cornerstone of human survival and development, exerting a profound influence on the economic development of nations and the trajectory of global progress. On one hand, the gradual depletion of non-renewable resources coupled with the rapid escalation of energy demand poses significant challenges [1–3]. On the other hand, the combustion of fossil fuels such as coal and petroleum leads to atmospheric pollution and the emission of toxic gases, including sulfides, nitrides, and carbon dioxide contributing to the greenhouse effect, all of which have severely impacted the global climate and environment. Currently, air pollution has emerged as a pressing global issue. Consequently, research and development regarding clean energy sources play a pivotal role in ensuring the sustainable development of national economies [4–8]. Efforts are continuously being made to explore various renewable energy sources, including wind, solar, hydro, and tidal power, and notable progress has been achieved in this domain [9–15]. However, these renewable energy sources, which rely on natural conditions, inherently possess certain drawbacks. These include the intermittency of power generation, discontinuity in generation periods, and the uncontrollability of generation intensity, resulting in an unstable electrical output. Therefore, there is a crucial need for energy storage devices that can rapidly store this intermittent and unstable clean energy, thereby enabling the establishment of a continuous and stable energy supply system through these storage solutions. In all kinds of energy storage systems, electric energy storage systems occupy a key position, and batteries and electrochemical capacitors have become indispensable energy storage devices [16–19]. Advanced electrode materials are the key components of electrochemical energy systems. Strategies for increasing their energy densities include tailoring the chemistry, structure, and components of the electrode materials [20–26]. Although tremendous effort has been devoted to this field of research, revolutionary energy storage devices with both high energy densities and power densities still remain a challenge [27–33].

At the same time, with the rapid growth of the global population and the accelerated development of industry, freshwater resources are becoming increasingly scarce and severely polluted [34–41]. It is reported that by 2030, the world will face a shortage of potable water resources, and concerns over the safety of drinking water have also gained widespread attention. Approximately 3.1 million people die annually from diseases caused by unsafe drinking water. Water resource issues impact food production, industrial output, and environmental quality, further affecting the industrialized economic development of countries [42–53]. Therefore, the effective treatment of water pollution, the desalination of seawater resources, and the purification of drinking water resources are crucial means to address the current challenges [54–68].

The aim of this Special Issue is to publish original research articles and review papers on chemistry research regarding advanced materials relevant to energy and environmental sustainability. This Special Issue contains twelve papers, including one comprehensive review and eleven research papers. The review paper by Chen et al. [69] discusses carbon dots derived from non-biomass waste. The authors introduce various preparation methods, diverse applications, and future challenges of carbon dots. In this Special Issue, several papers focus on energy storage and conversion materials. Liu et al. [70] develop a high-performance dual-ion battery using a silicon–graphene composite as the anode and expanded graphite as the cathode. In this design, the stress/strain induced by electrode volume change during charging and discharging can be suppressed and the obtained full Si@G//EG DIBs exhibit a high energy density of 367.84 Wh kg^{-1} at a power density of 855.43 W kg^{-1}. This work sheds some light on the practical applications of high-energy DIBs. Manganese molybdate has been regarded as a promising electrode material for supercapacitors. However, its low electrical conductivity mainly blocks its application in practice. Liu and Li et al. [71] synthesize phosphorus-doped $MnMoO_4 \cdot H_2O$ nanosheets by means of a hydrothermal method and use them as an electrode material in an asymmetric supercapacitor. Owing to the phosphorus–metal bonds and oxygen vacancies induced by phosphorus element doping, the charge storage and conductivity of the electrode are increased, thereby resulting in enhanced electrochemical properties with a high energy density of 41.9 Wh kg^{-1} under 666.8 W kg^{-1}. Xie et al. [72] study the effect of $[BMP]^+$ $[BF4]^-$ additives on the performance of $CsPbI_{1.2}Br_{1.8}$ solar cells. It is found that the additive could effectively reduce the phase segregation phenomenon of the $CsPbI_{1.2}Br_{1.8}$ films. Inerbaev et al. [73] present a calculation result demonstrating that doping $BaTiO_3$ with Rh could reduce the overpotential of oxygen evolution when it was used as a catalyst. Rh doping could expand the spectrum of absorbed light to the entire visible range. Gaur et al. [74] report using hen feathers as an adsorbent in aqueous media. Their results show that hen feathers exhibit high impressive adsorption efficiency towards Metanil Yellow dye. Liu et al. [75] develop a high-performance nanofiltration membrane which exhibits a rejection rate of over 99% for various dyes. The nanofiltration is prepared using TEMPO-oxidized cellulose nanofibers via the vacuum filtration method. Yang et al. [76] report the use of activated red mud particles as adsorbents for phosphorus adsorption and the possible mechanism is examined by means of morphology analysis, FTIR, EDS, and mineral composition analysis. Kuppadakkath et al. [77] demonstrate that modified BTA molecules show anion-responsive properties and that they can also be used as adsorbents for hazardous dyes in water. Ni et al. [78] reveal that the mechanism of degradation of the photosensitive pollutant tetracycline is promoted by GO, which offers reference value for research in wastewater treatment. Wang et al. [79] prepare a new zwitterionic polymer and use it to construct microfiltration membranes. Their experiment showed that the as-prepared membranes exhibit excellent efficiency in oil–water separation. Fu et al. [80] prepare a cobalt–iron bimetallic modified hydrogen-type mordenite by means of the ion exchange method, which shows superior DME carbonylation catalytic activity and stability. In addition, the possible reasons for the improvement are clarified.

In summary, this Special Issue presents the latest research on the chemistry of materials for energy and environmental sustainability. From rationally designed composite electrode materials for energy storage and effective additives for promoting solar cells to powerful adsorbents of hazardous dyes in water and versatile membranes for oil–water separation, these reports showcase the state-of-the art material tailoring in the energy and environmental sustainability field. The advances in this Special Issue may shed some new light on possible solutions to energy and environmental challenges.

Funding: This work was funded by the Dongying Science Development Fund.

Conflicts of Interest: The author declares no conflicts of interest.

References

1. Padhi, A.K.; Nanjundaswamy, K.S.; Goodenough, J.B. Phospho-olivines as positive-electrode materials for rechargeable lithium batteries. *J. Electrochem. Soc.* **1997**, *144*, 1188–1194. [CrossRef]
2. Liu, J.-H.; Wang, P.; Gao, Z.; Li, X.; Cui, W.; Li, R.; Ramakrishna, S.; Zhang, J.; Long, Y.-Z. Review on electrospinning anode and separators for lithium ion batteries. *Renew. Sustain. Energy Rev.* **2024**, *189*, 113939. [CrossRef]
3. Zang, X.; Li, L.; Meng, J.; Liu, L.; Pan, Y.; Shao, Q.; Cao, N. Enhanced zinc storage performance of mixed valent manganese oxide for flexible coaxial fiber zinc-ion battery by limited reduction control. *J. Mater. Sci. Technol.* **2021**, *74*, 52–59. [CrossRef]
4. Zhang, X.; Tang, Y.; Zhang, F.; Lee, C.-S. A Novel Aluminum–Graphite Dual-Ion Battery. *Adv. Energy Mater.* **2016**, *6*, 1502588. [CrossRef]
5. Guyomard, D.; Tarascon, J.M. Rocking-chair or Lithium-ion rechargeable Lithium batteries. *Adv. Mater.* **1994**, *6*, 408–412. [CrossRef]
6. Cao, N.; Guo, J.; Cai, K.; Xue, Q.; Zhu, L.; Shao, Q.; Gu, X.; Zang, X. Functionalized carbon fiber felts with selective superwettability and fire retardancy: Designed for efficient oil/water separation. *Sep. Purif. Technol.* **2020**, *251*, 117308. [CrossRef]
7. Liu, X.; Ma, X.; Liu, G.; Zhang, X.; Tang, X.; Li, C.; Zang, X.; Cao, N.; Shao, Q. Polyaniline spaced MoS_2 nanosheets with increased interlayer distances for constructing high-rate dual-ion batteries. *J. Mater. Sci. Technol.* **2024**, *182*, 220–230. [CrossRef]
8. Luo, P.; Zheng, C.; He, J.; Tu, X.; Sun, W.; Pan, H.; Zhou, Y.; Rui, X.; Zhang, B.; Huang, K. Structural Engineering in Graphite-Based Metal-Ion Batteries. *Adv. Funct. Mater.* **2021**, *32*, 2107277. [CrossRef]
9. Li, C.; Liu, B.; Jiang, N.; Ding, Y. Elucidating the charge-transfer and Li-ion-migration mechanisms in commercial lithium-ion batteries with advanced electron microscopy. *Nano Res. Energy* **2022**, *1*, 9120031. [CrossRef]
10. Yu, T.; Li, G.; Duan, Y.; Wu, Y.; Zhang, T.; Zhao, X.; Luo, M.; Liu, Y. The research and industrialization progress and prospects of sodium ion battery. *J. Alloys Compd.* **2023**, *958*, 170486. [CrossRef]
11. Ji, B.; Zhang, F.; Song, X.; Tang, Y. A Novel Potassium-Ion-Based Dual-Ion Battery. *Adv. Mater.* **2017**, *29*, 1700519. [CrossRef]
12. Zhao, W.; Ma, X.; Gao, L.; Wang, X.; Luo, Y.; Wang, Y.; Li, T.; Ying, B.; Zheng, D.; Sun, S.; et al. Hierarchical Architecture Engineering of Branch-Leaf-Shaped Cobalt Phosphosulfide Quantum Dots: Enabling Multi-Dimensional Ion-Transport Channels for High-Efficiency Sodium Storage. *Adv. Mater.* **2024**, *36*, 2305190. [CrossRef]
13. Shao, Q.; Tang, X.; Liu, X.; Qi, H.; Dong, J.; Liu, Q.; Ma, X.; Zhang, X.; Zang, X.; Cao, N. Hierarchical nanosheets-assembled hollow $NiCo_2O_4$ nanoboxes for high-performance asymmetric supercapacitors. *J. Energy Storage* **2023**, *73*, 108944. [CrossRef]
14. Zheng, C.; Wu, J.; Li, Y.; Liu, X.; Zeng, L.; Wei, M. High-Performance Lithium-Ion-Based Dual-Ion Batteries Enabled by Few-Layer $MoSe_2$/Nitrogen-Doped Carbon. *ACS Sustain. Chem. Eng.* **2020**, *8*, 5514–5523. [CrossRef]
15. Cao, N.; Chen, S.; Di, Y.; Li, C.; Qi, H.; Shao, Q.; Zhao, W.; Qin, Y.; Zang, X. High efficiency in overall water-splitting via Co-doping heterointerface-rich NiS_2/MoS_2 nanosheets electrocatalysts. *Electrochim. Acta* **2022**, *425*, 140674. [CrossRef]
16. Liu, X.; Ma, X.; Zhang, X.; Liu, G.; Li, C.; Liang, L.; Dong, J.; Tang, X.; Zang, X.; Cao, N.; et al. Insertion of $AlCl_3$ in graphite as both cation and anion insertion host for dual-ion battery. *J. Energy Storage* **2023**, *72*, 108687. [CrossRef]
17. Liu, W.; Gao, P.; Mi, Y.Y.; Chen, J.T.; Zhou, H.H.; Zhang, X.X. Fabrication of high tap density $LiFe_{0.6}Mn_{0.4}PO_4$/C microspheres by a double carbon coating-spray drying method for high rate lithium ion batteries. *J. Mater. Chem. A* **2013**, *1*, 2411–2417. [CrossRef]
18. Hou, H.; Qiu, X.; Wei, W.; Zhang, Y.; Ji, X. Carbon Anode Materials for Advanced Sodium-Ion Batteries. *Adv. Energy Mater.* **2017**, *7*, 1602898. [CrossRef]
19. Wei, C.; Liu, C.; Xiao, Y.; Wu, Z.; Luo, Q.; Jiang, Z.; Wang, Z.; Zhang, L.; Cheng, S.; Yu, C. SnF_2-induced multifunctional interface-stabilized $Li_{5.5}PS_{4.5}Cl_{1.5}$-based all-solid-state lithium metal batteries. *Adv. Funct. Mater.* **2024**, *34*, 2314306. [CrossRef]
20. Zang, X.; Zhou, C.; Shang, Q.; Yu, S.; Qin, Y.; Lin, X.; Cao, N. One-step synthesis of MoS_2 nanosheet arrays on 3D carbon fiber felts as a highly efficient catalyst for the hydrogen evolution reaction. *Energy Technol.* **2019**, *7*, 1900052. [CrossRef]
21. Luo, X.-F.; Yang, C.-H.; Peng, Y.-Y.; Pu, N.-W.; Ger, M.-D.; Hsieh, C.-T.; Chang, J.-K. Graphene nanosheets, carbon nanotubes, graphite, and activated carbon as anode materials for sodium-ion batteries. *J. Mater. Chem. A* **2015**, *3*, 10320–10326. [CrossRef]
22. Tan, H.; Chen, D.; Rui, X.; Yu, Y. Peering into Alloy Anodes for Sodium-Ion Batteries: Current Trends, Challenges, and Opportunities. *Adv. Funct. Mater.* **2019**, *29*, 1808745. [CrossRef]
23. Ma, X.; Liu, X.; Liu, G.; Tang, X.; Zhang, X.; Ma, Y.; Gao, Y.; Zang, X.; Cao, N.; Shao, Q. Superior dual-ion batteries enabled by mildly expanded graphite cathode and hierarchical MoS_2@C anode. *Electrochim. Acta* **2024**, *474*, 143568. [CrossRef]
24. Wang, Z.; Du, Z.; Wang, L.; He, G.; Parkin, I.P.; Zhang, Y.; Yue, Y. Disordered materials for high-performance lithium-ion batteries: A review. *Nano Energy* **2024**, *121*, 109250. [CrossRef]
25. Cao, N.; Zhang, X.; Li, Q.; Liu, X.; Ma, X.; Liu, G.; Tang, X.; Li, C.; Zang, X.; Shao, Q. The role of nitrogen-doping on the electrochemical behavior of MOF-derived carbons in ionic liquid electrolytes. *Diam. Relat. Mater.* **2023**, *139*, 110412. [CrossRef]
26. Zheng, P.; Sun, J.; Liu, H.; Wang, R.; Liu, C.; Zhao, Y.; Li, J.; Zheng, Y.; Rui, X. Microstructure Engineered Silicon Alloy Anodes for Lithium-Ion Batteries: Advances and Challenges. *Batter. Supercaps* **2023**, *6*, e202200481. [CrossRef]
27. Han, Y.; Qi, P.; Feng, X.; Li, S.; Fu, X.; Li, H.; Chen, Y.; Zhou, J.; Li, X.; Wang, B. In Situ Growth of MOFs on the Surface of Si Nanoparticles for Highly Efficient Lithium Storage: Si@MOF Nanocomposites as Anode Materials for Lithium-Ion Batteries. *ACS Appl. Mater. Interfaces* **2015**, *7*, 2178–2182. [CrossRef] [PubMed]
28. Niu, J.; Zhang, S.; Niu, Y.; Song, H.; Chen, X.; Zhou, J. Silicon-Based Anode Materials for Lithium-Ion Batteries. *Prog. Chem.* **2015**, *27*, 1275–1290.

29. Wang, S.; Jiao, S.; Tian, D.; Chen, H.-S.; Jiao, H.; Tu, J.; Liu, Y.; Fang, D.-N. A Novel Ultrafast Rechargeable Multi-Ions Battery. *Adv. Mater.* **2017**, *29*, 1606349. [CrossRef]
30. Cheng, F.Q.; Wan, W.; TAN, Z.; Huang, Y.Y.; Zhou, H.H.; Chen, J.T.; Zhang, X.X. High power performance of nano-LiFePO$_4$/C cathode material synthesized via lauric acid-assisted solid-state reaction. *Electrochim. Acta* **2011**, *56*, 2999–3005. [CrossRef]
31. Shao, Q.; Liu, X.; Dong, J.; Liang, L.; Zhang, Q.; Li, P.; Yang, S.; Zang, X.; Cao, N. Vulcanization conditions of bimetallic sulfides under different sulfur sources for supercapacitors: A review. *J. Electron. Mater.* **2023**, *52*, 1769–1784. [CrossRef]
32. Zhang, S.S.; Allen, J.L.; Xu, K.; Jow, T.R. Optimization of reaction condition for solid-state synthesis of LiFePO$_4$ -C composite cathodes. *J. Power Sources* **2005**, *147*, 234–240. [CrossRef]
33. Ding, X.; Zhou, Q.; Li, X.; Xiong, X. Fast-charging anodes for lithium ion batteries: Progress and challenges. *Chem. Commun.* **2024**, *60*, 2472–2488. [CrossRef] [PubMed]
34. Jaspal, D.; Malviya, A. Composites for wastewater purification: A review. *Chemosphere* **2020**, *246*, 125788. [CrossRef]
35. Yangui, A.; Abderrabba, M.; Sayari, A. Amine-modified mesoporous silica for quantitative adsorption and release of hydroxytyrosol and other phenolic compounds from olive mill wastewater. *J. Taiwan Inst. Chem. Eng.* **2017**, *70*, 111–118. [CrossRef]
36. Sharma, V.K.; Jinadatha, C.; Lichtfouse, E. Environmental chemistry is most relevant to study coronavirus pandemics. *Environ. Chem. Lett.* **2020**, *18*, 993–996. [CrossRef]
37. Sarkar, S.; Banerjee, A.; Halder, U.; Biswas, R.; Bandopadhyay, R. Degradation of Synthetic Azo Dyes of Textile Industry: A Sustainable Approach Using Microbial Enzymes. *Water Conserv. Sci. Eng.* **2017**, *2*, 121–131. [CrossRef]
38. Zare, E.N.; Motahari, A.; Sillanpää, M. Nanoadsorbents based on conducting polymer nanocomposites with main focus on polyaniline and its derivatives for removal of heavy metal ions/dyes: A review. *Environ. Res.* **2018**, *162*, 173–195. [CrossRef] [PubMed]
39. Bazoti, F.N.; Gikas, E.; Skaltsounis, A.L.; Tsarbopoulos, A. Development of a liquid chromatography–electrospray ionization tandem mass spectrometry (LC–ESI MS/MS) method for the quantification of bioactive substances present in olive oil mill wastewaters. *Anal. Chim. Acta* **2006**, *573*, 258–266. [CrossRef] [PubMed]
40. Al-Qodah, Z.; Al-Shannag, M.; Bani-Melhem, K.; Assirey, E.; Alananbeh, K.; Bouqellah, N. Biodegradation of olive mills wastewater using thermophilic bacteria. *Desalination Water Treat.* **2015**, *56*, 1908–1917. [CrossRef]
41. Tara, N.; Siddiqui, S.; Rathi, G.; Inamuddin, I.; Asiri, A.M. Nano-engineered adsorbent for removal of dyes from water: A review. *Curr. Anal. Chem.* **2019**, *16*, 14–40. [CrossRef]
42. Raiti, J.; Hafidi, A. Mixed micelles-mediated dephenolisation of table olive processing's wastewaters. *Water Sci. Technol.* **2015**, *72*, 2132–2138. [CrossRef] [PubMed]
43. Saeed, M.; Khan, I.; Adeel, M.; Akram, N.; Muneer, M. Synthesis of a CoO–ZnO photocatalyst for enhanced visible-light assisted photodegradation of methylene blue. *New J. Chem.* **2022**, *46*, 2224–2231. [CrossRef]
44. Sheng, W.; Shi, J.-L.; Hao, H.; Li, X.; Lang, X. Polyimide-TiO2 Hybrid Photocatalysis: Visible Light-Promoted Selective Aerobic Oxidation of Amines. *Chem. Eng. J.* **2020**, *379*, 122399. [CrossRef]
45. Meng, A.; Zhang, L.; Cheng, B.; Yu, J. Dual Cocatalysts in TiO2 Photocatalysis. *Adv. Mater.* **2019**, *31*, 1807660. [CrossRef] [PubMed]
46. Jamrah, A.; Al-Zghoul, T.M.; Darwish, M.M. A comprehensive review of combined processes for olive mill wastewater treatments. *Case Stud. Chem. Environ. Eng.* **2023**, *8*, 100493. [CrossRef]
47. Neffa, M.; Hanine, H.; Lekhlif, B.; Taourirt, M.; Habbari, K. Treatment of wastewaters olive mill by electrocoagulation and biological process. In Proceedings of the 2010: Proceedings from Linnaeus ECO-TECH'10, Kalmar, Sweden, 22–24 November 2010; pp. 295–304.
48. Hazra, S.; Dome, R.N.; Ghosh, S.; Ghosh, D. Protective effect of methanolic leaves extract of coriandrum sativum against metanil yellow induced lipid peroxidation in goat liver: An in vitro study. *Intern. J. Pharmacol. Pharmaceut. Sci.* **2016**, *3*, 34–41.
49. Ramchandani, S.; Das, M.; Joshi, A.; Khanna, S.K. Effect of oral and parenteral administration of metanil yellow on some hepatic and intestinal biochemical parameters. *J. Appl. Toxicol.* **1997**, *17*, 85–91. [CrossRef]
50. Rehman, K.; Fatima, F.; Waheed, I.; Akash, M.S.H. Prevalence of exposure of heavy metals and their impact on health consequences. *J. Cell. Biochem.* **2019**, *119*, 157–184. [CrossRef]
51. Roig, A.; Cayuela, M.L.; Sánchez-Monedero, M.A. An overview on olive mill wastes and their valorisation methods. *Waste Manag.* **2006**, *26*, 960–969. [CrossRef] [PubMed]
52. Sharma, G.; AlGarni, T.S.; Kumar, P.S.; Bhogal, S.; Kumar, A.; Sharma, S.; Naushad, M.; ALOthman, Z.A.; Stadler, F.J. Utilization of Ag$_2$O–Al$_2$O$_3$–ZrO$_2$ Decorated onto RGO as Adsorbent for the Removal of Congo Red from Aqueous Solution. *Environ. Res.* **2021**, *197*, 111179. [CrossRef] [PubMed]
53. Abhinaya, M.; Parthiban, R.; Kumar, P.S.; Vo, D.-V.N. A Review on Cleaner Strategies for Extraction of Chitosan and Its Application in Toxic Pollutant Removal. *Environ. Res.* **2021**, *196*, 110996. [CrossRef] [PubMed]
54. Xu, X.; Wang, W.; Zhou, W.; Shao, Z. Recent Advances in Novel Nanostructuring Methods of Perovskite Electrocatalysts for Energy-Related Applications. *Small Methods* **2018**, *2*, 1800071. [CrossRef]
55. Gupta, V.K.; Carrott, P.J.M.; Ribeiro Carrott, M.M.L.; Suhas. Low-cost adsorbents: Growing approach to wastewater treatment—A review. *Crit. Rev. Environ. Sci. Technol.* **2009**, *39*, 783–842. [CrossRef]
56. Khdair, I.A.; Abu-Rumman, G. Evaluation of the environmental pollution from olive mills wastewater. *Fresenius Environ. Bull.* **2017**, *26*, 2537–2540.

57. Chen, Y.-Z.; Zhang, R.; Jiao, L.; Jiang, H.-L. Metal-organic framework derived porous materials for catalysis. *Coord. Chem. Rev.* **2018**, *362*, 1–23. [CrossRef]
58. Ullah, S.; Al-Sehemi, A.G.; Mubashir, M.; Mukhtar, A.; Saqib, S.; Bustam, M.A.; Cheng, C.K.; Ibrahim, M.; Show, P.L. Adsorption Behavior of Mercury over Hydrated Lime: Experimental Investigation and Adsorption Process Characteristic Study. *Chemosphere* **2021**, *271*, 129504. [CrossRef]
59. Manna, S.; Saha, P.; Roy, D.; Sen, R.; Adhikari, B. Defluoridation potential of jute fibers grafted with fatty acyl chain. *Appl. Surf. Sci.* **2015**, *356*, 30–38. [CrossRef]
60. Lu, P.; Yang, G.; Tanaka, Y.; Tsubaki, N. Ethanol Direct Synthesis from Dimethyl Ether and Syngas on the Combination of Noble Metal Impregnated Zeolite with Cu/ZnO Catalyst. *Catal. Today* **2014**, *232*, 22–26. [CrossRef]
61. Saravanan, A.; Kumar, P.S.; Yaashikaa, P.R.; Karishma, S.; Jeevanantham, S.; Swetha, S. Mixed Biosorbent of Agro Waste and Bacterial Biomass for the Separation of Pb(II) Ions from Water System. *Chemosphere* **2021**, *277*, 130236. [CrossRef]
62. Sheng, W.; Shi, J.-L.; Hao, H.; Li, X.; Lang, X. Selective Aerobic Oxidation of Sulfides by Cooperative Polyimide-TiO$_2$ Photocatalysis and Triethylamine Catalysis. *J. Colloid Interface Sci.* **2020**, *565*, 614–622. [CrossRef] [PubMed]
63. Wang, D.; Yang, G.; Ma, Q.; Yoneyama, Y.; Tan, Y.; Han, Y.; Tsubaki, N. Facile Solid-State Synthesis of Cu–Zn–O Catalysts for Novel Ethanol Synthesis from Dimethyl Ether (DME) and Syngas (CO+H$_2$). *Fuel* **2013**, *109*, 54–60. [CrossRef]
64. Fan, Z.; Sun, K.; Wang, J. Perovskites for photovoltaics: A combined review of organic–inorganic halide perovskites and ferroelectric oxide perovskites. *J. Mater. Chem. A* **2015**, *3*, 18809–18828. [CrossRef]
65. Dissanayake, D.G.K.; Weerasinghe, D.U.; Thebuwanage, L.M.; Bandara, U.A.A.N. An environmentally friendly sound insulation material from post-industrial textile waste and natural rubber. *J. Build. Eng.* **2021**, *33*, 101606. [CrossRef]
66. Mittal, J. Permissible synthetic food dyes in India. *Resonance. J. Sci. Educ.* **2020**, *25*, 567–577.
67. Royer, S.; Duprez, D.; Can, F.; Courtois, X.; Batiot-Dupeyrat, C.; Laassiri, S.; Alamdari, H. Perovskites as substitutes of noble metals for heterogeneous catalysis: Dream or reality. *Chem. Rev.* **2014**, *114*, 10292–10368. [CrossRef]
68. Li, X.; San, X.; Zhang, Y.; Ichii, T.; Meng, M.; Tan, Y.; Tsubaki, N. Direct Synthesis of Ethanol from Dimethyl Ether and Syngas over Combined H-Mordenite and Cu/ZnO Catalysts. *ChemSusChem* **2010**, *3*, 1192–1199. [CrossRef]
69. Chen, W.; Yin, H.; Cole, I.; Houshyar, S.; Wang, L. Carbon dots derived from non-biomass waste: Methods, applications, and future perspectives. *Molecules* **2024**, *29*, 2441. [CrossRef] [PubMed]
70. Liu, G.; Liu, X.; Ma, X.; Tang, X.; Zhang, X.; Dong, J.; Ma, Y.; Zang, X.; Cao, N.; Shao, Q. High-performance dual-ion battery based on silicon–graphene composite anode and expanded graphite cathode. *Molecules* **2023**, *28*, 4280. [CrossRef] [PubMed]
71. Liu, Y.; Li, Y.; Liu, Z.; Feng, T.; Lin, H.; Li, G.; Wang, K. Uniform p-doped MnMoO$_4$ nanosheets for enhanced asymmetric supercapacitors performance. *Molecules* **2024**, *29*, 1988. [CrossRef]
72. Xie, H.; Li, L.; Zhang, J.; Zhang, Y.; Pan, Y.; Xu, J.; Yin, X.; Que, W. [BMP]$^+$[BF$_4$]$^-$-Modified CsPbI$_{1.2}$Br$_{1.8}$ solar cells with improved efficiency and suppressed photoinduced phase segregation. *Molecules* **2024**, *29*, 1476. [CrossRef]
73. Inerbaev, T.M.; Abuova, A.U.; Zakiyeva, Z.Y.; Abuova, F.U.; Mastrikov, Y.A.; Sokolov, M.; Gryaznov, D.; Kotomin, E.A. Effect of Rh doping on optical absorption and oxygen evolution reaction activity on BaTiO$_3$ (001) surfaces. *Molecules* **2024**, *29*, 2707. [CrossRef] [PubMed]
74. Gaur, B.; Mittal, J.; Shah, S.A.A.; Mittal, A.; Baker, R.T. Sequestration of an azo dye by a potential biosorbent: Characterization of biosorbent, adsorption isotherm and adsorption kinetic studies. *Molecules* **2024**, *29*, 2387. [CrossRef]
75. Liu, S.; Sun, M.; Wu, C.; Zhu, K.; Hu, Y.; Shan, M.; Wang, M.; Wu, K.; Wu, J.; Xie, Z.; et al. Fabrication of loose nanofiltration membrane by crosslinking tempo-oxidized cellulose nanofibers for effective dye/salt separation. *Molecules* **2024**, *29*, 2246. [CrossRef] [PubMed]
76. Yang, Z.; Li, L.; Wang, Y. Mechanism of phosphate desorption from activated red mud particle adsorbents. *Molecules* **2024**, *29*, 974. [CrossRef] [PubMed]
77. Kuppadakkath, G.; Jayabhavan, S.S.; Damodaran, K.K. Supramolecular gels based on c3-symmetric amides: Application in anion-sensing and removal of dyes from water. *Molecules* **2024**, *29*, 2149. [CrossRef]
78. Ni, K.; Chen, Y.; Xu, R.; Zhao, Y.; Guo, M. Mapping photogenerated electron–hole behavior of graphene oxide: Insight into a new mechanism of photosensitive pollutant degradation. *Molecules* **2024**, *29*, 3765. [CrossRef] [PubMed]
79. Wang, M.; Huang, T.; Shan, M.; Sun, M.; Liu, S.; Tang, H. Zwitterionic tröger's base microfiltration membrane prepared via vapor-induced phase separation with improved demulsification and antifouling performance. *Molecules* **2024**, *29*, 1001. [CrossRef] [PubMed]
80. Fu, G.; Dong, X. Enhanced stability of dimethyl ether carbonylation through pyrazole tartrate on tartaric acid-complexed cobalt–iron-modified hydrogen-type mordenite. *Molecules* **2024**, *29*, 1510. [CrossRef] [PubMed]

Disclaimer/Publisher's Note: The statements, opinions and data contained in all publications are solely those of the individual author(s) and contributor(s) and not of MDPI and/or the editor(s). MDPI and/or the editor(s) disclaim responsibility for any injury to people or property resulting from any ideas, methods, instructions or products referred to in the content.

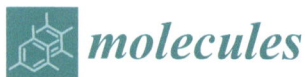 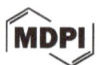

Article

Uniform P-Doped MnMoO$_4$ Nanosheets for Enhanced Asymmetric Supercapacitors Performance

Yu Liu [1], Yan Li [2,*], Zhuohao Liu [1], Tao Feng [1], Huichuan Lin [2], Gang Li [1] and Kaiying Wang [3,*]

[1] Institute of Energy Innovation, College of Materials Science and Engineering, Taiyuan University of Technology, Taiyuan 030024, China; liuyu0226@link.tyut.edu.cn (Y.L.); liuzhuohao0286@link.tyut.edu.cn (Z.L.); fengtao22657@163.com (T.F.); ligang02@tyut.edu.cn (G.L.)

[2] Key Laboratory of Light Field Manipulation and System Integration Applications in Fujian Province, School of Physics and Information Engineering, Minnan Normal University, Zhangzhou 363000, China; lhc1810@mnnu.edu.cn

[3] Department of Microsystems, University of South-Eastern Norway, 3184 Horten, Norway

* Correspondence: liyan1734@mnnu.edu.cn (Y.L.); kaiying.wang@usn.no (K.W.)

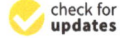

Citation: Liu, Y.; Li, Y.; Liu, Z.; Feng, T.; Lin, H.; Li, G.; Wang, K. Uniform P-Doped MnMoO$_4$ Nanosheets for Enhanced Asymmetric Supercapacitors Performance. *Molecules* **2024**, *29*, 1988. https://doi.org/10.3390/molecules29091988

Academic Editor: Qingguo Shao

Received: 2 April 2024
Revised: 23 April 2024
Accepted: 24 April 2024
Published: 26 April 2024

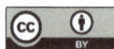

Copyright: © 2024 by the authors. Licensee MDPI, Basel, Switzerland. This article is an open access article distributed under the terms and conditions of the Creative Commons Attribution (CC BY) license (https://creativecommons.org/licenses/by/4.0/).

Abstract: Manganese molybdate has garnered considerable interest in supercapacitor research owing to its outstanding electrochemical properties and nanostructural stability but still suffers from the common problems of transition metal oxides not being able to reach the theoretical specific capacitance and lower electrical conductivity. Doping phosphorus elements is an effective approach to further enhance the electrochemical characteristics of transition metal oxides. In this study, MnMoO$_4$·H$_2$O nanosheets were synthesized on nickel foam via a hydrothermal route, and the MnMoO$_4$·H$_2$O nanosheet structure was successfully doped with a phosphorus element using a gas–solid reaction method. Phosphorus element doping forms phosphorus–metal bonds and oxygen vacancies, thereby increasing the charge storage and conductivity of the electrode material. The specific capacitance value is as high as 2.112 F cm^{-2} (1760 F g^{-1}) at 1 mA cm^{-2}, which is 3.2 times higher than that of the MnMoO$_4$·H$_2$O electrode (0.657 F cm^{-2}). The P–MnMoO$_4$//AC ASC device provides a high energy density of 41.9 Wh kg^{-1} at 666.8 W kg^{-1}, with an 84.5% capacity retention after 10,000 charge/discharge cycles. The outstanding performance suggests that P–MnMoO$_4$ holds promise as an electrode material for supercapacitors.

Keywords: asymmetric supercapacitor; MnMoO$_4$; nanosheets; phosphorus doping

1. Introduction

The swift growth of the worldwide economy has led to a rise in the extraction and utilization of fossil fuels like oil and coal. Consequently, nonrenewable energy reservoirs are progressively dwindling [1]. With the advancement and application of electrical energy, the imperative lies in creating high-performance electrical energy storage devices to minimize secondary energy wastage [2]. Supercapacitors, positioned between traditional capacitors and batteries, possess a blend of characteristics from both: high capacity, rapid charging and discharging, extended cycle life, and elevated energy density [3,4]. Supercapacitors are primarily categorized into double-layer capacitors (EDLCs) and pseudocapacitors (PCs) based on the charge storage mechanism [5,6]. Selecting the appropriate electrode materials is crucial for the practical implementation of energy storage supercapacitors. Carbon-based materials are commonly employed as electrodes in EDLCs, while transition metal oxides and conducting polymers are frequently utilized as electrode materials for pseudocapacitors. The capacitors with carbon-based electrode materials suffer from low energy storage and poor stability, which conducting polymer layer tends to detach from the substrate [7–9]. Therefore, transition metal oxides (TMOs) are favored by researchers because of their generally large theoretical specific capacitance and are often used as electrode materials in energy storage supercapacitors [10].

Transition metal oxides like Fe_3O_4, MnO_2, RuO_2, NiO, etc. are commonly employed as electrode materials in supercapacitors, but these unit transition metal oxides generally have the disadvantage in their actual specific capacitances being much smaller than the theoretical specific capacitances [11–14]. Therefore, research workers have focused on binary transition metal oxides, mainly including spinel cobaltates (XCo_2O_4, X = Ni, Mn, Zn, etc.) and molybdates ($YMoO_4$, Y = Ni, Co, Mn, etc.) [15]. Characterized by the low cost of abundant molybdenum ore resources and multiple oxidation valence states (+3–+6) for easy storage of charge, molybdate is well suited to supercapacitor cathode material [15,16]. Among them, manganese molybdate has good structural stability (compared to cobalt-based molybdates and nickel-based molybdates) due to its special structure and low cohesive energy [16,17]. Manganese molybdate boasts a high theoretical specific capacity (998 mAh g^{-1}), stemming from the synergistic effect of the two elements of Mo and Mn (molybdenum ions provide electronic conductivity and manganese ions provide redox activity) [18].

In order to make the actual specific capacitance of manganese molybdate as close as possible to the theoretical value, one approach is to synthesize nanoscale $MnMoO_4$ electrodes of a specific micromorphological structure. For instance, Mu et al. synthesized $MnMoO_4 \cdot nH_2O$ nanosheets on nickel foam using a one-step hydrothermal method, achieving a specific capacitance of 1271 F g^{-1} at a scan rate of 5 mV s^{-1} with 84.5% capacitance retention after 2000 charge/discharge cycles [19]. Doping P, S, and other anions in binary transition metal oxides has been demonstrated to enhance electrical conductivity and promote more extensive oxide reduction reactions, thereby enhancing the charge storage capacity of the electrode materials [20–22]. For instance, Meng et al. synthesized uniform P-doped Co–Ni–S nanosheet arrays as binder-free electrodes, exhibiting an ultra–high specific capacitance of 3677 F g^{-1} at 1 A g^{-1} and outstanding cycling stability (approximately 84% capacitance retention after 10,000 charge/discharge cycles) [21].

The electronic arrangement of the element phosphorus leads to multivalent, metal-like properties and better electrical conductivity of transition metal phosphides compared to transition metal oxides, due to the relatively narrow gap between their conduction and valence bands, and the excellent electrical conductivity is very favorable for electrochemical energy storage processes [23]. Transition metal phosphides can be regarded as phosphorus elements doped into transition metals and their oxides [24]. It is the gas–solid reaction method that the phosphine gas involved in the phosphorylation reaction makes the phosphorus element doped into the metal oxide. The advantage of this method is that the morphological structure of the phosphated product remains essentially the same as that of the precursor. However, because phosphine is highly toxic, the gas–solid reaction is generally chosen to decompose hypophosphite into phosphine gas by heating, which then participates in the phosphorylation reaction [25,26].

In this research, $MnMoO_4 \cdot H_2O$ nanosheets were initially synthesized directly on nickel foam using the hydrothermal method. Then, the prepared $MnMoO_4 \cdot H_2O$ nanosheets were subjected to phosphorus doping in a tube furnace using a gas–solid reaction method. Sodium hypophosphite was used as the phosphorus source, and the experimental parameters of the phosphorus source content, phosphorylation reaction temperature, and reaction time were optimized for phosphorylation.

2. Results and Discussion

2.1. Structure and Morphology Analysis

Figure 1 illustrates the preparation process of phosphorus-doped $MnMoO_4$ nanomaterials on NF. With the clean nickel foam immersed in a mixed solution of $MnSO_4 \cdot H_2O$ and $Na_2MoO_4 \cdot 2H_2O$ the first step of the hydrothermal reaction at 150 °C for 8 h yielded a nanosheet array of $MnMoO_4 \cdot H_2O$ grown on the nickel foam. The nickel foam that has gone through the first hydrothermal process and the sodium hypophosphite powder were placed into a tubular furnace side by side. Phosphorus element doping was achieved using the gas–solid reaction method, with $NaH_2PO_2·H_2O$ positioned upstream in an argon atmosphere and $MnMoO_4·H_2O$/NF positioned downstream.

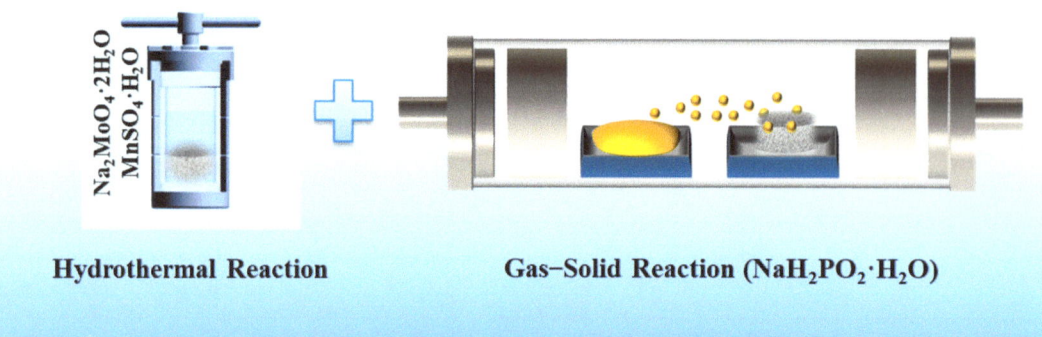

Figure 1. Diagram illustrating the preparation of P–$MnMoO_4$/NF.

The morphologies of the $MnMoO_4·H_2O$ and P–$MnMoO_4$ nanosheets were analyzed by SEM. Before phosphorylation, manganese molybdate presents as a dense, uniform, vertically aligned array of nanosheets on the surface of NF. The cores of $MnMoO_4·H_2O$ nanosheets present a regular morphology and crosslinking structure without aggregation (Figure 2a). This architecture minimizes the electrode material's inactive volume and enhances the electron conduction efficiency during electrochemical processes. Figure 2b shows that the phosphorus-doped manganese molybdate sample is vertically interconnected, and the addition of phosphorus does not change the original morphological structure of the samples. The skeleton of the nickel foam substrate is covered by a layer of uniformly dense nanosheets. Possibly due to the distribution at the edges of the nickel foam skeleton, some aggregates and nanoflowers appear, which have little effect on the overall morphology, and a small number of nanoflowers can increase the specific surface area and improve the electrochemical properties (Figure S1). However, the surface of the nanosheets becomes coarse, and the surface is covered with separated particles producing a large number of marginal sites of small size effects (Figure 2c). These alterations lead to an increased specific surface area of the P–$MnMoO_4$ nanosheets electrode material, enhancing the electrical contact with the electrolyte. Additionally, the incorporation of phosphorus elements enhances the overall electrical conductivity and promotes electrochemical activity.

The nanosheet structure of the P–$MnMoO_4$ nanomaterial was analyzed using TEM images. Figure 2d shows the TEM image of P–$MnMoO_4$, revealing a distinct nanosheet structure. Figure 2e shows the HRTEM image of P–$MnMoO_4$ with clear lattice fringes. The lattice distances of 0.240 nm, 0.282 nm, and 0.339 nm depicted in Figure 2f–h correspond to the (021), ($\bar{2}$10), and (110) planes of the $MnMoO_4·H_2O$ phase, respectively. Figure 2i shows the SAED pattern of P–$MnMoO_4$, indicating its polycrystalline nature with distinct spots and rings. The SAED pattern matches the ($\bar{2}$21), (110), and (010) planes of $MnMoO_4·H_2O$, indicating that a small amount of phosphorus doping does not affect the $MnMoO_4·H_2O$ nanosheet substrate. To ascertain the elemental composition of the experimental samples, EDS scans were conducted on the doped samples. Figure 2j shows the P–$MnMoO_4$ scanning the EDS diagram at the magnification surface. Mn, Mo, O, and P are evenly dispersed across the nickel foam's surface. The successful doping of phosphorus atoms into manganese molybdate was demonstrated.

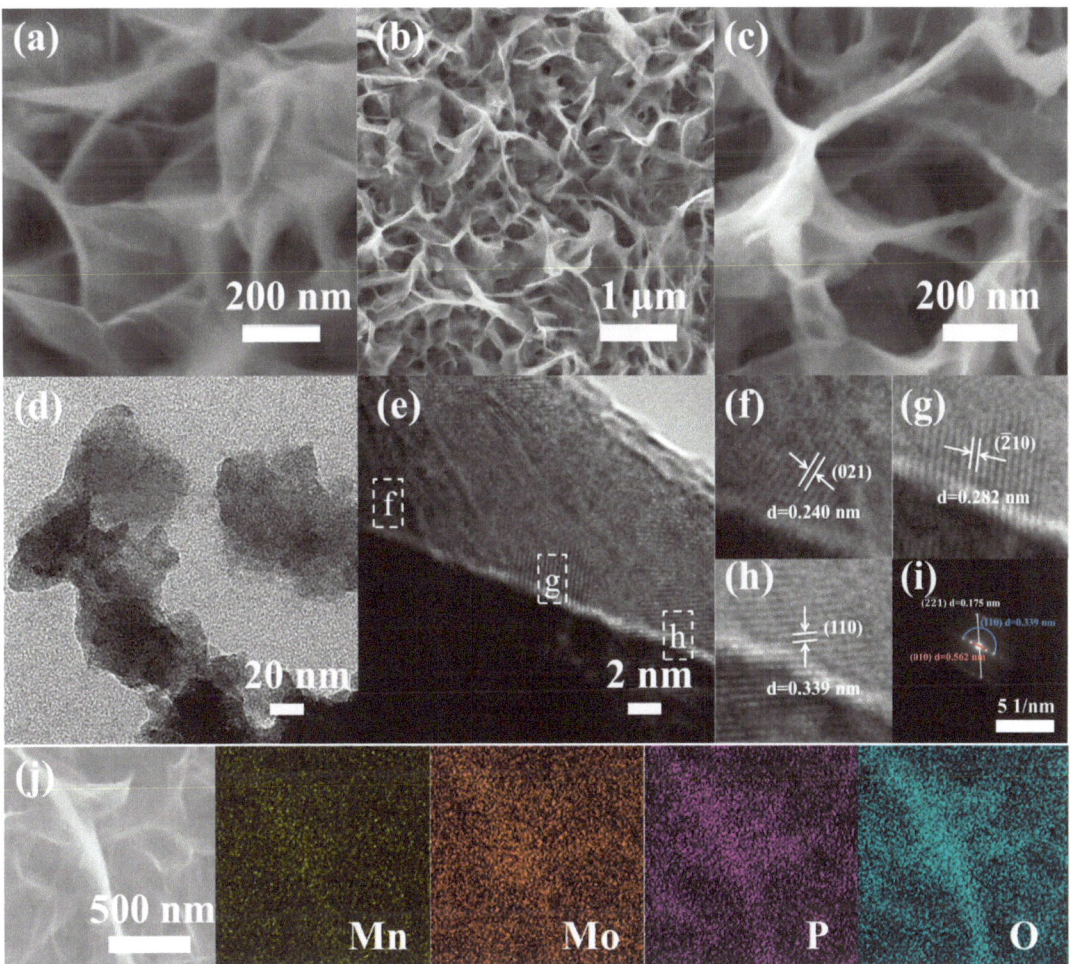

Figure 2. SEM images of (**a**) MnMoO$_4$·H$_2$O and (**b**,**c**) P–MnMoO$_4$; (**d**) TEM and (**e**–**h**) HRTEM images of P–MnMoO$_4$ and (**i**) the corresponding SAED pattern; and (**j**) EDS mapping of P–MnMoO$_4$.

To examine the crystal structure and composition of the samples, XRD analysis was conducted on the prepared MnMoO$_4$·H$_2$O and P–MnMoO$_4$ nanosheets, as depicted in Figure 3a. Because the X-ray diffraction peak of nickel is rather strong and the amount of MnMoO$_4$·H$_2$O grown in situ is low, the active material was first scraped off from the nickel foam, and the scraped nickel monomers were absorbed with a magnet for XRD testing. The diffraction peaks of MnMoO$_4$·H$_2$O grown in situ by the hydrothermal method are consistent with the standard triclinic MnMoO$_4$·H$_2$O (JCPDS card No.78–0220) [27]. Among them, the characteristic peaks with 2θ of 12.92°, 15.94°, 18.79°, 26.28°, and 31.98° correspond to the (001), (010), ($\bar{1}$10), (110), and (111) crystal plane diffractions of MnMoO$_4$·H$_2$O, respectively. Meanwhile, the high and fine diffraction peaks of MnMoO$_4$·H$_2$O indicate better crystallinity.

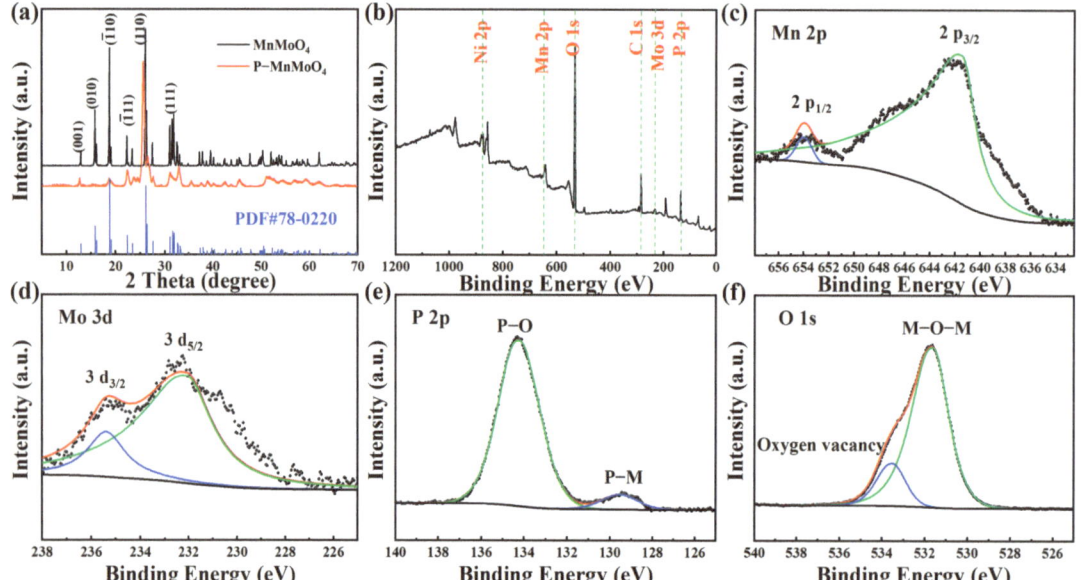

Figure 3. (a) XRD patters of MnMoO$_4$·H$_2$O and P–MnMoO$_4$, and (b) the XPS survey spectrum of the P–MnMoO$_4$, (c) Mn 2p, (d) Mo 3d, (e) P 2p, and (f) O 1s spectrum.

The diffraction pattern of P–MnMoO$_4$ did not change significantly, indicating that only a small amount of phosphorus was doped during the gas–solid reaction. The diffraction peaks of P–MnMoO$_4$ at 12.71°, 18.74°, 25.65°, and 31.87° correspond to the (001), ($\bar{1}$10), (110), and (111) crystal plane diffractions of MnMoO$_4$·H$_2$O, respectively. It shows that the structure of manganese molybdate is not changed after phosphorylation, which is consistent with the SEM results. The synthesized material is uniform in composition rather than being composite. The low and broad diffraction peaks of P–MnMoO$_4$ compared to those of MnMoO$_4$·H$_2$O indicate that poorer crystallinity was obtained. This difference may be caused by P doping, in which the larger radius P elements partially replace the original position of O, which may lead to a slight change in the crystallinity [28], and no additional diffraction peaks appeared, indicating that the doping of the P element did not change the original crystal structure.

To gain a more thorough insight into the elemental composition and chemical states of P–MnMoO$_4$ nanosheets, XPS analysis was performed. The XPS (Figure 3b) of P–MnMoO$_4$ demonstrated the existence of Mo, Mn, P, and O elements. The binding energy peaks at 653.73 eV and 641.40 eV are attributed to Mn 2p$_{1/2}$ and Mn 2p$_{3/2}$, respectively (Figure 3c). The energy gap between these two peaks is 12.33 eV, suggesting the presence of Mn^{2+} [29,30]. In Figure 3d, the binding energy peaks at 235.45 eV and 231.74 eV are attributed to Mo 3d$_{3/2}$ and Mo 3d$_{5/2}$, respectively. The energy gap between these two peaks is 3.71 eV, suggesting the presence of Mo^{6+} [31,32]. In Figure 3e, the P 2p core energy level spectrum reveals two peaks with binding energies of 134.14 eV and 129.48 eV, corresponding to the P–O bond (phosphide signal peak) and the phosphorus–metal bond, respectively [21,33]. The binding energy peaks at 533.25 eV and 531.60 eV in Figure 3f correspond to the characteristic peaks of the oxygen vacancies and metal–oxygen bonds, respectively [20,34]. There was no significant change observed in the chemical state in the P 2p spectra, suggesting the structural stability of the material. These findings further confirm the successful doping of elemental P into the MnMoO$_4$ nanosheets, which are also indicated by the results of the XRD test described previously.

2.2. Electrochemical Characterizations

Through prior research experience, the optimal hydrothermal reaction time and temperature conditions were determined for the preparation of the precursor $MnMoO_4 \cdot H_2O$ nanosheets using the hydrothermal method. The experimental conditions of 150 °C and 8 h are used to generate $MnMoO_4 \cdot H_2O$ nanosheets of favorable microscopic morphology and pore size for good contact between the electrolyte and active material [20,35]. In the gas–solid reaction method, the thermal decomposition of $NaH_2PO_2 \cdot H_2O$ produces PH_3 gas and water vapor present in the tube furnace. Driven by argon, PH_3 gas moves to the surface of manganese molybdate and reacts with it to form phosphoric acid. A small amount of phosphoric acid is gradually "acid dissociated" in the presence of water vapor to produce HPO_4^{2-} and $H_2PO_4^{-}$ in turn. Then, $H_2PO_4^{-}$ and OH^{-} undergo ion exchange on the surface of $MnMoO_{4-4x}$, OH^{-} diffuses outward, and $H_2PO_4^{-}$ penetrates inward slowly to realize the phosphorus doping. The specific reaction equations are as follows:

$$NaH_2PO_2 \cdot H_2O \rightarrow PH_3 \uparrow + Na_2HPO_4 + H_2O \uparrow \tag{1}$$

$$MnMoO_4 + xPH_3 = MnMoO_{4-4x} + xH_3PO_4 \tag{2}$$

$$H_2O + PO_4^{3-} = HPO_4^{2-} + OH^{-} \tag{3}$$

$$HPO_4^{2-} + H_2O = H_2PO_4^{-} + OH^{-} \tag{4}$$

In order to determine the optimal phosphorylation reaction conditions, three parameters were studied in terms of the amount of phosphorus source, phosphorylation temperature, and phosphorylation time, respectively. Subsequently, CV and GCD tests were performed to evaluate the impact of these parameters on the electrochemical properties resulting from the phosphorylation reaction. Figure 4a depicts the CV curves of the phosphorylated manganese molybdate electrode at 20 mV s^{-1} for varying phosphorus source quantities: 0.3 g, 0.6 g, 0.8 g, 1.0 g, and 1.3 g. Observably, the curve corresponding to a hypophosphite quantity of 0.8 g covers a larger enclosed area and demonstrates a higher capacitance area ratio. The mass ratio of the precursor to phosphorus source ranges from 1:10 to 1:40 or even higher [36,37]. From the preliminary experiments, the electrochemical properties of P–MnMoO$_4$/NF generated by the gas phase reaction were not significantly improved when the content of the phosphorus source (NaH_2PO_2) was lower than 0.3 g. The electrochemical properties of P–MnMoO$_4$/NF generated by the gas phase reaction were not significantly improved. If the content of the phosphorus source is too much and too high, it may lead to the accumulation of the phosphorus source (NaH_2PO_2) before the decomposition reaction, which leads to the ineffective improvement of the electrochemical performance and, at the same time, causes a large amount of phosphorus resources to be wasted. Figure 4b illustrates the GCD curves of the electrodes (0–0.5 V) following the phosphorylation of manganese molybdate with different phosphorus source amounts at 1 mA cm^{-2}. The amount of hypophosphite is 0.8 g for the longest discharge time and higher charging and discharging plateau voltage, so it is determined that 0.8 g is the optimal amount of sodium hypophosphite for the phosphorus source.

The effect of the phosphorylation temperature on the experimental results was studied based on the phosphorus source content of 0.8 g and the temperatures of 250 °C, 350 °C, 400 °C, and 450 °C, respectively. Figure 4c illustrates the CV plots of the three samples at different temperatures at a 20 mV s^{-1} scan rate. It can be seen that P–MnMoO$_4$ are pseudocapacitor materials at three different temperatures, but there is little difference in the wrapping area of the CV curves at 400 °C and 450 °C. Constant current charge and discharge are tested and shown in Figure 4d, in which the GCD curve of 400 °C has the longest discharge time, so the optimal phosphorylation reaction temperature is determined to be 400 °C. The experiments to determine the phosphorylation time were conducted under the condition of 0.8 g sodium hypophosphite and a reaction temperature of 400 °C. The reaction durations chosen were 1 h, 2 h, and 3 h, respectively. CV and GCD tests were conducted at identical scan rates and current densities, respectively (Figure 4e,f). The area enclosed by the CV curves is difficult to directly assess, indicating that the phosphorylation time has minimal impact on the electrochemical performance. The GCD curves were measured to quantitatively analyze the respective specific capacitance, and the optimal phosphorylation reaction time of 2 h was subsequently determined. In summary, the ideal parameters for the phosphorylation experiment were 0.8 g of sodium hypophosphite, a reaction temperature of 400 °C, and a reaction time of 2 h. The electrochemical performance of P–MnMoO$_4$ and MnMoO$_4$·H$_2$O prepared under the optimal experimental conditions was compared.

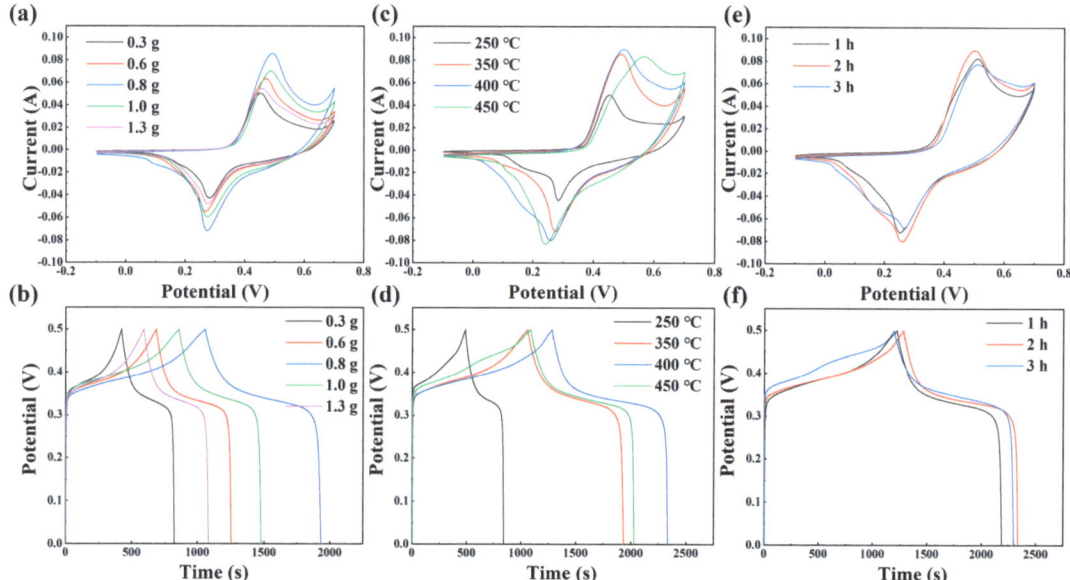

Figure 4. Comparison of the P–MnMoO$_4$ electrode under different experimental conditions: (**a**,**b**) CV curves at 20 mV s^{-1} and GCD curves at 1 mA cm^{-2} for different phosphorus source contents; (**c**,**d**) phosphorylation temperatures; (**e**,**f**) phosphorylation times.

We compared the electrochemical performance of the P–MnMoO$_4$ electrode (0.8 g, 400 °C, 2 h) prepared with the optimal parameters separately with that of the MnMoO$_4$·H$_2$O electrode. Detailed CV and GCD curves for the MnMoO$_4$·H$_2$O and P–MnMoO$_4$ electrode materials at different scan rates and current densities are shown in Figures S2 and S3. The area specific capacitances of the MnMoO$_4$·H$_2$O electrodes are 0.657, 0.634, 0.605, 0.550, 0.505, 0.451, and 0.400 F cm^{-2} at current densities of 1, 2, 3, 5, 10, 15, and 20 mA cm^{-2}. The CV curves of the P–MnMoO$_4$ electrode (0.8 g, 400 °C, 2 h) at various scanning rates exhibited minimal change in curve morphology, suggesting excellent reversibility of the electrode.

Figure 5a depicts the CV curves of the P–MnMoO$_4$ and MnMoO$_4$·H$_2$O electrodes within the potential range of −0.1 to 0.7 V at a scanning rate of 20 mV s^{-1}. The enclosed area of the CV curve for the P–MnMoO$_4$ electrode exceeds that of the MnMoO$_4$·H$_2$O electrode, indicating that P–MnMoO$_4$ can store more charge and has better electrochemical performance, mainly attributed to the addition of phosphorus elements. Both CV curves exhibit a pair of well-defined redox peaks, indicative of Faraday reactions associated with electrochemical capacitance. In Figure 5b, the GCD curves of the P–MnMoO$_4$ and MnMoO$_4$·H$_2$O electrodes are shown, measured at 1 mA cm^{-2}. The discharge time of the P–MnMoO$_4$ electrode (1054 s) notably surpasses that of the MnMoO$_4$·H$_2$O electrode (327 s). At 1 mA cm^{-2}, the specific capacitance of P–MnMoO$_4$ is 2.112 F cm^{-2}, approximately 3.2 times greater than that of the MnMoO$_4$·H$_2$O electrode (0.657 F cm^{-2}). The two electrodes both exhibit charge/discharge plateaus, indicating the pseudocapacitive characteristics of the active material. In Figure 5c, Nyquist plots of the P–MnMoO$_4$ and MnMoO$_4$·H$_2$O electrodes are displayed, with the inset illustrating the equivalent circuit diagram. Since both materials are grown on nickel foam, the contact resistance is minimal and manifests at the intersection of the impedance curve with the horizontal axis. The radius of the curvature of P–MnMoO$_4$ in the high-frequency region is smaller than that of MnMoO$_4$·H$_2$O, indicating a reduced charge transfer resistance. In the low-frequency region, a linear trend with a slope close to 1 represents the Warburg impedance, reflecting the efficiency of electrolyte ion transfer at the electrode surface and in solution. The findings indicate that the internal resistance (R_s = 0.198 Ω) and charge transfer resistance (R_{ct} = 0.735 Ω) of P–MnMoO$_4$ are lower than those of MnMoO$_4$·H$_2$O (internal resistance (R_s = 1.121 Ω) and charge transfer resistance (R_{ct} = 5.398 Ω)), attributed to the incorporation of phosphorus to enhance the overall conductivity of the electrode material.

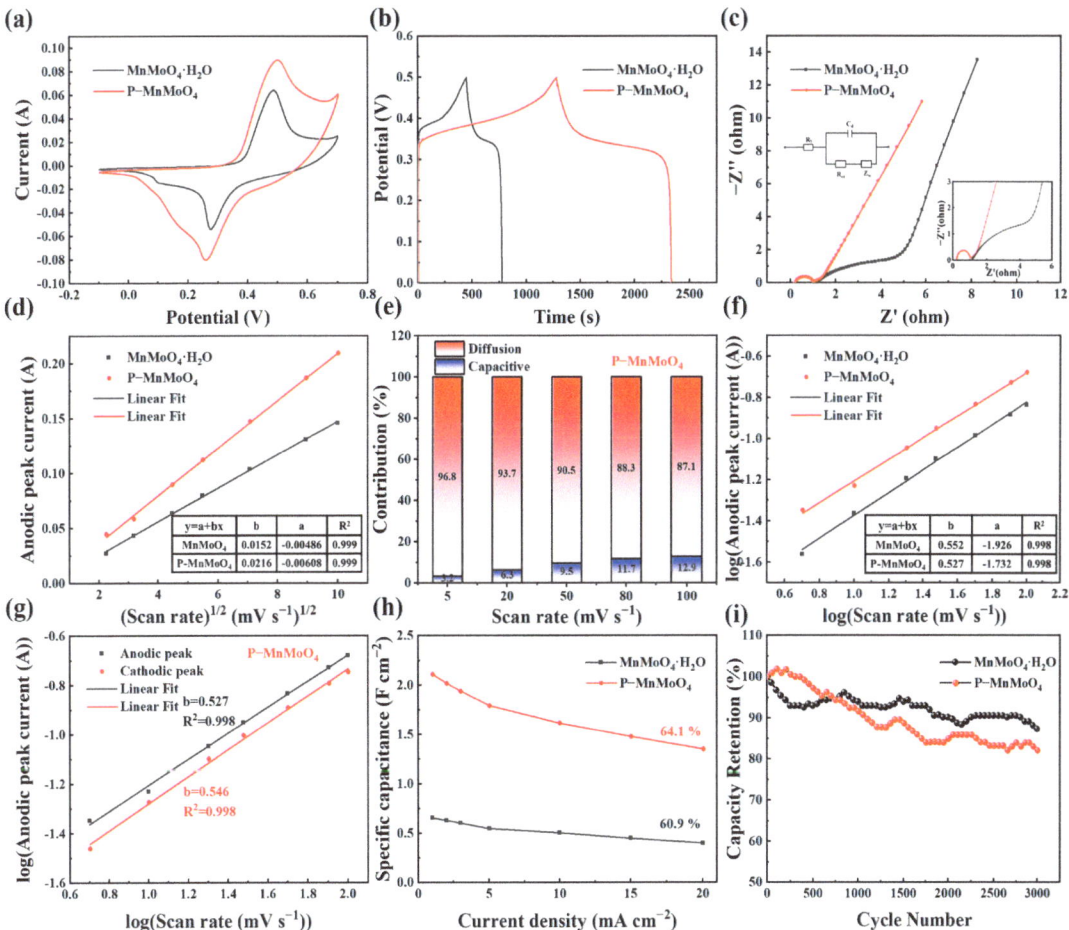

Figure 5. Comparison of MnMoO$_4$·H$_2$O and P–MnMoO$_4$: (**a**) CV curves at 20 mV s^{-1}; (**b**) GCD curves at 1 mA cm^{-2}; (**c**) Nyquist plots (insets show the corresponding high-magnified EIS and equivalent circuit); (**d**) relationship between the peak anode current and square root of the sweep rate; (**e**) proportions of capacitive and diffusion-controlled contributions at various scan rates of the P–MnMoO$_4$ electrode; (**f**) relationship between log (|i|) and log (v); (**g**) the log (|i|) versus log (v) plots of the cathodic and anodic peak current responses of the P–MnMoO$_4$ electrode; (**h**) rate capability; (**i**) stability test.

Figure 5d shows that the corresponding currents of the redox peaks of the P–MnMoO$_4$ and MnMoO$_4$·H$_2$O electrodes are roughly linear with the one-half order of the sweep speed. It shows that the energy storage of the P–MnMoO$_4$ and MnMoO$_4$·H$_2$O electrodes is mainly carried out by the redox reaction inside the electrode material, not only by the surface redox reaction [38]. The P–MnMoO$_4$ electrode has a larger slope of the fitted line (b = 0.0216), indicating a high ion migration rate. Indirectly, it is proven that the phosphorus element is doped into the interior of MnMoO$_4$·H$_2$O and participates in the redox reaction, possibly forming oxygen vacancies or phosphorus atoms replacing oxygen atoms. Figure 5e shows the contribution rates of the surface-controlled and diffusion-controlled capabilities of the P–MnMoO$_4$ electrode at different scan rates. As the scan rates increase, the surface-controlled capabilities become more prominent due to the suppression of ion diffusion [39]. However, at 100 mV s^{-1}, the diffusion-controlled reaction capacitance remains dominant at 87.3%, indicating that the fast redox reaction process of the P–MnMoO$_4$ electrode in electrochemical reactions is less affected by the scan rate, corresponding to the high ion migration rate. Figure 5f illustrates the fitting line of log (i) versus log (v) collected from the CV curve of various electrodes. The constant of the P–MnMoO$_4$ electrode is 0.527, closer to 0.5, revealing that the P–MnMoO$_4$ electrode is a typical diffusion-controlled Faraday reaction. In Figure 5g, the fitting b values of the oxidation and reduction peaks of the P–MnMoO$_4$ electrode are displayed, both approaching 0.5. This suggests excellent reversibility in the redox reaction of the P–MnMoO$_4$ electrode, facilitating rapid and reversible electron transfer at the interface between the electrode material and the electrolyte.

Area-specific capacitances for the P–MnMoO$_4$ and MnMoO$_4$·H$_2$O electrodes were computed from the GCD curves at various current densities (Figure 5h). As the current density increased, the specific capacitance of both the P–MnMoO$_4$ and MnMoO$_4$·H$_2$O electrodes decreased. Due to the rapid decrease in the charge/discharge time at higher charge/discharge rates, the movement of ions is restricted and the ions cannot reach the interior of the electrode material in a short time, and the redox and ion intercalation reactions occur incompletely [40]. As the current density increased from 1 mA cm^{-2} to 20 mA cm^{-2}, the specific capacitance retention of the P–MnMoO$_4$ electrode was 64.1%, which was higher than that of the MnMoO$_4$·H$_2$O electrode (60.9%). The P–MnMoO$_4$ and MnMoO$_4$·H$_2$O electrodes were charged and discharged 3000 times at 5 mA cm^{-2} (Figure 5i). After 3000 charge/discharge cycles, the specific capacitance retention rate of P–MnMoO$_4$ was 82.1%, slightly lower than that of the MnMoO$_4$·H$_2$O electrode (87.3%). The nanosheet morphology of the P–MnMoO$_4$ electrode material does not change after long-term cycling (Figure S4). The decrease in capacity retention after multiple charge/discharge cycles is mainly due to the possible slight exfoliation of the nanosheet structure of the electrode material and the change in electrolyte concentration during long cycling. Nonetheless, the specific capacity after cycling of the P–MnMoO$_4$ electrode remains higher than the specific capacity before cycling of the MnMoO$_4$·H$_2$O electrode. Overall, the P–MnMoO$_4$ electrode material still demonstrates favorable cycling stability.

2.3. P–MnMoO$_4$//AC ASC Testing

To evaluate P–MnMoO$_4$'s practical utility, we constructed an asymmetric supercapacitor device with P–MnMoO$_4$ serving as the positive electrode and activated carbon (AC) as the negative electrode, 2 M KOH as the electrolyte, and cellulose paper as the diaphragm (Figure 6a). Detailed CV and GCD curves for commercial activated carbon (AC) anode electrode materials are given in Figure S5, and the CV curves are quasi-rectangular in shape, which is a double electric layer capacitance characteristic. In the three-electrode test regime, Figure 6b shows the CV curves measured at 20 mV s^{-1} for P–MnMoO$_4$ and activated carbon, respectively. The absence of overlap between the individual CV curve regions of the positive and negative electrodes within the potential window confirms the precise alignment of the two electrodes during the assembly of the asymmetric supercapacitor [41]. To establish the voltage window of the device, we expanded the voltage range of the CV curve from 0–0.8 V to 0–1.8 V at a scan rate of 20 mV s^{-1} (Figure 6c). There was no significant polarization in the 0–1.6 V range, and the P–MnMoO$_4$//AC device was CV tested at scan rates of 10 to 100 mV s^{-1} during this voltage window (Figure 6d). As the scan rate increases, all CV curve shapes do not change due to the increase in scan speed, and they are irregularly rectangular in shape. Both pseudocapacitors and double-layer capacitors contribute to this asymmetric supercapacitor device [42]. Figure 6e shows the GCD curve that indicates the maximum voltage window, which is obtained by incrementing the voltage from 0 to 0.8 V with a step of 0.2 V at 5 mA cm^{-2}. If the GCD test is performed above the 1.6 V voltage window, it will cause the device to remain in the charging state rather than be discharged, and a higher voltage window will not be achieved. The CV and GCD tests incremented the voltage window, and the final test results were consistent, identifying the device voltage window as 0–1.6 V. Figure 6f shows the variation of the GCD curve of P–MnMoO$_4$//AC as the current density increases from 5 mA cm^{-2} to 30 mA cm^{-2} within the voltage range of 0–1.6 V. The symmetrical shapes of the CV and GCD curves of the devices tested at different scanning speeds and current densities indicate that the two electrode materials are well matched and have excellent charge/discharge reversibility [38].

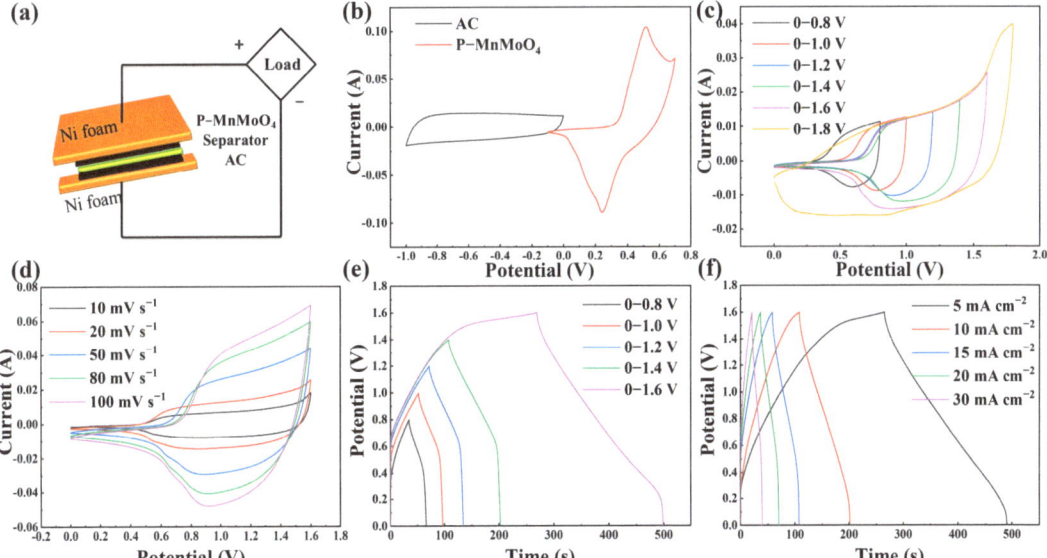

Figure 6. (a) Schematic representation of the assembled hybrid P–MnMoO$_4$//AC supercapacitor; (b) CV curves for the positive and negative electrodes at 20 mV s^{-1}; (c) CV curves at different voltage windows (20 mV s^{-1}); (d) CV curves, (e) GCD curves at different voltage windows (5 mA cm^{-2}); (f) GCD curves.

The power and energy density of the P–MnMoO$_4$//AC ASC device can be computed using Equations (7) and (8). The energy density of P–MnMoO$_4$//AC was 41.9, 34.8, 27.6, 25.3, and 21.2 Wh kg^{-1} for power densities of 666.8, 1348.8, 2015.4, 2751.7, and 4128.3 W kg^{-1}, respectively. The capacity retention of the P–MnMoO$_4$//AC ASC device was 84.5% after 10,000 cycles, and the Coulombic efficiency remained nearly 100% throughout each charge/discharge cycle, with the initial increase in capacity during the cycling period likely attributable to the activation process of the electrode material (Figure 7). When compared to other asymmetric supercapacitors comprising MnMoO$_4$ material and activated carbon, the P–MnMoO$_4$//AC supercapacitor demonstrates superior energy density at equivalent power densities and exhibits outstanding cycling stability (Table S1). The results imply the possibility of practical applications of phosphorus-doped manganese molybdate in energy storage devices.

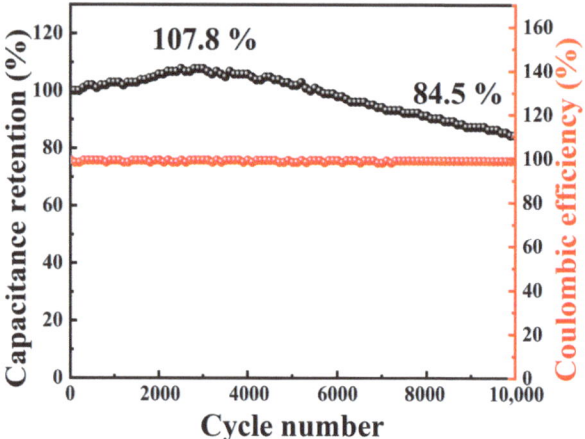

Figure 7. Cycling performance of the P–MnMoO$_4$//AC ASC device.

3. Materials and Methods

3.1. Chemicals and Materials

The reagents included Na$_2$MoO$_4$·2H$_2$O, MnSO$_4$·H$_2$O, NaH$_2$PO$_2$·H$_2$O, anhydrous ethanol, KOH, HCl, CH$_3$COCH$_3$, NF, commercial active carbon, acetylene black, polyvinylidene fluoride (PVDF), and N–methyl pyrrolidone, purchased from Sinopharm Chemical Reagents Co. Ltd. (Shanghai, China). The 1 mm thick Ni foams were trimmed into pieces measuring 1 cm × 1.5 cm for ease of handling. Subsequently, they were immersed in 1 M HCl solution and acetone for ultrasonic cleaning for 15 min to eliminate NiO and organic contaminants from the surface. Afterwards, the pretreated Ni foams underwent thorough rinsing with deionized water and ethanol before being vacuum-dried at 60 °C for 12 h. All reagents utilized were of analytical grade and necessitated no further purification.

3.2. Synthesis of MnMoO$_4$·H$_2$O Precursors and P–MnMoO$_4$

In a typical synthesis, 2 mmol of Na$_2$MoO$_4$·2H$_2$O and 2 mmol of MnSO$_4$·H$_2$O were dissolved separately in 40 mL of deionized water. The mixed solution and clean Ni foam were then transferred into a 100 mL stainless steel autoclave and placed in a blast-drying oven at 150 °C for 8 h. After the reaction was completed, the samples were cooled to room temperature, gently rinsed with deionized water to prevent detachment of the grown MnMoO$_4$·H$_2$O from the nickel foam, and subsequently dried at 60 °C for 12 h.

The doping of the phosphorus element was achieved using a gas–solid reaction method. MnMoO$_4$·H$_2$O/NF and NaH$_2$PO$_2$·H$_2$O were placed in the porcelain boat, with NaH$_2$PO$_2$·H$_2$O positioned upstream and MnMoO$_4$·H$_2$O/NF downstream. Then, it was placed in a tube furnace, heated with argon gas to a certain temperature for a certain period of time, and then cooled to room temperature to obtain P–MnMoO$_4$/NF. In this paper, we proposed the optimization of the experimental parameters of the phosphorus source (0.3 g, 0.6 g, 0.8 g, 1.0 g, and 1.3 g); phosphating temperature (250 °C, 350 °C, 400 °C, and 450 °C); and phosphating time (1 h, 2 h, and 3 h) to generate P–MnMoO$_4$. The mass of active material on NF of the MnMoO$_4$·H$_2$O and P–MnMoO$_4$ (0.8 g, 400 °C, 2 h) samples was about 1 mg cm^{-2} and 1.2 mg cm^{-2}, respectively, measured by an electronic balance.

3.3. P–MnMoO$_4$//AC Asymmetric Supercapacitor Assembly

Activated carbon (AC), conductive carbon black, and polyvinylidene fluoride (PVDF) were mixed in a mass ratio of 8:1:1 and combined with an appropriate amount of N–methylpyrrolidone. The mixture was stirred into a paste at room temperature and then uniformly applied to clean Ni foam to prepare the negative electrode of the device. This asymmetric device was assembled at room temperature and in air and used for the two-electrode test. The amount of AC required was calculated according to Equation (5) [43]:

$$\frac{m^+}{m^-} = \frac{C^- \times \Delta V^-}{C^+ \times \Delta V^+} \quad (5)$$

where m (g), C (F cm^{-2}), and ΔV (V) represent the mass of electrode material, specific capacitance, and potential window, respectively.

3.4. Characterization of Materials

The nanostructured morphologies of the samples were examined using a scanning electron microscope (SEM, ZEISS Gemini 300, Jena, Germany). Elemental mapping imaging was performed using energy dispersive X-ray spectroscopy (EDS, Horiba EMAX Energy, EX-350, Kyoto, Japan). Transmission electron microscopy (TEM), high-resolution transmission electron microscopy (HRTEM), and selected area electron diffraction (SAED) images were obtained with a FEI-TALOS-F200X (Thermo Fisher Scientific, Waltham, MA, USA). The crystal structure of the samples was analyzed using an X-ray powder diffractometer (XRD, Empyrean, Malvern Panalytical B.V, Almelo, The Netherlands) with graphite monochromatic Cu Kα irradiation. The chemical compositions of the nanocomposites were analyzed using X-ray photoelectron spectroscopy (XPS, American Thermo Fisher Scientific K-Alpha, USA).

3.5. Electrochemical Measurements

All electrochemical measurements were performed using an electrochemical workstation (CHI 660D). Samples of MnMoO$_4$·H$_2$O and P–MnMoO$_4$ electrode materials prepared on Ni foam were directly used as working electrodes for the three-electrode test, and Pt net and Hg/HgO electrodes were used as counter and reference electrodes in 2 M KOH aqueous electrolytes. The specific capacitance of the single and full electrode devices were calculated using Equation (6) [44]:

$$C_s = \frac{I \times \Delta t}{m \times \Delta V} \quad (6)$$

where I (A) is the discharge current, Δt (s) is the discharge time, m (g) is the mass loading of the active material, ΔV is the operating voltage, and C_s (F g^{-1}) is the mass ratio capacitance. When its m (g) is replaced with the effective area of the electrode, Equation (6) can be used for the calculation of the area ratio capacitance (F cm^{-2}).

To calculate the energy and power density of the asymmetric supercapacitor, the following Equations (7) and (8) were used [45]:

$$E = \frac{1}{7.2}CV^2 \quad (7)$$

$$P = \frac{3600E}{\Delta t} \quad (8)$$

where E (Wh kg^{-1}) is the energy density, P (W kg^{-1}) stands for the power density, C (F g^{-1}) is the specific capacitance, V(V) is the operating voltage window, and Δt (s) is the discharge time.

4. Conclusions

In this research, MnMoO$_4$·H$_2$O nanosheets were initially synthesized on nickel foam via a hydrothermal approach, followed by the introduction of phosphorus into the MnMoO$_4$·H$_2$O nanosheets using a gas–solid reaction method. The experimental parameters of the phosphorus source content, reaction temperature, and reaction duration were optimized for phosphorylation. The phosphorylated manganese molybdate nanosheets were characterized and electrochemically measured. The P–MnMoO$_4$ of the preferred electrochemical properties were achieved when the phosphorus source content was 0.8 g, the heating temperature was 400 °C, and the heating time was 2 h. At l mA cm^{-2}, the specific capacitance of P–MnMoO$_4$ was 2.112 F cm^{-2}, approximately 3.2 times greater than that of the MnMoO$_4$·H$_2$O electrode. Following 3000 charge/discharge cycles at 5 mA cm^{-2}, the specific capacitance of P–MnMoO$_4$ remained at approximately 82.1% of its initial value. Phosphorus doping enhances the charge storage, conductivity, and ion migration rate of MnMoO$_4$ while preserving the nanosheet morphology of MnMoO$_4$. P–MnMoO$_4$//AC devices provide a high energy density of 41.9 Wh kg^{-1} at a power density of 666.8 W kg^{-1}, with 84.5% capacity retention after 10,000 charge/discharge cycles. This work shows that the P–MnMoO$_4$ material is a potential electrode material with extensive applications in building high-performance energy storage devices.

Supplementary Materials: The following Supplementary Materials can be downloaded at https://www.mdpi.com/article/10.3390/molecules29091988/s1: Figure S1. SEM images of (a,b) NF, (c,d) MnMoO$_4$·H$_2$O, and (e,f) P–MnMoO$_4$; Figure S2. (a) CV curve of MnMoO$_4$·H$_2$O; (b) GCD curve; Figure S3. (a) CV curve of P–MnMoO$_4$; (b) GCD curve; Figure S4. (a–c) SEM images of the P–MnMoO$_4$ electrode material after charge/discharge cycles; Figure S5. (a) CV curve of activated carbon; (b) GCD curve; Table S1. Performance comparison of the hybrid supercapacitor based on the MnMoO$_4$ electrode material with other reported devices. Refs. [46–51] are cited in the Supplementary Materials.

Author Contributions: Conceptualization, K.W. and G.L.; Methodology, K.W. and Y.L. (Yan Li); Data curation, K.W. and Y.L. (Yan Li); Writing–original draft, Y.L. (Yu Liu) and Z.L.; Writing–review and editing Y.L. (Yu Liu), Y.L. (Yan Li), T.F. and H.L.; Supervision, K.W. and G.L. All authors have read and agreed to the published version of the manuscript.

Funding: This research was financially supported by the National Natural Science Foundation of China (Grant Nos. U1810204, 61901293, 22002083, 61975072, 12174173, and 21905099); Natural Science Foundation of Shanxi Province, China (Grant No. 201901D111099); Natural Science Foundation of Fujian Province, grant numbers 2022H0023, 2022J02047, and 2022G02006; and the University Science and Technology Innovation Project of Shanxi Province (Grant No.2019L0316). The author K.W. acknowledges the research grants from EEA (European Economic Area)-Norway-Romania Project Graftid, RO-NO-2019-0616 and EEA-Poland-NOR/POLNORCCS/PhotoRed/0007/2019-00.

Institutional Review Board Statement: Not applicable.

Informed Consent Statement: Not applicable.

Data Availability Statement: The data presented in this study are available in the article.

Conflicts of Interest: The authors declare no conflicts of interest.

References

1. Zou, C.; Zhao, Q.; Zhang, G.; Xiong, B. Energy revolution: From a fossil energy era to a new energy era. *Nat. Gas Ind. B* **2016**, *3*, 1–11. [CrossRef]
2. Raza, W.; Ali, F.; Raza, N.; Luo, Y.; Kim, K.-H.; Yang, J.; Kumar, S.; Mehmood, A.; Kwon, E.E. Recent advancements in supercapacitor technology. *Nano Energy* **2018**, *52*, 441–473. [CrossRef]
3. Libich, J.; Máca, J.; Vondrák, J.; Čech, O.; Sedlaříková, M. Supercapacitors: Properties and applications. *J. Energy Storage* **2018**, *17*, 224–227. [CrossRef]
4. Yang, H.; Kannappan, S.; Pandian, A.S.; Jang, J.H.; Lee, Y.S.; Lu, W. Graphene supercapacitor with both high power and energy density. *Nanotechnology* **2017**, *28*, 445401. [CrossRef] [PubMed]
5. Chodankar, N.R.; Pham, H.D.; Nanjundan, A.K.; Fernando, J.F.S.; Jayaramulu, K.; Golberg, D.; Han, Y.K.; Dubal, D.P. True Meaning of Pseudocapacitors and Their Performance Metrics: Asymmetric versus Hybrid Supercapacitors. *Small* **2020**, *16*, e2002806. [CrossRef] [PubMed]
6. Lim, E.; Jo, C.; Lee, J. A mini review of designed mesoporous materials for energy-storage applications: From electric double-layer capacitors to hybrid supercapacitors. *Nanoscale* **2016**, *8*, 7827–7833. [CrossRef] [PubMed]
7. Han, Y.; Dai, L. Conducting Polymers for Flexible Supercapacitors. *Macromol. Chem. Phys.* **2019**, *220*, 1800355. [CrossRef]
8. Najib, S.; Erdem, E. Current progress achieved in novel materials for supercapacitor electrodes: Mini review. *Nanoscale Adv.* **2019**, *1*, 2817–2827. [CrossRef]
9. Zhang, Y.; Mei, H.-X.; Cao, Y.; Yan, X.-H.; Yan, J.; Gao, H.-L.; Luo, H.-W.; Wang, S.-W.; Jia, X.-D.; Kachalova, L.; et al. Recent advances and challenges of electrode materials for flexible supercapacitors. *Coord. Chem. Rev.* **2021**, *438*, 213910. [CrossRef]

10. Dai, M.; Zhao, D.; Wu, X. Research progress on transition metal oxide based electrode materials for asymmetric hybrid capacitors. *Chin. Chem. Lett.* **2020**, *31*, 2177–2188. [CrossRef]
11. Movassagh-Alanagh, F.; Bordbar-Khiabani, A.; Ahangari-Asl, A. Fabrication of a ternary PANI@Fe$_3$O$_4$@CFs nanocomposite as a high performance electrode for solid-state supercapacitors. *Int. J. Hydrogen Energy* **2019**, *44*, 26794–26806. [CrossRef]
12. Ryu, I.; Kim, D.; Choe, G.; Jin, S.; Hong, D.; Yim, S. Monodisperse RuO$_2$ nanoparticles for highly transparent and rapidly responsive supercapacitor electrodes. *J. Mater. Chem. A* **2021**, *9*, 26172–26180. [CrossRef]
13. Zheng, D.; Zhao, F.; Li, Y.; Qin, C.; Zhu, J.; Hu, Q.; Wang, Z.; Inoue, A. Flexible NiO micro-rods/nanoporous Ni/metallic glass electrode with sandwich structure for high performance supercapacitors. *Electrochim. Acta* **2019**, *297*, 767–777. [CrossRef]
14. Zhong, R.; Xu, M.; Fu, N.; Liu, R.; Zhou, A.A.; Wang, X.; Yang, Z. A flexible high-performance symmetric quasi-solid supercapacitor based on Ni-doped MnO$_2$ nano-array @ carbon cloth. *Electrochim. Acta* **2020**, *348*, 136209. [CrossRef]
15. Liang, R.; Du, Y.; Xiao, P.; Cheng, J.; Yuan, S.; Chen, Y.; Yuan, J.; Chen, J. Transition Metal Oxide Electrode Materials for Supercapacitors: A Review of Recent Developments. *Nanomaterials* **2021**, *11*, 1248. [CrossRef] [PubMed]
16. Zhu, Z.; Sun, Y.; Li, C.; Yang, C.; Li, L.; Zhu, J.; Chou, S.; Wang, M.; Wang, D.; Li, Y. Mini review: Progress on micro/nanoscale MnMoO$_4$ as an electrode material for advanced supercapacitor applications. *Mater. Chem. Front.* **2021**, *5*, 7403–7418. [CrossRef]
17. Watcharatharapong, T.; Minakshi Sundaram, M.; Chakraborty, S.; Li, D.; Shafiullah, G.M.; Aughterson, R.D.; Ahuja, R. Effect of Transition Metal Cations on Stability Enhancement for Molybdate-Based Hybrid Supercapacitor. *ACS Appl. Mater. Interfaces* **2017**, *9*, 17977–17991. [CrossRef] [PubMed]
18. Li, L.; Wang, L.; Zhang, C. Hierarchical MnMoO$_4$@nitrogen-doped carbon core-shell microspheres for lithium/potassium-ion batteries. *J. Alloys Compd.* **2022**, *893*, 162336. [CrossRef]
19. Mu, X.; Zhang, Y.; Wang, H.; Huang, B.; Sun, P.; Chen, T.; Zhou, J.; Xie, E.; Zhang, Z. A high energy density asymmetric supercapacitor from ultrathin manganese molybdate nanosheets. *Electrochim. Acta* **2016**, *211*, 217–224. [CrossRef]
20. Fu, H.; Wang, M.; Ma, Q.; Wang, M.; Ma, X.; Ye, Y. MnMoO$_4$-S nanosheets with rich oxygen vacancies for high-performance supercapacitors. *Nanoscale Adv.* **2022**, *4*, 2704–2712. [CrossRef]
21. Meng, Y.; Sun, P.; He, W.; Teng, B.; Xu, X. Uniform P doped Co-Ni-S nanostructures for asymmetric supercapacitors with ultra-high energy densities. *Nanoscale* **2019**, *11*, 688–697. [CrossRef] [PubMed]
22. Zhang, Q.; Feng, L.; Liu, Z.; Jiang, L.; Lan, T.; Zhang, C.; Liu, K.; He, S. High Rate Performance Supercapacitors Based on N, O Co-Doped Hierarchical Porous Carbon Foams Synthesized via Chemical Blowing and Dual Templates. *Molecules* **2023**, *28*, 6994. [CrossRef] [PubMed]
23. Yu, J.; Li, Z.; Liu, T.; Zhao, S.; Guan, D.; Chen, D.; Shao, Z.; Ni, M. Morphology control and electronic tailoring of Co$_x$A$_y$ (A = P, S, Se) electrocatalysts for water splitting. *Chem. Eng. J.* **2023**, *460*, 141674. [CrossRef]
24. Shi, Y.; Zhang, B. Recent advances in transition metal phosphide nanomaterials: Synthesis and applications in hydrogen evolution reaction. *Chem. Soc. Rev.* **2016**, *45*, 1529–1541. [CrossRef] [PubMed]
25. Guo, S.; Tang, Y.; Xie, Y.; Tian, C.; Feng, Q.; Zhou, W.; Jiang, B. P-doped tubular g-C$_3$N$_4$ with surface carbon defects: Universal synthesis and enhanced visible-light photocatalytic hydrogen production. *Appl. Catal. B Environ.* **2017**, *218*, 664–671. [CrossRef]
26. Liu, Q.; Tian, J.; Cui, W.; Jiang, P.; Cheng, N.; Asiri, A.M.; Sun, X. Carbon nanotubes decorated with CoP nanocrystals: A highly active non-noble-metal nanohybrid electrocatalyst for hydrogen evolution. *Angew. Chem. Int. Ed. Engl.* **2014**, *53*, 6710–6714. [CrossRef]
27. Xu, J.; Sun, Y.; Lu, M.; Wang, L.; Zhang, J.; Qian, J.; Liu, X. Fabrication of hierarchical MnMoO$_4$·H$_2$O@MnO$_2$ core-shell nanosheet arrays on nickel foam as an advanced electrode for asymmetric supercapacitors. *Chem. Eng. J.* **2018**, *334*, 1466–1476. [CrossRef]
28. Guan, D.; Shi, C.; Xu, H.; Gu, Y.; Zhong, J.; Sha, Y.; Hu, Z.; Ni, M.; Shao, Z. Simultaneously mastering operando strain and reconstruction effects via phase-segregation strategy for enhanced oxygen-evolving electrocatalysis. *J. Energy Chem.* **2023**, *82*, 572–580. [CrossRef]
29. Cao, Y.; Li, W.; Xu, K.; Zhang, Y.; Ji, T.; Zou, R.; Yang, J.; Qin, Z.; Hu, J. MnMoO$_4$·4H$_2$O nanoplates grown on a Ni foam substrate for excellent electrochemical properties. *J. Mater. Chem. A* **2014**, *2*, 20723–20728. [CrossRef]
30. Gao, L.; Chen, G.; Zhang, L.; Yan, B.; Yang, X. Engineering pseudocapacitive MnMoO$_4$@C microrods for high energy sodium ion hybrid capacitors. *Electrochim. Acta* **2021**, *379*, 138185. [CrossRef]
31. Nti, F.; Anang, D.A.; Han, J.I. Facile room temperature synthesis and application of MnMoO$_4$·0.9 H$_2$O as supercapacitor electrode material. *Mater. Lett.* **2018**, *217*, 146–150. [CrossRef]
32. Wei, H.; Yang, J.; Zhang, Y.; Qian, Y.; Geng, H. Rational synthesis of graphene-encapsulated uniform MnMoO$_4$ hollow spheres as long-life and high-rate anodes for lithium-ion batteries. *J. Colloid Interface Sci.* **2018**, *524*, 256–262. [CrossRef] [PubMed]
33. Xing, T.; Ouyang, Y.; Chen, Y.; Zheng, L.; Wu, C.; Wang, X. P-doped ternary transition metal oxide as electrode material of asymmetric supercapacitor. *J. Energy Storage* **2020**, *28*, 101248. [CrossRef]
34. Chen, Y.; Yang, W.; Gao, S.; Sun, C.; Li, Q. Synthesis of Bi$_2$MoO$_6$ nanosheets with rich oxygen vacancies by postsynthesis etching treatment for enhanced photocatalytic performance. *ACS Appl. Nano Mater.* **2018**, *1*, 3565–3578. [CrossRef]
35. Saravanakumar, B.; Ramachandran, S.P.; Ravi, G.; Ganesh, V.; Sakunthala, A.; Yuvakkumar, R. Transition mixed-metal molybdates (MnMoO$_4$) as an electrode for energy storage applications. *Appl. Phys. A* **2018**, *125*, 6. [CrossRef]
36. Shi, Y.; Li, M.; Yu, Y.; Zhang, B. Recent advances in nanostructured transition metal phosphides: Synthesis and energy-related applications. *Energy Environ. Sci.* **2020**, *13*, 4564–4582. [CrossRef]

37. Zong, Q.; Liu, C.; Yang, H.; Zhang, Q.; Cao, G. Tailoring nanostructured transition metal phosphides for high-performance hybrid supercapacitors. *Nano Today* **2021**, *38*, 101201. [CrossRef]
38. Yu, Z.; Zhang, N.; Li, G.; Ma, L.; Li, T.; Tong, Z.; Li, Y.; Wang, K. Funnel-shaped hierarchical NiMoO$_4$@Co$_3$S$_4$ core-shell nanostructure for enhanced supercapacitor performance. *J. Energy Storage* **2022**, *51*, 104511. [CrossRef]
39. Li, H.; Xuan, H. Hierarchical design of Ni(OH)$_2$/MnMoO$_4$ composite on reduced graphene oxide/Ni foam for high-performances battery-supercapacitors hybrid device. *Int. J. Hydrogen Energy* **2021**, *46*, 38198–38211. [CrossRef]
40. Han, X.; Yang, Y.; Zhou, J.J.; Ma, Q.; Tao, K.; Han, L. Metal-Organic Framework Templated 3D Hierarchical ZnCo$_2$O$_4$@Ni(OH)$_2$ Core-Shell Nanosheet Arrays for High-Performance Supercapacitors. *Chemistry* **2018**, *24*, 18106–18114. [CrossRef]
41. Sivaprakash, P.; Kumar, K.A.; Muthukumaran, S.; Pandurangan, A.; Dixit, A.; Arumugam, S. NiF$_2$ as an efficient electrode material with high window potential of 1.8 V for high energy and power density asymmetric supercapacitor. *J. Electroanal. Chem.* **2020**, *873*, 114379. [CrossRef]
42. Ruan, Y.; Lv, L.; Li, Z.; Wang, C.; Jiang, J. Ni nanoparticles@Ni–Mo nitride nanorod arrays: A novel 3D-network hierarchical structure for high areal capacitance hybrid supercapacitors. *Nanoscale* **2017**, *9*, 18032–18041. [CrossRef] [PubMed]
43. Li, D.; Liu, H.; Liu, Z.; Huang, Q.; Lu, B.; Wang, Y.; Wang, C.; Guo, L. Copper Oxide Nitrogen-Rich Porous Carbon Network Boosts High-Performance Supercapacitors. *Metals* **2023**, *13*, 981. [CrossRef]
44. Yesuraj, J.; Elumalai, V.; Bhagavathiachari, M.; Samuel, A.S.; Elaiyappillai, E.; Johnson, P.M. A facile sonochemical assisted synthesis of α-MnMoO$_4$/PANI nanocomposite electrode for supercapacitor applications. *J. Electroanal. Chem.* **2017**, *797*, 78–88. [CrossRef]
45. Xie, Z.; Liu, L.; Li, Y.; Yu, D.; Wei, L.; Han, L.; Hua, Y.; Wang, C.; Zhao, X.; Liu, X. Synthesis of core-shell structured Ni$_3$S$_2$@MnMoO$_4$ nanosheet arrays on Ni foam for asymmetric supercapacitors with superior performance. *J. Alloys Compd.* **2021**, *874*, 159860. [CrossRef]
46. Prabakaran, P.; Arumugam, G.; Ramu, P.; Selvaraj, M.; Assiri, M.A.; Rokhum, S.L.; Arjunan, S.; Rajendran, R. Construction of hierarchical MnMoO$_4$ nanostructures on Ni foam for high-performance asymmetric supercapacitors. *Surf. Interfaces* **2023**, *40*, 103086. [CrossRef]
47. Senthilkumar, B.; Selvan, R.K.; Meyrick, D.; Minakshi, M. Synthesis and Characterization of Manganese Molybdate for Symmetric Capacitor Applications. *Int. J. Electrochem. Sci.* **2015**, *10*, 185–193. [CrossRef]
48. Appiagyei, A.B.; Asiedua-Ahenkorah, L.; Bathula, C.; Kim, H.-S.; Han, S.S.; Rao, K.M.; Anang, D.A. Rational design of sucrose-derived graphitic carbon coated MnMoO4 for high performance asymmetric supercapacitor. *J. Energy Storage* **2023**, *58*, 106383. [CrossRef]
49. Bhagwan, J.; Hussain, S.K.; Krishna, B.V.; Yu, J.S. Facile synthesis of MnMoO$_4$@ MWCNT and their electrochemical performance in aqueous asymmetric supercapacitor. *J. Alloys Compd.* **2021**, *856*, 157874. [CrossRef]
50. Pallavolu, M.R.; Banerjee, A.N.; Nallapureddy, R.R.; Joo, S.W. Urea-assisted hydrothermal synthesis of MnMoO$_4$/MnCO$_3$ hybrid electrochemical electrode and fabrication of high-performance asymmetric supercapacitor. *J. Mater. Sci. Technol.* **2022**, *96*, 332–344. [CrossRef]
51. Feng, X.; Huang, Y.; Chen, M.; Chen, X.; Li, C.; Zhou, S.; Gao, X. Self-assembly of 3D hierarchical MnMoO$_4$/NiWO$_4$ microspheres for high-performance supercapacitor. *J. Alloys Compd.* **2018**, *763*, 801–807. [CrossRef]

Disclaimer/Publisher's Note: The statements, opinions and data contained in all publications are solely those of the individual author(s) and contributor(s) and not of MDPI and/or the editor(s). MDPI and/or the editor(s) disclaim responsibility for any injury to people or property resulting from any ideas, methods, instructions or products referred to in the content.

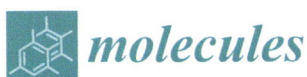

Article

Effect of Rh Doping on Optical Absorption and Oxygen Evolution Reaction Activity on BaTiO$_3$ (001) Surfaces

Talgat M. Inerbaev [1,2], Aisulu U. Abuova [1,*], Zhadyra Ye. Zakiyeva [1], Fatima U. Abuova [1], Yuri A. Mastrikov [3], Maksim Sokolov [3], Denis Gryaznov [3,*] and Eugene A. Kotomin [3]

[1] Department of Technical Physics, L.N. Gumilyov Eurasian National University, Astana 010000, Kazakhstan; talgat.inerbaev@gmail.com (T.M.I.); jadira.zakieva@mail.ru (Z.Y.Z.); abuova_fu@enu.kz (F.U.A.)
[2] Vernadsky Institute of Geochemistry and Analytical Chemistry, Russian Academy of Science, 119991 Moscow, Russia
[3] Institute of Solid State Physics, University of Latvia, LV-1063 Riga, Latvia; yuri@umd.edu (Y.A.M.); makcsokolov@gmail.com (M.S.); kotomin@latnet.lv (E.A.K.)
* Correspondence: aisulu-us1980@ya.ru (A.U.A.); denis.gryaznov@cfi.lu.lv (D.G.)

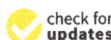

Abstract: In the present work, we investigate the potential of modified barium titanate (BaTiO$_3$), an inexpensive perovskite oxide derived from earth-abundant precursors, for developing efficient water oxidation electrocatalysts using first-principles calculations. Based on our calculations, Rh doping is a way of making BaTiO$_3$ absorb more light and have less overpotential needed for water to oxidize. It has been shown that a TiO$_2$-terminated BaTiO$_3$ (001) surface is more promising from the point of view of its use as a catalyst. Rh doping expands the spectrum of absorbed light to the entire visible range. The aqueous environment significantly affects the ability of Rh-doped BaTiO$_3$ to absorb solar radiation. After Ti→Rh replacement, the doping ion can take over part of the electron density from neighboring oxygen ions. As a result, during the water oxidation reaction, rhodium ions can be in an intermediate oxidation state between 3+ and 4+. This affects the adsorption energy of reaction intermediates on the catalyst's surface, reducing the overpotential value.

Keywords: electrocatalysis; photocatalysis; energy storage and conversion; electrode materials; water splitting

Citation: Inerbaev, T.M.; Abuova, A.U.; Zakiyeva, Z.Y.; Abuova, F.U.; Mastrikov, Y.A.; Sokolov, M.; Gryaznov, D.; Kotomin, E.A. Effect of Rh Doping on Optical Absorption and Oxygen Evolution Reaction Activity on BaTiO$_3$ (001) Surfaces. *Molecules* **2024**, *29*, 2707. https://doi.org/10.3390/molecules29112707

Academic Editor: Qingguo Shao

Received: 16 April 2024
Revised: 28 May 2024
Accepted: 3 June 2024
Published: 6 June 2024

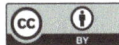

Copyright: © 2024 by the authors. Licensee MDPI, Basel, Switzerland. This article is an open access article distributed under the terms and conditions of the Creative Commons Attribution (CC BY) license (https://creativecommons.org/licenses/by/4.0/).

1. Introduction

The growing demand for environmentally friendly and cost-effective energy sources has led to intensive research into various renewable energy sources. In this regard, photo-electrochemical hydrogen generation through water splitting has emerged as a promising avenue due to its affordability and environmental friendliness. In 1972, Honda and Fujishima first reported hydrogen production through photochemical water splitting using the semiconductor TiO$_2$ [1]. Since then, this phenomenon has been extensively studied, and numerous materials and water-splitting systems have been developed. In the process of photoelectrochemical (PEC) water splitting, hydrogen is produced from water by using sunlight and specialized semiconductors called PEC materials. These materials directly split water molecules into hydrogen and oxygen using light energy.

An integrated PEC system consists of light absorbers, electrocatalysts for the hydrogen evolution reaction and the oxygen evolution reaction (OER), electrolytes, and membranes. This system can be used to efficiently produce hydrogen fuel from sunlight, especially through the photo-electrolysis of water, generating sustainable hydrogen and oxygen. However, the key to achieving viable PEC solar water splitting lies in carefully selecting semiconductive electrode materials. These materials must have low band gaps and exceptional stability and be inexpensive. This strategic choice allows for the absorption of a greater amount of visible light, thereby enhancing the overall efficiency of the process.

Perovskite-based materials are widely regarded as highly efficient photocatalysts for water splitting due to their adjustable electronic properties [2–6]. In addition, perovskite materials comprise environmentally benign and inexpensive elements abundant on Earth [7,8]. Recently, there has been increased focus on using perovskites as cost-effective catalysts for water electrolysis due to a deeper comprehension of the rapport between electronic structure and reactivity [9,10]. As a new category of perovskite derivatives, layered Ruddlesden–Popper perovskites are currently attracting growing research attention [11,12].

$BaTiO_3$, utilized as a crystal in non-linear optics, dielectric ceramics, and piezoelectric materials, is among the ferroelectric oxides that have been the subject of extended scientific inquiry [13]. The optical band gap of pristine $BaTiO_3$ is 3.2–3.4 eV, much larger than the activation energy of 1.23 eV required for water splitting [14]. Therefore, the use of bare titania for solar energy harvesting is not efficient. Band gap excitation requires ultraviolet irradiation (UV); however, UV light accounts for only 4% of the solar spectrum compared to the 45% that is visible. So, any shift in optical response to the visible range will have a profound positive effect on the photocatalytic efficiencies of $BaTiO_3$ materials.

There have been reports of water electrolysis using $BaTiO_3$ electrodes [15,16]. Ni-supported $BaTiO_3$ exhibits activity for CO_2 reformation [17], Pd-modified $BaTiO_3$ efficiently catalyzes NO_x reduction [18], and Cr-modified $BaTiO_3$ catalyzes the reduction of nitrobenzene and aniline [19]. Several methods are used for enhancing the electronic properties of barium titanate for electrocatalysts application. Catalyst performance could be, in principle, improved using different promoters like W, Mn, and Fe [20–22]. According to a theoretical study [23], Fe_{Ti} and Ni_{Ti} substitutions increased electrical conductivity and reduced overpotentials for the OER. Xie et al. [24] revealed experimentally that applying a 2% Mo doping to $BaTiO_3$ results in a reduction in the optical bandgap that activates its photocatalytic performance. Eu-doped $BaTiO_3$ nanoparticles show remarkable electrochemical performance towards the oxygen evolution reaction (OER) and excellent stability over 2000 cyclic voltammetry cycles [25].

Rh doping is one of the most effective methods that enables one to produce a visible-light-responsive photocatalyst [26–28]. Related to $BaTiO_3$, rhodium-doped $SrTiO_3$ exhibits remarkable photocatalytic efficiency in the process of H_2 evolution from an aqueous methanol solution under visible light irradiation, outperforming all other visible-light-activated oxide photocatalysts [27]. Bhat et al. [29] suggested that Rh-doped $BaTiO_3$ resulted in the formation of mid-gap electronic states, causing a reduction in the band gap of $BaTiO_3$ while simultaneously avoiding the formation of recombination centers. As seen from the studies mentioned above, the research on Rh-modified impacts on the catalyst properties of $BaTiO_3$ is limited and requires more detailed consideration. In light of these novel findings, in the current article, we investigate the degree to which a minor modification can be made to the chemical composition of the surface of barium titanate ($BaTiO_3$) to tune its catalytic reactivity. This study focuses on the optical absorption and catalytic performance towards OER of pure and Rh-modified tetragonal $BaTiO_3$ structures.

2. Theoretical Surface and Thermodynamic Model
2.1. Structure Models

In this work, the tetragonal $BaTiO_3$ phase, which is not energetically favorable at a temperature of zero but exists at room temperature, was used in the modeling conducted. Initial crystal structure was taken from the Materials Project database [30]. To make the (001) surface models of $BaTiO_3$, slabs with eleven layers of TiO_2 and BaO that are symmetric concerning the mirror plane were used. The end of one of these slabs had BaO planes for the crystal and was a supercell containing 108 atoms. The second slab terminated in TiO_2 planes containing 112 atoms. The (001) surface was chosen because it is the most energetically favorable for both TiO_2 and BaO terminations [31]. A vacuum layer measuring 15 Å thick was applied perpendicular to the slabs to avoid artificial interactions between the slab and its periodic images.

Even though these slabs are not stoichiometric, they maintain symmetry when the Ba/Ti atoms are substituted with Rh on the outermost layer, preventing the system from having a dipole moment. Due to periodic boundary conditions, this dipole moment may significantly distort the calculated energy values of the systems. These two slab ends (TiO_2 and BaO) are the only possible terminations of (001) surfaces for the $BaTiO_3$ perovskite lattice structure, as shown in Figure 1. Replacing the Ba atoms on a BaO-terminated surface results in the doping atom formally entering the Rh_{Ba}^{2+} state. Experimentally, Rh^{3+} and Rh^{4+} ions have been detected when $BaTiO_3$ is doped [32], so neutral OH groups were added to the surface to change Rh_{Ba}^{2+} into Rh_{Ba}^{3+}. The present study focuses on the TiO_2-terminated surface because it has recently been shown that the BaO-terminated surface is also unstable under operating conditions [23].

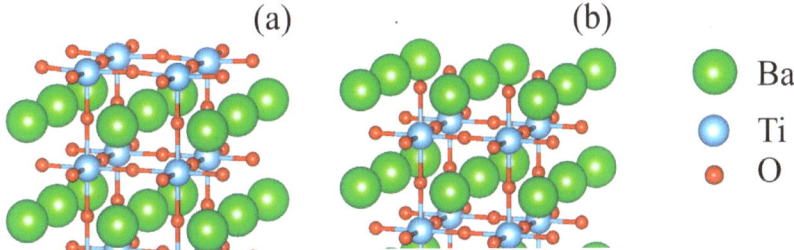

Figure 1. (a) TiO_2- and (b) BaO-terminated (001) surfaces of tetragonal $BaTiO_3$.

2.2. Thermodynamic Description

Under the standard conditions (T = 298 K, p = 1 bar, pH = 0), the equilibrium thermodynamic potential for water oxidation required to produce oxygen ($H_2O \rightarrow 1/2 O_2 + 4H^+ + 4e^-$) is 1.23 V vs RHE (the reference electrode is further omitted for brevity). In practice, a potential above 1.23 V is required for this reaction. For heterogeneous catalysts, this additional potential is referred to as the overpotential η.

The catalytic oxygen evolution reaction (OER) via water oxidation is divided into four fundamental reaction steps, wherein each step entails the exchange of an electron–proton pair (where * denotes the adsorption site of the catalyst) [33,34]:

$$2H_2O + * \rightleftharpoons OH^* + H_2O + H^+ + e^- \tag{1a}$$

$$OH^* + H_2O \rightleftharpoons O^* + H_2O + H^+ + e^- \tag{1b}$$

$$O^* + H_2O \rightleftharpoons OOH^* + H^+ + e^- \tag{1c}$$

$$OOH^* \rightleftharpoons * + O_2 + H^+ + e^- \tag{1d}$$

Using the normal (computational) hydrogen electrode approach, the reaction free energy ΔG of the charge transfer reaction $H^* \rightleftharpoons * + H^+ + e^-$ under standard ambient conditions is equal to the ΔG of the $H^* \rightleftharpoons * + 1/2 H_2$ reaction. The reactions' Gibbs free energy for steps ΔG_1, ΔG_2, ΔG_3, and ΔG_4 in Equation (1) can be expressed as

$$\begin{aligned}
\Delta G_1 &= \Delta G_{OH} - eU + \Delta G_{H+}(pH) \\
\Delta G_2 &= \Delta G_O - \Delta G_{OH} - eU + \Delta G_{H+}(pH) \\
\Delta G_3 &= \Delta G_{OOH} - \Delta G_O - eU + \Delta G_{H+}(pH) \\
\Delta G_4 &= 4.92[eV] - \Delta G_{OOH} - eU + \Delta G_{H+}(pH)
\end{aligned} \tag{2}$$

where U is the potential measured against a normal hydrogen electrode (NHE) under standard conditions. The free energy change of the protons relative to the NHE at non-zero pH is represented by the Nernst equation as $\Delta G_{H+}(pH) = -k_B T \ln(10) \times pH$. The Gibbs free energy differences in Equation (2) include zero-point energy (ZPE) and enthropy corrections according to $\Delta G_i = \Delta E_i - T\Delta S_i + \Delta ZPE_i - eU$. Entropic contributions under standard conditions were taken from the CRC Handbook [35]. The Supporting Information for Ref. [34] also includes these values. Energy differences ΔE_i calculated relative to H_2O and H_2 (at $U = 0$ and pH = 0) are approximated as follows:

$$\Delta E_{OH} = E(OH^*) - E(*) - \left[E(H_2O) - \tfrac{1}{2}E(H_2)\right]$$
$$\Delta E_O = E(O^*) - E(*) - [E(H_2O) - E(H_2)] \qquad (3)$$
$$\Delta E_{OOH} = E(OOH^*) - E(*) - \left[2E(H_2O) - \tfrac{3}{2}E(H_2)\right]$$

The theoretical overpotential can then be readily defined as

$$\eta = max[\Delta G_i]/e - 1.23 \text{ (V)} \qquad (4)$$

The overpotential represented by Equation (4) is simply a thermodynamic quantity. Due to the lack of activation barriers, experimentally determined overpotential values cannot be directly compared with theoretical ones. In addition, experiments are usually carried out using electrodes containing nanoparticles of the used material, whose active surface's exact value is difficult to determine.

3. Results and Discussion

3.1. Effect of Doping on Ground-State Electronic Properties

Geometry modification. The computed lattice parameters for the bulk tetragonal $BaTiO_3$ are a_0 = 4.0381 Å and c_0 = 4.0999 Å. Several of the experimental data that are accessible are comparable to our findings: a_0 falls within the range of 3.9860 Å to 3.9905 Å, and c_0 spans from 4.0170 Å to 4.0412 Å [36–40].

The TiO_2-terminated surface replacement of Ti^{4+} with Rh^{4+} leads to slight distortion of the lattice, as shown in Figure 2a–c. Each surface Ti^{4+} ion is surrounded by four neighboring surface oxygen ions (O1) and one nearest-subsurface oxygen (O2). All Ti^{4+}-O1 distances are the same and are 2.2027 Å, while the Ti^{4+}-O2 bond lengths are 1.9086 Å. After the $Ti^{4+} \rightarrow Rh^{4+}$ substitution, the Rh_{Ti}^{4+}-O1 bond lengths are 2.1046 Å, and the Rh_{Ti}^{4+}-O2 distance is 2.3089 Å. Substitution energy, $Ti^{4+} \rightarrow Rh^{4+}$, is calculated as follows:

$$E_{def} = (E(\text{Rh-doped}) + E(\text{Ti}) - E(\text{undoped}) - E(\text{Rh}))/2,$$

where E(undoped) and E(Rh-doped) are the calculated energies of the pristine and doped slabs, and E(Ti) and E(Rh) are the energies per atom for metals *hcp*-Ti and *bcc*-Rh. The calculations yield the value E_{def} = 7.212 eV per Rh atom. This value is typical for this type of substitution. Thus, the previously calculated value of the $Ti^{4+} \rightarrow Ru^{4+}$ substitution energy is 6.424 eV per Ru atom [41].

In the case of $Ba^{2+} \rightarrow Rh^{3+} + OH^-$ substitution, a much stronger distortion of the surface structure occurs. After geometry optimization, Rh_{Ba}^{3+} ions are displaced, moving from the surface layer deep in the slab to the subsurface layer, forming bonds with oxygen ions in this layer (Figure 2d–f). In this case, in the next atomic layer under the Rh^{3+} ion, Ba^{2+} is present. This finding shows that even if there were a BaO-terminated surface, the doping ion Rh_{Ba}^{3+} would not be on the surface layer. This would make this site less likely to be able to catalyze water-splitting reactions.

Electronic density of states. The HSE06-calculated electronic structures of the doped and undoped models are schematically summarized in Figure 3. Figure 3 presents the total (TDOS) and partial densities of states of the bare and doped TiO_2- and BaO-terminated surfaces. For both bare surfaces, the O-2p states predominately form a valence band, whereas the Ti-4d states form the conduction band minimum. The O-2p→Ti-3d transitions thus determine optical absorption for undoped $BaTiO_3$. The calculated band gaps for the undoped models are 2.8 eV and 3.0 eV for the TiO_2- and BaO-terminated surfaces, respectively. The different stoichiometries of the studied models account for this variation in the calculated bandgap values. However, the bandgap values obtained from the DOS calculations do not coincide with the results of the optical spectra calculations, which will be shown below when analyzing the optical absorption spectra.

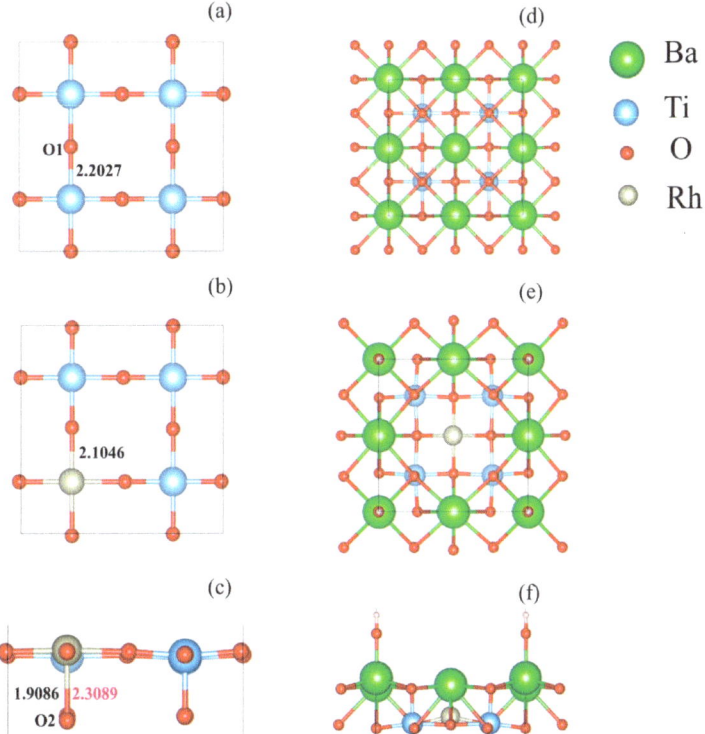

Figure 2. (**Left**): Top view of the outermost layer of TiO$_2$-terminated (**a**) undoped and (**b**) Rh-doped surfaces. The numbers indicate the distance (Å) between the (**a**) Ti and (**b**) Rh atoms and the nearest surface oxygen atoms (O1). (**c**) Side view of a doped TiO$_2$-terminated surface (Ba ions omitted); the numbers indicate the interatomic distance between the metal atoms (Ti: black, Rh: pink) and subsurface oxygen (O2). (**Right**): Top view of the two upper layers of BaO-terminated (**d**) undoped and (**e**) Rh-doped surfaces. Side view of a doped BaO-terminated surface (**f**).

Doping the TiO$_2$-terminated surface results in additional levels due to the Rh-4d states appearing in the band gap (Figure 3b). The Rh^{4+} ion also changes the electronic states of the oxygen atoms that are closest to it. This causes the O-2p peaks to appear in the calculated DOS near the valence band maximum. This effect also results in an additional reduction in the band gap. When doping a BaO-terminated surface, in addition to the Rh-4d states in the bandgap, the Ti-3d states appear near the minimum of the conduction band; titanium ions close to the Rh ion in the subsurface layer give rise to these states. As Rh^{4+} shifts from the surface to the layer below, it breaks the bonds between the dopant and the surface oxygen ions. This creates more O-2p-induced peaks in the DOS near the top of the valence band (Figure 3d).

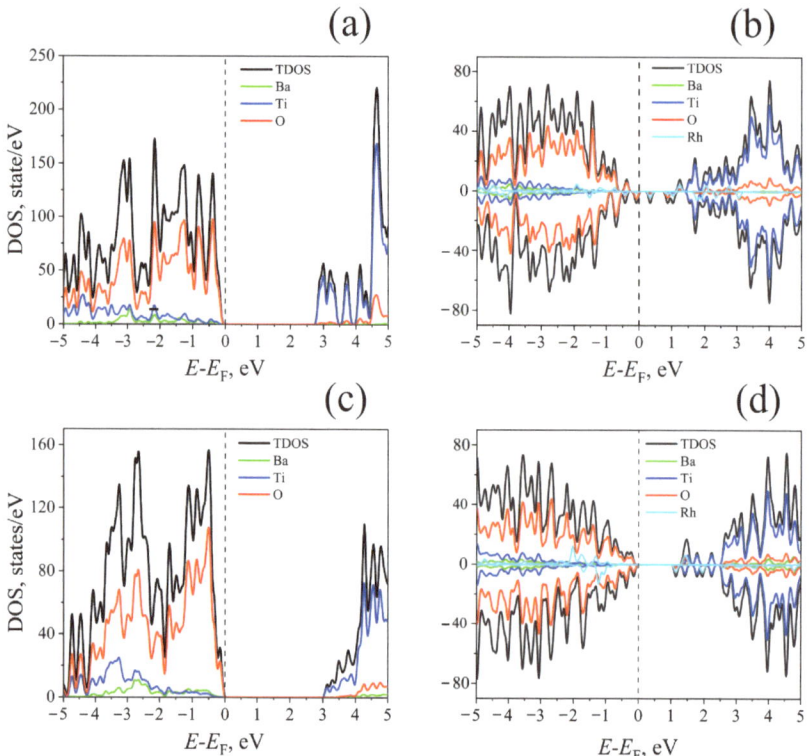

Figure 3. Total and partial densities of states for bare and doped TiO_2- and BaO-terminated surfaces. Top: (**a**) undoped TiO_2-terminated surface; (**b**) Rh-doped TiO_2-terminated surface. The contribution of the surface nearest to the oxygen atoms of Rh, O(Rh), is highlighted. Bottom: (**c**) undoped BaO-terminated surface; (**d**) Rh-doped BaO-terminated surface. E_F: Fermi energy.

3.2. Optical Absorption

The effect of doping on optical absorption is shown in Figure 4. Both dry and wet surfaces are considered. The presence of Rh^{4+} ions (Figure 4a) on the TiO_2-terminated surface substantially changes the optical absorption spectrum due to the DOS changes discussed above. Although the DOS calculations for an undoped surface yield a band gap of 2.8 eV, the optical absorption threshold is 3.35 eV (370 nm). This difference exists because for optical transitions of the O-2p→Ti-3d type in the energy range of 2.8–3.1 eV, the oscillator strengths calculated using Equation (8) are equal to zero or assume negligibly small values. As a result, the optical absorption threshold value for the undoped structure is in good agreement with experimental data [32]. The spin-down O-2p→Rh-4d transitions on a Rh-doped surface absorb light in the long-wavelength range. In the short-wavelength range, optical absorption occurs due to the O-2p→Ti-3d transitions. The optical absorption peak at 900 nm is suppressed in the aqueous environment and the absorption at 450 nm is significantly reduced. In this case, optical absorption increases in the 500–550 nm range. A comparison of the calculated data and the experimental results obtained after the 2 mol% doping of $BaTiO_3$ is presented [42]. The agreement between the theoretical and experimental results can be considered good since modeling shows that in the case of replacing the surface Ti^{4+} ion with Rh_{Ti}^{4+}, optical absorption occurs in a wide range of frequencies of electromagnetic radiation. Up to this stage, our model does not consider the role that Rh^{4+} ions inside the slab might play in optical absorption. In this case, these ions would not be on the sample's surface, and aqueous media would not affect their electronic states. Below, we present an analysis and its results for the situation when the Rh ions reside inside the slab.

The optical absorption threshold value for the BaO-terminated surface is the same as that found by directly estimating the bandgap value from the DOS calculation and amounts to 415 nm (2.99 eV). The optical absorption at longer wavelengths is also due to the O-2p→Rh-4d and O-2p→Ti-3d transitions. In this case, in contrast to the TiO$_2$-terminated surface, in the 400–520 nm wavelength range (2.4–3.1 eV), there is a contribution from the Rh-4d→Ti-3d transitions. This finding agrees with experimental data [32]. The transitions discussed here suggest that the electronic transitions from the Rh^{3+} ions to the conduction band are possible, even though Rh^{4+} usually plays the role of a trapping center [43].

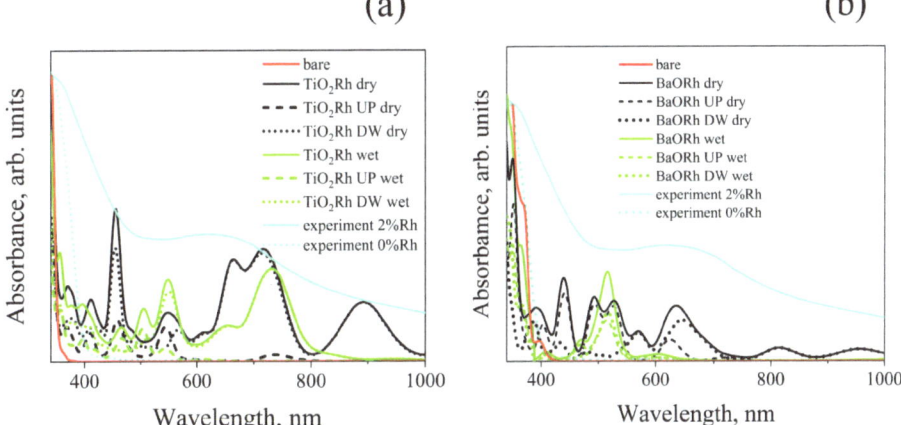

Figure 4. Optical absorption of undoped and Rh-doped (**a**) TiO$_2$- and (**b**) BaO-terminated surfaces. Black and blue lines correspond to dry and wet surfaces, respectively. The solid lines illustrate total optical absorption, while dashed and dotted lines correspond to the contributions of spin-up (UP) and spin-down (DW) electronic states. Orange lines refer to experimental data adapted from Ref. [32].

Since the BaO-terminated surface was probably unstable but we knew that the Rh^{3+} ions help with optical absorption, we also looked at a model where the Rh ions were put inside the BaO-terminated slab instead of the slab surface. To ensure the Rh^{3+} oxidation state was obtained, neutral OH groups were added to the surface.

The results of geometry optimization, DOS, and optical absorption calculations are presented in Figure 5. Figure 5a shows how the atomic structure changes when rhodium is added after the structure's geometry has been optimized. As in the case of the BaO-terminated surface (Figure 2e,f), the Rh$_{Ba}^{3+}$ ion is shifted towards the TiO$_2$ plane. Unlike in the previous case, the displacement occurs in a direction parallel to the surface plane since the lattice parameters in this direction are lower than those perpendicular to the direction. The DOS analysis (Figure 5b) shows that the nature of the bottom of the conduction band is due to the Rh-4d and Ti-3d levels. The Ti-3d states are localized on Ti atoms located near Rh. So, optical absorption (Figure 5c) begins at 550 nm (2.25 eV) and is caused by transitions from O-2p to Rh-4d for the spin-down states. Furthermore, at wavelengths of approximately 500 nm (2.5 eV) and shorter, Rh-4d→Ti-3d transitions are possible. Thus, the experimentally observed Rh-4d→Ti-3d transitions [32] are most likely caused by Rh^{3+} ions inside the sample.

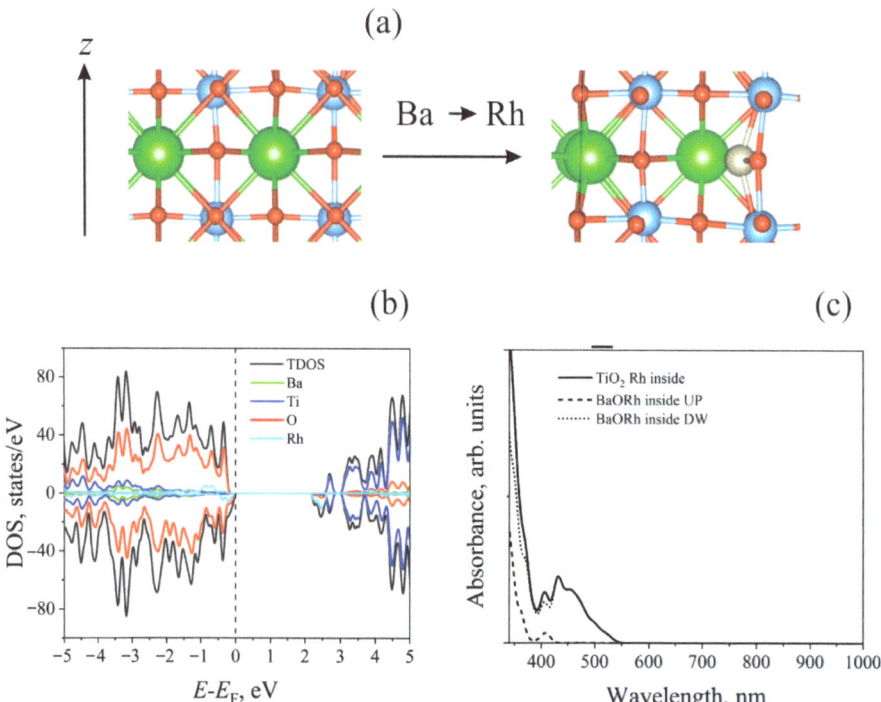

Figure 5. (a) Change in the arrangement of ions in the slab after Ba was replaced with Rh; (b) electronic DOS for relaxed slab; (c) optical absorption spectrum for the model investigated. Dashed and dotted lines represent optical absorption by spin-up and spin-down states. The solid line illustrates total absorption.

3.3. OER over Pristine and Rh-Modified BaTiO$_3$

The above results indicate that Rh doping dramatically improves the ability of BaTiO$_3$ to absorb sunlight in the visible range. The TiO$_2$-terminated surface is also more stable regarding the Ti^{4+}→Rh^{4+} change, while the Ba-terminated surface's Rh^{3+} ion position is less stable. It was previously shown that the TiO$_2$-terminated surface is stable under operating conditions. In contrast, the BaO-terminated surface is unstable concerning Ba dissolution at a wide range of pH values and potentials [32]. Based on these results, we evaluated the reaction-free energy profile for the OER on the TiO$_2$-terminated surface of BaTiO$_3$, as described in the Models Section 2.

Figure 6 displays the free energies of water oxidation reactions on a pure and Rh-modified TiO$_2$-terminated BaTiO$_3$ surface at zero potential and equilibrium potential of 1.23 V vs RHE. (Equation (1)). The oxidation reaction of a single water molecule is considered both on a dry surface and considering the influence of the aqueous environment. On a bare TiO$_2$-terminated surface, an overpotential of 1.18 V was found when the surface was dry. This value is close to the earlier-reported one calculated on the same surface, equal to 1.22 V [23]. Due to the aqueous environment, this value reduced to 1.08 V. For the Rh-modified surface, the overpotential values were 0.45 and 0.23 V for dry and wet surfaces, respectively, which implies that Rh doping improves catalytic activity. The obtained values are close to those for NiO$_x$ films, in which cerium was used as a dopant and gold was employed as a metal support [44].

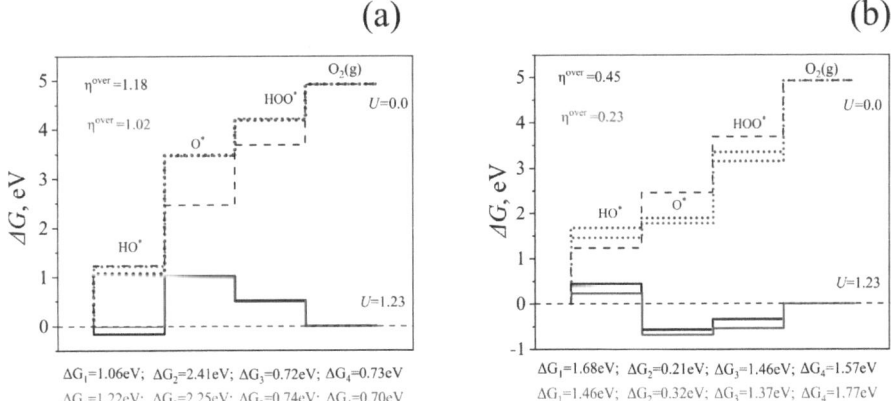

Figure 6. Standard free energy diagram for the OER at zero potential ($U = 0$, dotted lines) and equilibrium potential for oxygen evolution ($U = 1.23$ V, solid lines) at pH = 0 and T = 298 K. Black and blue lines show data for dry and wet surfaces, respectively. Dashed lines correspond to the ideal catalyst.

Since the efficiency of the photocatalyst in the process of the water oxidation reaction is determined by the energies of the interaction of intermediate reaction products with the surface (Equation (1)), it is necessary to analyze the oxidation states of active sites during the water-splitting process. The results regarding the Bader analysis and the spin states of active sites on the surface of the catalyst and the intermediate reaction products are given in Table 1. The number of active sites on the surface also includes the nearest neighboring ions, O1 and O2, since their charges and spin states change on the doped surface during the reactions represented by Equation (1).

Table 1. TiO$_2$-terminated surface. Calculated Bader charges q (in $|e|$) and local magnetic moments (in μ_B) for the Ti (undoped surface) and Rh (doped surface) empty sites and as well as sites occupied by O, OH, and OOH.

		TiO$_2$ Surface							
		Empty site (*)		OH*		O*		OOH*	
	Species	q	μ	q	μ	q	μ	q	μ
Dry	Ti	2.15	0	2.25	0	2.10	0	2.22	0
	O1	−1.18	0	−1.15	0	−1.15	0	−1.13	0
	O2	−1.22	0	−1.24	0	−1.19	0	−1.24	0
	Adsorbant	-	-	−0.49	0	−0.74	0.53	−0.31	0.14
Wet	Ti	2.24	0	2.24	0	2.12	0	2.21	0
	O1	−1.22	0	−1.16	0	−1.19	0	−1.15	0
	O2	−1.23	0	−1.24	0	−1.22	0	−1.24	0
	Adsorbant	-	-	−0.52	0	−0.91	0.48	−0.35	0.13
		TiO$_2$:Rh surface							
Dry	Rh	1.51	1.59	1.77	0.85	1.73	1.04	1.64	0.73
	O1	−1.06	0.17	−1.04	0.11	−1.03	0.129	−1.02	0.13
	O2	−1.11	0.15	−1.20	0.03	−1.19	0.014	−1.18	0.01
	Adsorbant	-	-	−0.37	0.86	−0.33	1.04	−0.19	0.28
Wet	Rh	1.49	1.60	1.76	0.84	1.73	1.08	1.63	0.74
	O1	−1.08	0.17	−1.08	0.11	−1.05	0.14	−1.05	0.13
	O2	−1.10	0.15	−1.11	0.03	−1.20	0.019	−1.20	0.01
	Adsorbant	-	-	−0.43	0.84	−0.46	1.08	−0.23	0.29

In the case of an unmodified TiO$_2$-terminated surface, the charge and spin states of the catalyst ions change slightly during the oxidation of water, both in the case of dry and wet surfaces. The active site of a titanium ion is always in the 4+ oxidation state, and its nearest neighbors are in the O^{2-} state. An aqueous environment noticeably affects only the intermediate reaction product O*, reflected in a decrease in overpotential at this reaction step. In a sense, the electronic Ti^{4+} ion is too rigid in terms of its properties and cannot adjust its electronic structure to optimize the water-splitting process. Surface modification with Rh solves this problem.

When replacing the surface titanium ion with rhodium, the dopant also affects its nearest neighboring O1 and O2 ions. The data in Table 1 show that as the absolute value of the Bader charge on the O1 and O2 ions decreases, a non-zero magnetic moment also appears on these ions. This indicates a charge transfer from the O1 and O2 ions to the dopant. The spin state of the Rh ion also shows that it is not in the 4+ oxidation state since in this latter case its formal magnetic moment is 1 μ_B in the low-spin state ($4d^5$). The present calculations suggested a value of 1.59 μ_B for the spin magnetic moment of Rh, which means Rh is in the 3+ oxidation state; i.e., the formal magnetic moment is 2 μ_B in the intermediate spin state. This deviation from the formal value is associated with the charge transfer from O1 and O2 to the doping cation. During the oxidation of water, the magnetic moment of Rh is 1.04 (O*) and decreases to 0.85 (OH*) and 0.75 (OOH*) μ_B. This can be interpreted as the oxidation state of Rh undergoing a change from 3+ (O*) to 4+ (OH* and OOH*).

Because of the water oxidation reaction, the oxidation state and spin magnetic moment of the ions on the catalyst surface change, and the reaction intermediates change with them. The ability of Rh and the surrounding ions on the surface to change their electronic properties leads to more efficient water oxidation. The influence of the aqueous environment significantly affects the behavior of OH* species, which, in turn, leads to a decrease in the overpotential.

Figure 7 shows how the electronic charge density redistributes between the dry TiO_2-terminated surface and the reaction intermediates. The charge transfer ΔQ can be calculated using the formula given below:

$$\Delta Q = Q_{SA} - Q_S - Q_A, \tag{5}$$

Here, Q_{SA}, Q_S, and Q_A represent the spatial charge density distributions for systems wherein the intermediate reaction products are adsorbed on the surface of the catalyst, the bare catalyst surface, and the adsorbed species treated separately from the catalyst, respectively. The oxygen atoms of the adsorbed species are mainly responsible for the charge transfer. These findings are summarized in Table 1.

We compared the geometry of optimized undoped and doped TiO_2-terminated catalyst surfaces with adsorbed reaction intermediates. Table 2 summarizes the distances between the adsorbents and the surface. In all cases, doping decreases the distance between the adsorbent and the catalyst surface, except for OOH species adsorption. There is a significant difference between the undoped and doped surfaces in regard to the orientation of the adsorbed OH group. In the case of adsorption on an undoped surface, the angle TiÔH = 128°, while in the case of a doped surface, the OH group is directed perpendicular to the surface, and RhÔH = 180°.

To illustrate the effect of an aqueous environment, we calculated the spatial distribution of charge density difference between wet and dry TiO_2-terminated surfaces; this distribution was calculated as follows:

$$\Delta Q = Q_{wet} - Q_{dry} \tag{6}$$

Figure 8 illustrates the obtained results. The aqueous environment leads to a transfer of electron density from surface oxygen ions to titanium ions. In an aqueous environment, the doped structure experiences a decrease in the electron density on Rh.

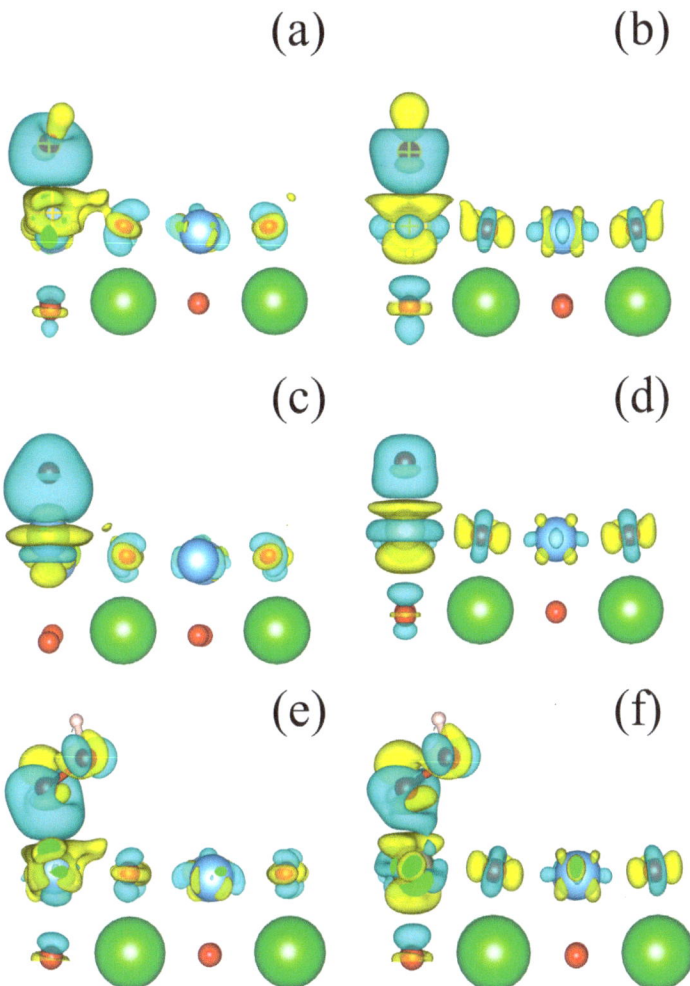

Figure 7. Equation (5) calculates the charge transfer between the TiO$_2$-termiated catalyst surface and the intermediate reaction products. A side view of the surface of the top two layers is presented. OH adsorbed on (**a**) undoped and (**b**) Rh-doped surfaces; O adsorbed on (**c**) undoped and (**d**) Rh-doped surfaces; and HOO adsorbed on (**e**) undoped and (**f**) Rh-doped surfaces. The yellow and blue clouds indicate the isocontours of positive and negative values of the electron charge density, respectively.

Table 2. Distance (Å) between adsorbents and undoped and doped TiO$_2$-terminated catalysts' surfaces.

Surface	Adsorbant		
	O	OH	OOH
Undoped	1.655	1.836	2.055
Rh-doped	1.754	1.897	1.902

Although the predicted overpotential values are small, in practice, implementing an electrode with such indicators will take much work. Here, we consider the ideal case of doping wherein all Rh ions are located on the surface of BaTiO$_3$ at 1.8 at.% doping. In practice, a significant portion of the doping atoms will occupy sites inside the nanoparticles.

When the degree of doping is raised to increase the concentration of surface Rh ions, the hexagonal BaTiO$_3$ phase forms [32]. The catalytic properties of the hexagonal phase still need to be studied.

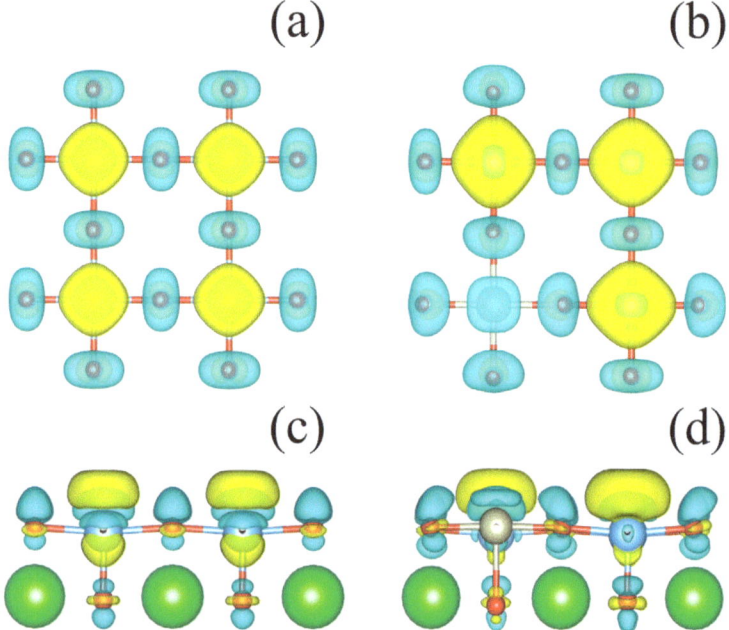

Figure 8. Equation (6) calculates the charge transfer between wet and dry TiO$_2$-termiated catalyst surfaces. Top view of the upper layer of the (**a**) undoped and (**b**) Rh-doped surfaces; side view of the two upper layers of the (**c**) undoped and (**d**) Rh-doped surfaces. The yellow and blue clouds indicate the isocontours of positive and negative values of the electron charge density, respectively.

Optimizing catalyst activity hinges on the discovery of a catalyst with a significantly larger surface area and a higher concentration of dopant atoms. These things are very important for making the tetragonal phase of BaTiO$_3$ doped with Rh function as efficiently as possible. Ref. [32] serves as a valuable guide for determining the optimal doping level. The results show that adding 8 mol% Rh changes 85% of the tetragonal BaTiO$_3$ phase into a hexagonal structure. When synthesizing BaTiO$_3$ crystals with a Rh content below the specified level, grinding the crystals becomes necessary. This process enhances the working surface area of the catalyst, thereby increasing the likelihood of detecting Rh atoms on the surfaces of the resulting nanoparticles. By following this procedure, we can secure the most efficient catalyst based on BaTiO$_3$ doped with Rh.

4. Computational Details

All the calculations were performed with the ab initio plane wave computer code VASP [45,46] using the projector-augmented plane wave (PAW) formalism [47]. Optimization of the geometry of the studied models and calculation of the thermodynamics of the water-splitting reaction were carried out using the GGA-PBE (Perdew–Burke–Ernzerhof) exchange correlation functional [48]. The on-site Coulomb correlation of d-electrons was taken into account by employing Hubbard corrections in the Dudarev parametrization [49] with a $U_{\text{eff}} = U_c - J$ value of 2.6 eV for titanium [50]. We must admit, on the basis of our test calculations, that the application of the U_{eff}-parameter to Ti/Rh does not change the main conclusions/results regarding the surface free energy diagrams. Contrarily, the calculations of optical properties require accurate electronic band structures. We therefore applied the hybrid HSE06 density functional to calculate the electronic density of states and optical absorption from the DFT+U optimized charge density [51]. The optical properties were analyzed based on the transition dipole moment matrix elements:

$$D_{\sigma,ij} = e\left\langle \psi_{\sigma,i}^{KS} \middle| r \middle| \psi_{\sigma,j}^{KS} \right\rangle \quad (7)$$

for transitions between the initial state (σ,i) and final state (σ,j) calculated on the basis of Kohn–Sham orbitals $\psi_{\sigma,i}^{KS}$, where σ is a spin index, i(j) labels orbitals, and e is an elementary charge. The transition dipole moment was used for calculating oscillator strength:

$$f_{\sigma,ij} = \frac{4\pi m \nu_{\sigma,ij}}{3e^2 \hbar} |D_{\nu,ij}|^2, \quad (8)$$

where m and $\hbar$ are the electron mass and Planck constant, respectively, and abd $\nu_{\sigma,ij}$ is the frequency of transition between the ith and jth states. Using the oscillator strengths and assuming a lack of spin–orbit coupling, the absorption spectra can then be determined as follows: $\alpha(\nu) = \alpha_\alpha(\nu) + \alpha_\beta(\nu)$, where $\alpha_\sigma(\nu) = \sum_{ij} f_{\sigma,ij} \delta(\nu - \nu_{\sigma,ij})$.

The thermodynamic corrections for the solvation effect were calculated using VASPsol [52], allowing us to consider surface wetting through the water continuum model and distinguish between dry and wet conditions. If the continuum model applied, the wet conditions were stated. The Monkhorst–Pack grid-sampling mesh used for the bulk calculations had dimensions of 2 × 2 × 2, and that for the slab calculations had dimensions of 2 × 2 × 1, with a cutoff energy value of 520 eV. The charge distribution on the ions was studied using Bader topological analysis [42]. All calculations were carried out while taking spin polarization into account, except in the case of bare undoped slabs. It has been shown that it is important to consider spin polarized electronic structures since adsorbed species have a spin moment [53].

5. Conclusions

The viability of the Rh-modified TiO_2-terminated $BaTiO_3$ (001) surface for developing efficient water oxidation catalysts to be used as photoanodes in PEC systems was examined using first-principles calculations. According to our results, Rh doping has a double effect on the properties of $BaTiO_3$. On the one hand, doping causes the material under study to absorb sunlight in almost the entire visible range. On the other hand, the surface Rh ion acts as an excellent catalytic center, significantly lowering the overpotential values of the electrochemical reaction. It has been shown that considering the aqueous environment influences both effects.

Author Contributions: Conceptualization, D.G., A.U.A., E.A.K. and Y.A.M.; methodology, A.U.A. and F.U.A.; software, T.M.I. and D.G.; validation, M.S., Y.A.M. and Z.Y.Z.; formal analysis, A.U.A. and T.M.I.; investigation, Z.Y.Z., Y.A.M., A.U.A. and Y.A.M.; resources, Y.A.M., T.M.I. and E.A.K.; writing—original draft preparation, T.M.I.; writing—review and editing, Y.A.M. and Ł.A.K.; visualization, A.U.A.; supervision, T.M.I.; project administration, F.U.A.; funding acquisition, T.M.I. All authors have read and agreed to the published version of the manuscript.

Funding: This work was carried out with the financial support of the Ministry of Science and Higher Education of the Republic of Kazakhstan: AP14869492 "Development of nanocrystalline metal oxide catalysts for hydrogen production". EK thanks M-Era.NET project HetCat. The calculations were partly performed at the High-Performance Computing Center Stuttgart (HLRS) within the project DEFTD 12939. YM and DG thank the Latvian Council of Science, project No. lzp-2021/1-0203. The work by T.M.I. was performed under the state assignment of GEOKHI RAS. T.I. also thanks the Center for Computational Materials Science (IMR, Tohoku University) for providing access to the supercomputing system used to perform the simulations. The Institute of Solid-State Physics, University of Latvia (Latvia), as a Center of Excellence, has received funding from the European Union's Horizon 2020 Framework Program H2020-WIDESPREAD-01-2016-2017-Teaming Phase2 under grant agreement No. 739508, project CAMART[2].

Institutional Review Board Statement: Not applicable.

Informed Consent Statement: Not applicable.

Data Availability Statement: Data are contained within the article.

Conflicts of Interest: There are no conflicts to declare.

References

1. Fujishima, A.; Honda, K. Electrochemical photolysis of water at a semiconductor electrode. *Nature* **1972**, *238*, 37–38. [CrossRef] [PubMed]
2. Kudo, A.; Miseki, Y. Heterogeneous photocatalyst materials for water splitting. *Chem. Soc. Rev.* **2009**, *38*, 253–278. [CrossRef] [PubMed]
3. Suntivich, J.; May, K.J.; Gasteiger, H.A.; Goodenough, J.B.; Shao-Horn, Y. A perovskite oxide optimized for oxygen evolution catalysis from molecular orbital principles. *Science* **2011**, *334*, 1383–1385. [CrossRef]
4. Castelli, I.E.; Landis, D.D.; Thygesen, K.S.; Dahl, S.; Chorkendorff, I.; Jaramillo, T.F.; Jacobsen, K.W. New cubic perovskites for one-and two-photon water splitting using the computational materials repository. *Energy Environ. Sci.* **2012**, *5*, 9034–9043. [CrossRef]
5. Luo, J.; Im, J.-H.; Mayer, M.T.; Schreier, M.; Nazeeruddin, M.K.; Park, N.-G.; Tilley, S.D.; Fan, H.J.; Grätzel, M. Water photolysis at 12.3% efficiency via perovskite photovoltaics and Earth-abundant catalysts. *Science* **2014**, *345*, 1593–1596. [CrossRef] [PubMed]
6. Xu, X.; Wang, W.; Zhou, W.; Shao, Z. Recent Advances in Novel Nanostructuring Methods of Perovskite Electrocatalysts for Energy-Related Applications. *Small Methods* **2018**, *2*, 1800071. [CrossRef]
7. Royer, S.; Duprez, D.; Can, F.; Courtois, X.; Batiot-Dupeyrat, C.; Laassiri, S.; Alamdari, H. Perovskites as substitutes of noble metals for heterogeneous catalysis: Dream or reality. *Chem. Rev.* **2014**, *114*, 10292–10368. [CrossRef] [PubMed]
8. Fan, Z.; Sun, K.; Wang, J. Perovskites for photovoltaics: A combined review of organic–inorganic halide perovskites and ferroelectric oxide perovskites. *J. Mater. Chem. A* **2015**, *3*, 18809–18828. [CrossRef]
9. Mefford, J.T.; Rong, X.; Abakumov, A.M.; Hardin, W.G.; Dai, S.; Kolpak, A.M.; Johnston, K.P.; Stevenson, K.J. Water electrolysis on $La_{1-x}Sr_xCoO_{3-\delta}$ perovskite electrocatalysts. *Nat. Commun.* **2016**, *7*, 11053. [CrossRef] [PubMed]
10. Rong, X.; Parolin, J.; Kolpak, A.M. A fundamental relationship between reaction mechanism and stability in metal oxide catalysts for oxygen evolution. *Acs Catal.* **2016**, *6*, 1153–1158. [CrossRef]
11. Tang, J.; Xu, X.; Tang, T.; Zhong, Y.; Shao, Z. Perovskite-Based Electrocatalysts for Cost-Effective Ultrahigh-Current-Density Water Splitting in Anion Exchange Membrane Electrolyzer Cell. *Small Methods* **2022**, *6*, 2201099. [CrossRef] [PubMed]
12. Xu, X.; Pan, Y.; Zhong, Y.; Ran, R.; Shao, Z. Ruddlesden–Popper perovskites in electrocatalysis. *Mater. Horiz.* **2020**, *7*, 2519–2565. [CrossRef]
13. Buscaglia, V.; Buscaglia, M.T.; Canu, G. $BaTiO_3$-based ceramics: Fundamentals, properties and applications. *Encycl. Mater. Tech. Ceram. Glas.* **2021**, *3*, 311–344.
14. Wemple, S. Polarization Fluctuations and the Optical-Absorption Edge in $BaTiO_3$. *Phys. Rev. B* **1970**, *2*, 2679. [CrossRef]
15. Kennedy, J.H.; Frese, K.W. Photo-oxidation of water at barium titanate electrodes. *J. Electrochem. Soc.* **1976**, *123*, 1683. [CrossRef]
16. Nasby, R.; Quinn, R.K. Photoassisted electrolysis of water using a $BaTiO_3$ electrode. *Mater. Res. Bull.* **1976**, *11*, 985–992. [CrossRef]
17. Hayakawa, T.; Suzuki, S.; Nakamura, J.; Uchijima, T.; Hamakawa, S.; Suzuki, K.; Shishido, T.; Takehira, K. CO_2 reforming of CH_4 over Ni/perovskite catalysts prepared by solid phase crystallization method. *Appl. Catal. A Gen.* **1999**, *183*, 273–285. [CrossRef]
18. Ko, S.; Tang, X.; Gao, F.; Wang, C.; Liu, H.; Liu, Y. Selective catalytic reduction of NOx with NH3 on Mn, Co-BTC-derived catalysts: Influence of thermal treatment temperature. *J. Solid State Chem.* **2022**, *307*, 122843. [CrossRef]
19. Srilakshmi, C.; Saraf, R.; Prashanth, V.; Rao, G.M.; Shivakumara, C. Structure and catalytic activity of Cr-doped $BaTiO_3$ nanocatalysts synthesized by conventional oxalate and microwave assisted hydrothermal methods. *Inorg. Chem.* **2016**, *55*, 4795–4805. [CrossRef]
20. Upadhyay, S.; Shrivastava, J.; Solanki, A.; Choudhary, S.; Sharma, V.; Kumar, P.; Singh, N.; Satsangi, V.R.; Shrivastav, R.; Waghmare, U.V. Enhanced photoelectrochemical response of $BaTiO_3$ with Fe doping: Experiments and first-principles analysis. *J. Phys. Chem. C* **2011**, *115*, 24373–24380. [CrossRef]
21. Nageri, M.; Kumar, V. Manganese-doped $BaTiO_3$ nanotube arrays for enhanced visible light photocatalytic applications. *Mater. Chem. Phys.* **2018**, *213*, 400–405. [CrossRef]
22. Demircivi, P.; Simsek, E.B. Visible-light-enhanced photoactivity of perovskite-type W-doped $BaTiO_3$ photocatalyst for photodegradation of tetracycline. *J. Alloys Compd.* **2019**, *774*, 795–802. [CrossRef]
23. Artrith, N.; Sailuam, W.; Limpijumnong, S.; Kolpak, A.M. Reduced overpotentials for electrocatalytic water splitting over Fe- and Ni-modified $BaTiO_3$. *Phys. Chem. Chem. Phys.* **2016**, *18*, 29561–29570. [CrossRef] [PubMed]
24. Xie, P.; Yang, F.; Li, R.; Ai, C.; Lin, C.; Lin, S. Improving hydrogen evolution activity of perovskite $BaTiO_3$ with Mo doping: Experiments and first-principles analysis. *Int. J. Hydrogen Energy* **2019**, *44*, 11695–11704. [CrossRef]
25. Tanwar, N.; Upadhyay, S.; Priya, R.; Pundir, S.; Sharma, P.; Pandey, O. Eu-doped $BaTiO_3$ perovskite as an efficient electrocatalyst for oxygen evolution reaction. *J. Solid State Chem.* **2023**, *317*, 123674. [CrossRef]

26. Maeda, K. Rhodium-doped barium titanate perovskite as a stable p-type semiconductor photocatalyst for hydrogen evolution under visible light. *ACS Appl. Mater. Interfaces* **2014**, *6*, 2167–2173. [CrossRef] [PubMed]
27. Konta, R.; Ishii, T.; Kato, H.; Kudo, A. Photocatalytic activities of noble metal ion doped $SrTiO_3$ under visible light irradiation. *J. Phys. Chem. B* **2004**, *108*, 8992–8995. [CrossRef]
28. Nishioka, S.; Maeda, K. Hydrothermal synthesis of rhodium-doped barium titanate nanocrystals for enhanced photocatalytic hydrogen evolution under visible light. *RSC Adv.* **2015**, *5*, 100123–100128. [CrossRef]
29. Bhat, D.K.; Bantawal, H.; Shenoy, U.S. Rhodium doping augments photocatalytic activity of barium titanate: Effect of electronic structure engineering. *Nanoscale Adv.* **2020**, *2*, 5688–5698. [CrossRef]
30. Jain, A.; Ong, S.P.; Hautier, G.; Chen, W.; Richards, W.D.; Dacek, S.; Cholia, S.; Gunter, D.; Skinner, D.; Ceder, G. Commentary: The Materials Project: A materials genome approach to accelerating materials innovation. *APL Mater.* **2013**, *1*, 011002. [CrossRef]
31. Eglitis, R.; Vanderbilt, D. Ab initio calculations of $BaTiO_3$ and $PbTiO_3$ (001) and (011) surface structures. *Phys. Rev. B* **2007**, *76*, 155439. [CrossRef]
32. Shi, K.; Zhang, B.; Liu, K.; Zhang, J.; Ma, G. Rhodium-Doped Barium Titanate Perovskite as a Stable p-Type Photocathode in Solar Water Splitting. *ACS Appl. Mater. Interfaces* **2023**, *15*, 47754–47763. [CrossRef] [PubMed]
33. Man, I.C.; Su, H.-Y.; Calle-Vallejo, F.; Hansen, H.A.; Martínez, J.I.; Inoglu, N.G.; Kitchin, J.; Jaramillo, T.F.; Nørskov, J.K.; Rossmeisl, J. Universality in oxygen evolution electrocatalysis on oxide surfaces. *ChemCatChem* **2011**, *3*, 1159–1165. [CrossRef]
34. García-Mota, M.; Bajdich, M.; Viswanathan, V.; Vojvodic, A.; Bell, A.T.; Nørskov, J.K. Importance of correlation in determining electrocatalytic oxygen evolution activity on cobalt oxides. *J. Phys. Chem. C* **2012**, *116*, 21077–21082. [CrossRef]
35. Haynes, W.M. *CRC Handbook of Chemistry and Physics*, 93rd ed.; CRC Press: Boca Raton, FL, USA, 2012.
36. Shirane, G.; Danner, H.; Pepinsky, R. Neutron Diffraction Study of Orthorhombic $BaTi_3$. *Phys. Rev.* **1957**, *105*, 856–860. [CrossRef]
37. Yasuda, N.; Murayama, H.; Fukuyama, Y.; Kim, J.; Kimura, S.; Toriumi, K.; Tanaka, Y.; Moritomo, Y.; Kuroiwa, Y.; Kato, K.; et al. X-ray diffractometry for the structure determination of a submicrometre single powder grain. *J. Synchrotron Radiat.* **2009**, *16*, 352–357. [CrossRef]
38. Al-Shakarchi, E.K.; Mahmood, N.B. Three Techniques Used to Produce $BaTiO_3$ Fine Powder. *J. Mod. Phys.* **2011**, *2*, 9. [CrossRef]
39. Buttner, R.H.; Maslen, E.N. Structural parameters and electron difference density in $BaTiO_3$. *Acta Crystallogr. Sect. B* **1992**, *48*, 764–769. [CrossRef]
40. Xiao, C.J.; Jin, C.Q.; Wang, X.H. Crystal structure of dense nanocrystalline $BaTiO_3$ ceramics. *Mater. Chem. Phys.* **2008**, *111*, 209–212. [CrossRef]
41. Inerbaev, T.M.; Hoefelmeyer, J.D.; Kilin, D.S. Photoinduced Charge Transfer from Titania to Surface Doping Site. *J. Phys. Chem. C* **2013**, *117*, 9673–9692. [CrossRef]
42. Bader, R.F.W. *Atoms in Molecules. A Quantum Theory*; Oxford University Press, Oxford, UK, 1990.
43. Iwashina, K.; Kudo, A. Rh-Doped $SrTiO_3$ Photocatalyst Electrode Showing Cathodic Photocurrent for Water Splitting under Visible-Light Irradiation. *J. Am. Chem. Soc.* **2011**, *133*, 13272–13275. [CrossRef] [PubMed]
44. Ng, J.W.D.; García-Melchor, M.; Bajdich, M.; Chakthranont, P.; Kirk, C.; Vojvodic, A.; Jaramillo, T.F. Gold-supported cerium-doped NiOx catalysts for water oxidation. *Nat. Energy* **2016**, *1*, 16053. [CrossRef]
45. Kresse, G.; Joubert, D. From ultrasoft pseudopotentials to the projector augmented-wave method. *Phys. Rev. B* **1999**, *59*, 1758. [CrossRef]
46. Kresse, G.; Furthmüller, J. Efficient iterative schemes for ab initio total-energy calculations using a plane-wave basis set. *Phys. Rev. B* **1996**, *54*, 11169. [CrossRef] [PubMed]
47. Blöchl, P.E. Projector augmented-wave method. *Phys. Rev. B* **1994**, *50*, 17953. [CrossRef] [PubMed]
48. Perdew, J.P.; Burke, K.; Ernzerhof, M. Generalized gradient approximation made simple. *Phys. Rev. Lett.* **1996**, *77*, 3865. [CrossRef] [PubMed]
49. Dudarev, S.L.; Botton, G.A.; Savrasov, S.Y.; Humphreys, C.J.; Sutton, A.P. Electron-energy-loss spectra and the structural stability of nickel oxide: An LSDA+U study. *Phys. Rev. B* **1998**, *57*, 1505–1509. [CrossRef]
50. Maldonado, F.; Jácome, S.; Stashans, A. Codoping of Ni and Fe in tetragonal $BaTiO_3$. *Comput. Condens. Matter* **2017**, *13*, 49–54. [CrossRef]
51. Heyd, J.; Scuseria, G.E.; Ernzerhof, M. Hybrid functionals based on a screened Coulomb potential. *J. Chem. Phys.* **2003**, *118*, 8207–8215. [CrossRef]
52. Mathew, K.; Sundararaman, R.; Letchworth-Weaver, K.; Arias, T.A.; Hennig, R.G. Implicit solvation model for density-functional study of nanocrystal surfaces and reaction pathways. *J. Chem. Phys.* **2014**, *140*, 084106. [CrossRef]
53. Mom, R.V.; Cheng, J.; Koper, M.T.M.; Sprik, M. Modeling the Oxygen Evolution Reaction on Metal Oxides: The Infuence of Unrestricted DFT Calculations. *J. Phys. Chem. C* **2014**, *118*, 4095–4102. [CrossRef]

Disclaimer/Publisher's Note: The statements, opinions and data contained in all publications are solely those of the individual author(s) and contributor(s) and not of MDPI and/or the editor(s). MDPI and/or the editor(s) disclaim responsibility for any injury to people or property resulting from any ideas, methods, instructions or products referred to in the content.

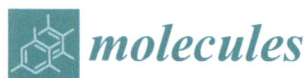 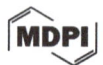

Article

Mapping Photogenerated Electron–Hole Behavior of Graphene Oxide: Insight into a New Mechanism of Photosensitive Pollutant Degradation

Kaijie Ni [1,*], Yanlong Chen [1], Ruiqi Xu [1], Yuming Zhao [2] and Ming Guo [1,*]

[1] College of Chemistry and Materials Engineering, Zhejiang Agriculture and Forestry University, Hangzhou 311300, China
[2] Department of Chemistry, Memorial University of Newfoundland, St. John's, NL A1B 3X7, Canada
* Correspondence: nikaijie@zafu.edu.cn (K.N.); guoming@zafu.edu.cn (M.G.)

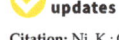

Citation: Ni, K.; Chen, Y.; Xu, R.; Zhao, Y.; Guo, M. Mapping Photogenerated Electron–Hole Behavior of Graphene Oxide: Insight into a New Mechanism of Photosensitive Pollutant Degradation. *Molecules* **2024**, *29*, 3765. https://doi.org/10.3390/molecules29163765

Academic Editor: Qingguo Shao

Received: 9 July 2024
Revised: 6 August 2024
Accepted: 6 August 2024
Published: 8 August 2024

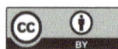

Copyright: © 2024 by the authors. Licensee MDPI, Basel, Switzerland. This article is an open access article distributed under the terms and conditions of the Creative Commons Attribution (CC BY) license (https://creativecommons.org/licenses/by/4.0/).

Abstract: The use of graphene oxide (GO) photogenerated electron–hole (e–h$^+$) pairs to degrade pollutants is a novel green method for wastewater treatment. However, the interaction between photosensitive pollutants and a GO–light system remains unclear. In this work, the mechanism of degradation of photosensitive pollutant tetracycline (TC) promoted by GO photogenerated e–h$^+$ pairs was studied. Our studies encompassed the determination of TC removal kinetics, analysis of active substances for TC degradation, identification of degradation products, and computational modeling. Clear evidence shows that a new reaction mechanism of enhanced adsorption and induced generation of reactive oxygen species (ROS) was involved. This mechanism was conducive to significantly enhanced TC removal. Kinetic studies showed a first-order behavior that can be well described by the Langmuir–Hinshelwood model. Radical scavenging experiments confirmed that $^1O_2$, $\bullet O_2^-$, and holes (h$^+$) were the main active substances for TC degradation. Electron spin resonance analysis indicated that photoexcited TC molecules may transfer electrons to the conduction band of GO to induce the generation of additional ROS. A major transformation product (m/z 459) during TC degradation was identified with liquid chromatography–mass spectrometry. Density functional theory calculation indicated a stronger adsorption between TC and GO under photoirradiation. This mechanism of photo-enhanced adsorption and synergistic induced generation of ROS provides a new strategy for the removal of emerging pollutants in water. Overall, the new mechanism revealed in this work expands the knowledge of applying GO to wastewater treatment and is of great reference value for research in this field.

Keywords: graphene oxide; photogenerated electron and hole; photosensitive pollutants; tetracycline removal; degradation pathway

1. Introduction

Graphene has received unprecedented attention due to its unique properties and highly promising application [1–3]. Graphene oxide (GO), a common precursor for graphene preparation, has additional oxygen-containing functional groups in its structure. These oxygenated groups are covalently bound to the base surfaces (epoxies and hydroxyl groups) and/or edges (carbonyl and carboxyl groups) of GO [4,5], which in turn disrupt the perfect lattice structure of graphene and change the hybrid state of some carbon atoms from sp^2 to sp^3. As such, GO attains a relatively large energy gap to exhibit semiconducting properties [6]. Compared with pristine graphene, the covalent oxygenated functional groups present in GO lead to significant structure defects. This is concomitant with some loss in electrical conductivity [7], which limits the direct application of GO in electrically active materials. However, at the same time, the polar oxygen functional groups of GO render it strongly hydrophilic. This gives GO good dispersibility in many solvents, particularly in water, which is important for processing and further derivatization [8].

Usually, GO has larger surface areas than pristine graphite, because the oxygen groups of GO expand the interplanar space. The specific surface area of drying GO reported in the literature ranges from 30 to 295 $m^2 \cdot g^{-1}$ depending on the oxygen contents [9]. Because of its unique properties, GO has been actively researched in modern optoelectronics, ranging from supercapacitors [10] to lithium-ion batteries [11], flexible electronic devices [12], and biomedicines [13]. Moreover, the extended π-conjugated units in the GO structure result in photosensitivity; upon photoexcitation, a π-electron in the sp^2 domain is promoted to the π* orbital, populating the conduction band with an electron and creating a hole in the valence band. The photochemistry taking place at the sp^2 domains of GO can be specifically tailored to achieve photocatalytic performance [14]. In addition, the abundant oxygen-containing functional groups of GO make it show strong hydrophilicity. Consequently, GO serves as an ideal nanomaterial to induce photochemical reactivity in aqueous environments.

To date, most of the studies published on the performance of GO in removing contaminants focus on the aspect of photocatalytic degradation of organic pollutants, in which GO was used together with metal [15–22] or non-metal [23–27] catalysts. In these studies, GO was used as a photocatalyst carrier to promote the dispersion of nanoparticles and to enhance the separation efficiency of photogenerated $e–h^+$ pairs of the photocatalyst for improved photocatalytic efficiency [28]. Conversely, undoped single GO materials are rarely addressed in the field of photocatalytic degradation of organic pollutants [29–32]. Nevertheless, some studies have already pointed to this possibility. For example, GO was found to change into reduced GO under light conditions, producing photodegraded products such as carbon dioxide and polycyclic aromatic hydrocarbons [33,34]. Pedrosa et al. reported that GO prepared by the Brodie method shows a high degree of $e–h^+$ separation efficiency and can degrade 95% phenol under light irradiation [35]. Recently, Zou et al. demonstrated GO under simulated sunlight irradiation can promote the rapid degradation (95%) of paracetamol (APAP) within 10 min. Their studies revealed that the main active substance for the degradation of APAP comes from the photogenic holes (h^+) of GO [36]. These studies demonstrate that the photoreactivity of GO can significantly impact the fate and transformation of numerous environmental pollutants. However, the use of the photoreactivity of GO for the degradation of emerging pollutants has not yet been fully explored. More fundamental studies are warranted to acquire a deep understanding of the interplay between GO's adsorptivity and photoactivity before the potential of GO can be fully unlocked in environmental applications.

Antibiotics represent important emerging contaminants of global concern [37]. TC is one of the most commonly used photosensitive antibiotics in modern medicine [38]. Nowadays, TC is frequently detected in wastewater. The continuous release of TC into the environment is surely an issue of serious environmental and health consequences [39]. Removal of TC from aquatic environments is an urgent task to carry out, but traditional municipal wastewater treatment technologies are ineffective in addressing this issue. TC and other photosensitive antibiotics are chemically stable and not susceptible to biodegradation. The use of photoactive GO to degrade pollutants is an important green technique for wastewater treatment. Since this method only involves GO and photons, it can effectively avert secondary pollution caused by using toxic metal-based photocatalysts. In addition, the electronic and bandgap properties of GO can be regulated through further oxidation or reduction, which are useful for the design of novel highly efficient photocatalysts. To this end, we have recently conducted a series of investigations of the interactions of GO with TC under various conditions. We proposed that GO can act as a dual-functional nanomaterial to promote the efficient removal of antibiotic pollutants from water. On one hand, GO has been known to be an effective adsorbent of antibiotics such as TC [40]. On the other hand, GO may possess the ability to photocatalytically degrade TC, which is evidenced by previous literature reports on the combined use of GO with other photocatalysts to promote the photodegradation of TC [41]. This manuscript, hence, adds new knowledge about the concerted effects of the adsorptive and photoactive sites in GO on the removal of photosensitive pollutants. The prepared GO was fully characterized. The removal of

TC by GO under various conditions was performed. Radical scavenging experiments and ESR analysis were conducted. The degradation pathway of TC was proposed based on the LC/MS results. Finally, DFT calculation was used to reveal the adsorption of TC on GO under photoirradiation conditions. A new mechanism of pollutant removal promoted by GO photogenerated e–h$^+$ pairs was disclosed.

2. Results and Discussion

2.1. Characterization

The prepared GO was characterized by a range of spectroscopic and microscopic analyses (Figure S1). The FT-IR spectrum shows the presence of O–H (3400 cm^{-1}), C=O (1725 cm^{-1}), C–O (1630 cm^{-1}), C–OH (1225 cm^{-1}), and C–O (1040 cm^{-1}) functional groups (Figure S1a), indicating that various oxygen-containing groups were introduced. The XRD patterns of the prepared GO (Figure S1) show a strong and sharp diffraction peak at $2\theta = 9.2°$, which corresponds to a layer spacing of 0.97 nm and matches that of typical GO. Pure graphite has been reported to generate a diffraction peak at $2\theta = 26°$ [42], but it was not observed in our measurement. The absence of this peak suggests that water molecules and OFGs (such as carboxyl, hydroxyl, and epoxy groups) were inserted in layers of graphite during the oxidation process, thus destroying the sp2 π-conjugated structure. Raman spectroscopy is an effective tool for the characterization of carbon materials. The Raman spectrum of our prepared GO shows two characteristic graphitic bands, the G band at around 1580 cm^{-1} and the D band at 1350 cm^{-1} (Figure S1). The G band is associated with sp^2 C=C bond stretching, while the D band is due to the vibrations of sp^3 carbon atoms. Typically, graphite shows strong and sharp G bands and insignificant D bands as a feature of highly graphitized materials with fewer defects. The Raman spectrum of our prepared GO shows significant D and G bands and the intensity ratio of ID/IG is 0.87. This result confirms that the chemical oxidation treatment destroyed the integrated layers and introduced large amounts of defects on the surface of graphite. According to TEM imaging characterization (see the inset of Figure S1b), the prepared GO is lamellar on the microscopic scale. The results indicated that the GO takes a multi-layer architecture through aggregation rather than being single-layered. GO dispersed in water was analyzed by the UV-Vis absorption method. Figure S1d shows the absorption spectrum of GO, which has the strongest absorption band present at 231 nm, due to the π→π* transition of the aromatic C=C bonds in the graphitic domain. A noticeable shoulder band appears around 310 nm, which can be assigned to n→π* transitions of various oxygen-containing functional groups, especially the carbonyl group. The UV-Vis absorption features of our GO are consistent with those reported in the literature [43].

2.2. Removal of TC Promoted by GO under Light

The results of GO-induced removal of TC under xenon lamp irradiation as well as relevant control experiments are shown in Figure 1a. The degradation rate of TC under light alone is insignificant. It can also be seen that the addition of natural graphite to TC solution does not cause much photodegradation of TC, indicating that graphite does not have any photocatalytic effect. Graphite contains only sp^2 carbons in its structure and does not have effective adsorption sites for TC. Moreover, graphite has a zero band gap and, hence, cannot effectively induce any photocatalytic effects.

The TC removal curve of GO shows that 40% of TC in the test solution was removed within one hour under dark conditions. After one hour, the curve does not significantly change, indicating that the process has reached equilibrium. The rapid removal effect is because GO has a high specific surface area and a large number of active adsorption sites such as those oxygen-containing groups characterized by IR analysis. Under dark conditions, the removal of TC from water is primarily due to the adsorption of TC on the surface of GO. Our analysis shows that the equilibrium adsorption of TC by GO is about 235 mg·g^{-1}, which is consistent with previous reports [40].

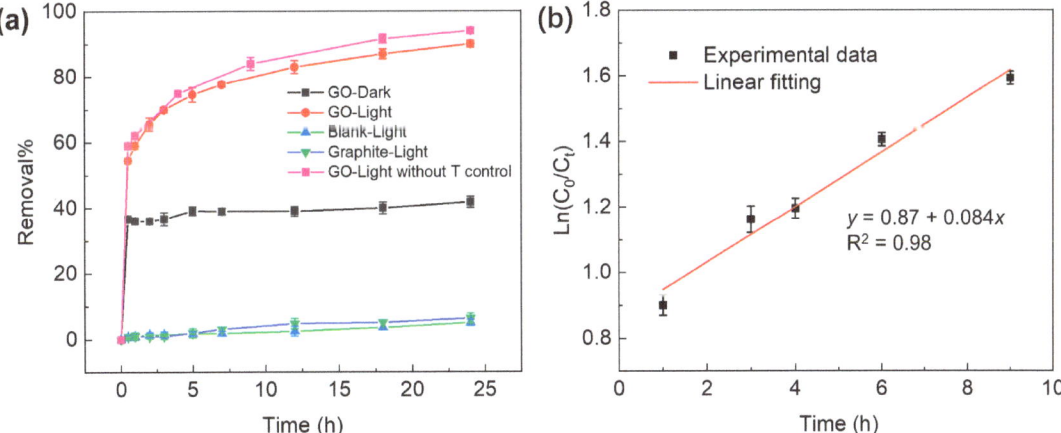

Figure 1. (**a**) TC removal by GO and graphite under dark or xenon lamp irradiation. (**b**) TC removal kinetic in the GO–light system. Initial conditions: [GO] = 200 mg·L^{-1}, [TC] = 100 mg·L^{-1}.

TC removal performance under light shows a stark contrast to that measured under dark conditions. As shown in Figure 1a (red color), the TC removal rate rapidly reaches 55% within one hour and then continues to increase. Eventually, the removal rate achieves 90%, which is more than double the value determined under dark conditions. The kinetics of TC removal under light irradiation without temperature control (pink color) showed a higher TC removal rate compared to that with the temperature maintained at room temperature (red color). A comparison of these results indicates that thermal effects delivered by the magnitude of the irradiance of the xenon light incident contribute to enhanced TC removal. In our experiments, the TC removal rate was determined by monitoring the absorbance at 356 nm, a characteristic absorption peak of TC. The removal kinetics of TC in this GO–light system is shown by the plot in Figure 1b. The linear correlation between Ln(C_0/C_t) and time in this plot discloses a first-order behavior.

To test the applicability of the GO–light system, the influence of various TC concentrations (30 to 200 mg·L^{-1}) on the removal effect of TC was investigated. The removal rate of low-concentration TC (30 to 70 mg·L^{-1}) in the GO–light system largely reached the maximum within one hour (Figure S2). The kinetics of TC removal in the GO–light system are well described by the Langmuir–Hinshelwood model expressed as Equation (1) [44]:

$$\frac{1}{r_0} = \frac{1}{k_r} + \frac{1}{k_r k_a C_0} \tag{1}$$

where r_0 is the initial reaction rate and k_r is the reaction rate constant. k_a is the equilibrium constant and C_0 is the initial TC concentration. For the batch reactor, the initial reaction rate r_0 can be obtained from the change of concentration in Equation (2) with time (the first 60 min in this work):

$$\frac{dC}{dt} = -r \tag{2}$$

where r is the instantaneous removal rate of TC and C is the instantaneous concentration of TC.

Figure 2a shows the linear fitting of the kinetics data. The high correlation coefficient (R^2 = 0.99) indicates that the photocatalytic removal of TC in the GO–light system can be well described by the Langmuir–Hinshelwood model. In addition, we evaluated the effect of GO dose (30, 60, 100, 200, 400 mg·L^{-1}) on TC removal efficiency at an initial TC concentration of 100 mg·L^{-1}. As shown in Figure 2b, with a gradual increase in added GO, the efficiency of TC removal of the GO–light system increases proportionally, and the TC removal rate within one hour achieves 36%, 43%, 55%, and 73%, respectively. After one hour, the removal rate increases much less significantly as a function of time, indicating that the TC removal in this time domain is slow and approaches equilibrium. The increased removal rate can be attributed to a larger surface area and more active sites [45].

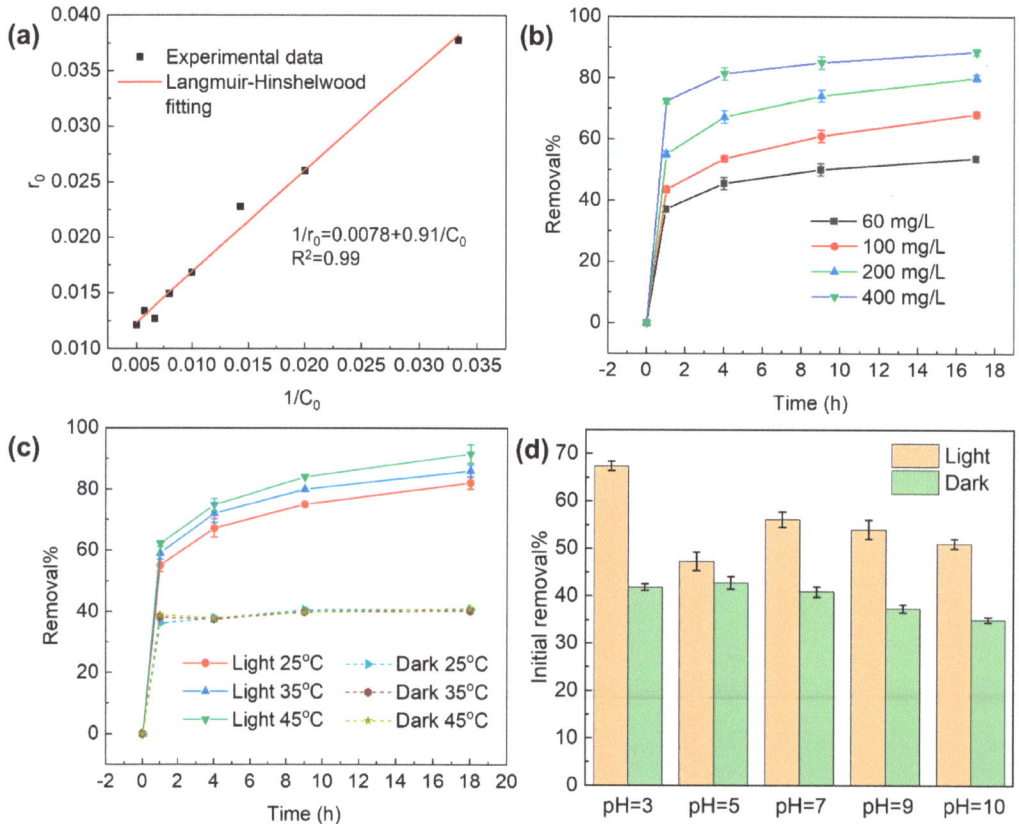

Figure 2. (**a**) Correlation of the TC initial concentration (35 to 200 mg·L^{-1}) and r_0 of the initial reaction rate by the Langmuir–Hinshelwood model. (**b**) Effect of GO dose on TC removal performance. (**c**) Effect of temperature on TC removal performance. (**d**) Removal of TC under dark and light conditions in different acidic and basic conditions (pH = 3–10).

The effect of temperature on the performance of GO in TC removal is shown in Figure 2c. The effect of temperature on the adsorption removal of TC is small in dark conditions, but much larger in light. The removal rate of TC is also found to gradually increase with increasing temperature. When the temperature is changed from 25 to 45 °C, the removal rate of TC is increased by about 10% within one hour. It is likely that at elevated temperature, the surface of GO becomes more adsorptive for TC and the photocatalytic effects of GO are further enhanced.

The effect of pH on the removal of TC by the GO–light system is depicted in Figure 2d. Under dark conditions, the adsorption performance of GO toward TC gradually decreases with increasing pH. Under acidic conditions (pH < 3.3), TC is mainly positively charged in water, which can be captured by GO through the electrostatic attraction and hydrogen-bonding interactions. When the pH is above 3.3, TC changes into a zwitterionic or negatively charged form. The electrostatic attraction between TC and GO is accordingly reduced and can even be changed into electrostatic repulsion [40]. However, the removal rate of TC decreased by only 6.8% when the pH changed from 2 to 10. It is possible that other non-covalent forces, such as van der Waals, dipole interactions, and hydrogen bonding, come into play to compensate for the loss of electrostatic attraction at higher pH values. Under light, the effect of pH becomes more significant. At pH 3, the removal rate of TC reaches a maximum of 67%, which is 16% higher than that at pH 10. The results indicated that acidic conditions are more favorable for the removal of TC in the GO–light system.

2.3. Effects of Radical and Hole Inhibitors on TC Removal Efficiency and ESR Analysis

Studies have shown that GO is prone to photoreaction under light and may be involved in the production of electron–hole pairs [33]. In this study, radical scavenging experiments were performed to examine the mechanism of TC removal by the GO–light system. EDTA-2Na, FFA, SOD, and isopropyl alcohol were chosen as radical scavengers in our experiments, as they can effectively interact with the reactive species generated during photoactivation of GO; specifically, EDTA-2Na is a hole scavenger [46], FFA is a superoxide radical scavenger [47], SOD is a superoxide radical scavenger [48], and isopropyl alcohol is a hydroxyl radical scavenger [49]. As shown in Figure 3, the presence of EDTA-2Na results in a significant reduction in TC removal efficiency, confirming that holes are involved in the photocatalytic degradation of TC on GO. It is worth noting that EDTA-2Na was also found to show a somewhat inhibitive effect on TC removal under dark conditions (Figure 3a); however, the extent is not as significant as in light. The inhibitive effect observed in the dark can be explained by the fact that EDTA-2Na and TC make competitive adsorption on the GO surface, hence, attenuating TC removal efficiency. The significant inhibition of TC removal by EDTA-2Na under light can, therefore, be attributed to both the photogenerated holes in GO and the competitive adsorption of EDTA-2Na.

The presence of FFA and SOD also significantly inhibits the removal of TC, attesting to the fact that singlet oxygen ($^1O_2$) and the superoxide radical ($\bullet O_2^-$) play important roles in the degradation of TC under irradiation. However, the introduction of isopropyl alcohol (hydroxyl radical scavenger) to the system does not result in significantly inhibited TC removal. It is, therefore, reasonable to conclude that hydroxyl radicals are not significantly produced during the photoexcitation of GO.

The reactive oxygen species (ROS) involved in the photodegradation of TC were investigated by ESR analysis. In this work, DMPO was used as a spin trap to detect hydroxyl radicals and superoxide radicals, TEMP was used to detect singlet oxygen, and TEMPO was used to detect holes [50,51]. As shown in Figure 3c, the TEMP–$^1O_2$ signal was recorded by ESR after GO was irradiated by a xenon lamp in water. The signals acquired after 5 min irradiation are of much stronger intensity than those after 3 min irradiation. The presence of $\bullet O_2^-$ was also detected. In Figure 3d, the signals of $\bullet O_2^-$ show significant enhancement in intensity when the irradiation time is increased from 3 min to 5 min. These results suggest that $^1O_2$ and $\bullet O_2^-$ are the active species involved in the removal of TC by the GO–light system. In our ESR analysis, $\bullet OH$ signals were also detected, but they were not particularly obvious and only observable from the noisy baseline (Figure 3e). The weak signals suggest that $\bullet OH$ is not sufficiently produced through photoexcitation of the GO, and, hence, plays only a minor role in the TC removal process. TEMPO can produce a triplet ESR signal by itself, and this ESR signal intensity would be weakened by reaction with h^+, forming spin-adducts of (TEMPO–h^+) [52]. In other words, the weakening of TEMPO signals indicates the generation of h^+. As shown in Figure 3f, the intensity of the peak produced by TEMPO noticeably decreased after light irradiation, corroborating that holes are generated in the GO–light system. Overall, the results of our ESR studies agree with the different inhibitory removal effects observed for EDTA-2Na, FFA, SOD, and isopropyl alcohol on TC as shown in Figure 3a.

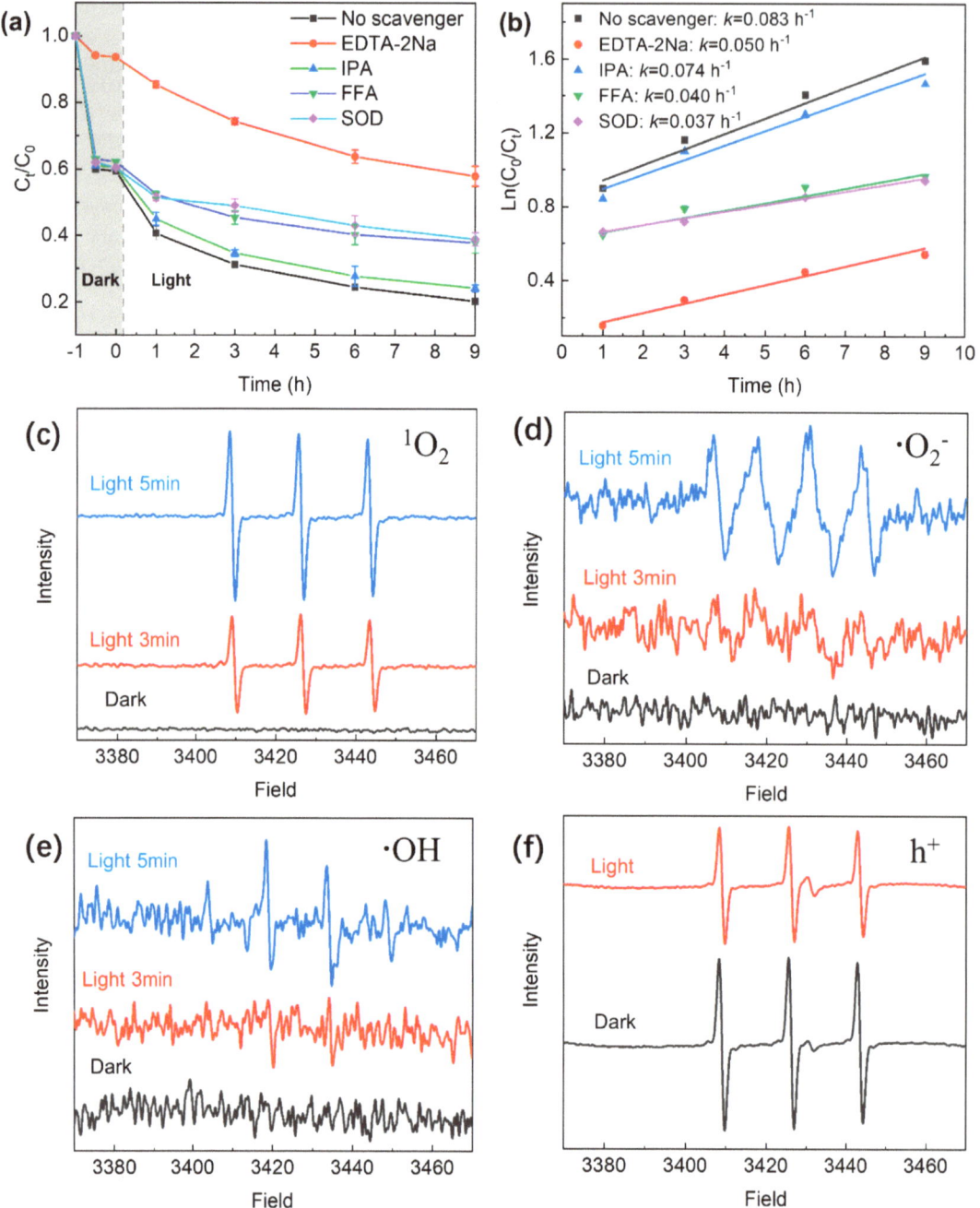

Figure 3. (**a**) Effect of various scavengers on TC removal in the GO–light system. (**b**) First-order kinetic plots for the scavenger-involved reactions. ESR spectra of free radicals and holes trapped by TEMP ($^1O_2$), TEMPO (h^+) and DMPO ($\bullet O_2^-$ and $\bullet OH$) under xenon lamp irradiation: in aqueous dispersion for trapping $^1O_2$ (**c**); in methanol dispersion for trapping $\bullet O_2^-$ (**d**); in aqueous dispersion for trapping $\bullet OH$ (**e**); in aqueous dispersion for trapping h^+ (**f**).

Studies have demonstrated that the TC molecule is sensitive to various light sources in aqueous solutions [53–55]. For example, Hu et al. reported that TC can be effectively photodegraded on the surface of TiO_2 under visible light irradiation. This reactivity was rationalized by the fact that TC with photosensitivity may form a complex with the surface of TiO_2 to generate superoxide free radicals through the absorption of visible light [55]. In our work, the ESR spin-trap technique was used to analyze the production of ROS in TC solution by GO under light irradiation. As shown in Figure 4, both $^1O_2$ and $\bullet O_2^-$ were noticeably detected under light conditions. Interestingly, the concentration of $^1O_2$ and $\bullet O_2^-$ generated by GO in TC solution increased by about 1/3 compared with that in clean water, while the generation of $\bullet OH$ remained largely unchanged compared with that in clean water (Figure 4d). No ROS were detected in the TC solution in the absence of GO under the same light conditions. These results suggest that the interactions of GO and TC under photoirradiation contribute to increased $^1O_2$ and $\bullet O_2^-$ generation. GO has a large surface area and contains abundant oxygen-containing groups and sp^2 carbon domains on its surface to give strong adsorption performance for TC [40]. The adsorption of TC molecules on GO is facilitated by various non-covalent forces (e.g., electrostatic attraction, van der Waals forces, and hydrogen-bonding interactions). TC is a photosensitive molecule. Upon photoirradiation, the excited-state TC can inject electrons to the conduction band of GO, which in turn promotes the formation of more $^1O_2$ and $\bullet O_2^-$.

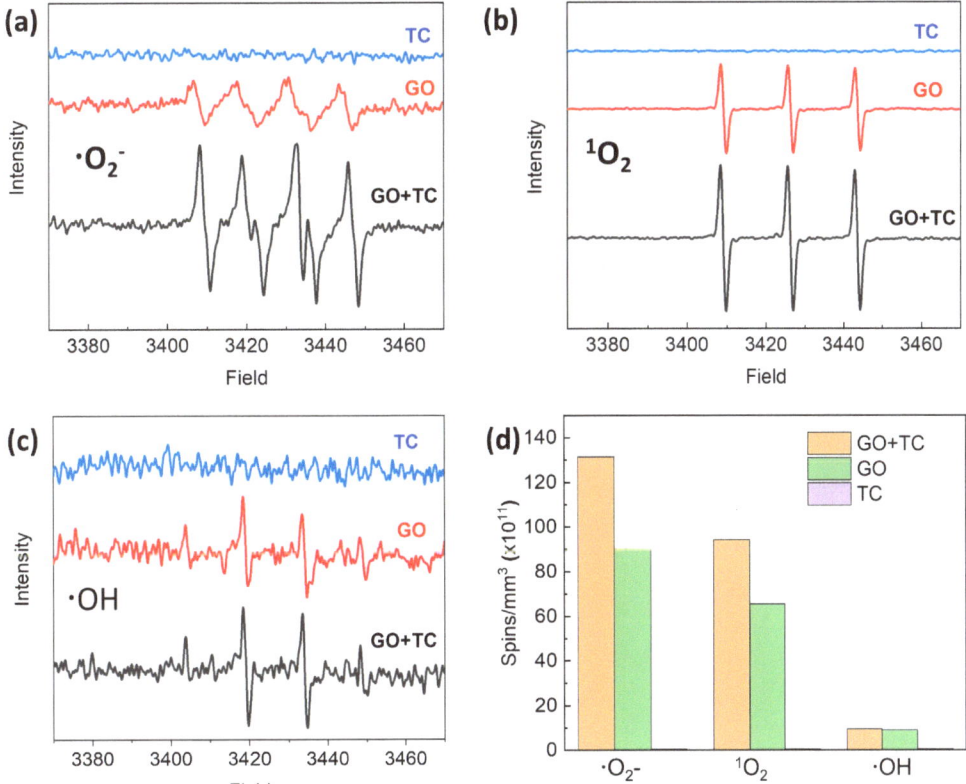

Figure 4. ESR spectra of radicals trapped by DMPO ($\bullet O_2^-$ and $\bullet OH$), TEMP ($^1O_2$), and TEMPO (h^+) in GO aqueous dispersion under xenon lamp irradiation: (**a**) for trapping $^1O_2$, (**b**) for trapping $\bullet O_2^-$, (**c**) for trapping h^+, and (**d**) quantitative comparison of $\bullet O_2^-$, $\bullet OH$, and $^1O_2$ produced by GO, TC, and [GO + TC], respectively.

2.4. TC Degradation Mechanism in GO–Light System

Aqueous samples of TC were analyzed by UV-Vis in TC solutions treated by GO (see Figure 5). The absorption spectra show that TC generates two main absorption peaks at 275 nm and 357 nm. The absorption at 357 nm is due to the aromatic rings B-D in TC, including enols and developed chromophores. The absorption at 275 nm is mainly related to the acyl-amino and hydroxyl groups on aromatic ring A [56]. These characteristic absorption bands were found to gradually decrease with increasing reaction time, suggesting that TC was gradually removed from aqueous solution. Compared to dark conditions, the absorption peak at 275 nm under photoirradiation shows a significant blue shift (Figure 5) as the reaction progresses. This observation is indicative of degradation of the TC structure, and the degradation of TC most likely occurred on the aromatic ring A part due to the attack by the generated ROS (e.g., $^1O_2$, $\bullet O_2^-$) and the reaction with holes. In fact, in the radical scavenging experiments, the addition of $^1O_2$ and hole scavengers significantly inhibited the blue shift of the 275 nm absorption peak (Figure 5b,c), whereas the addition of hydroxyl radical traps little inhibited the blue shift of the peak (Figure 5d). These experimental results further confirm that $^1O_2$ and holes directly participate in the photocatalytic degradation of TC, but hydroxyl radical is only minorly involved.

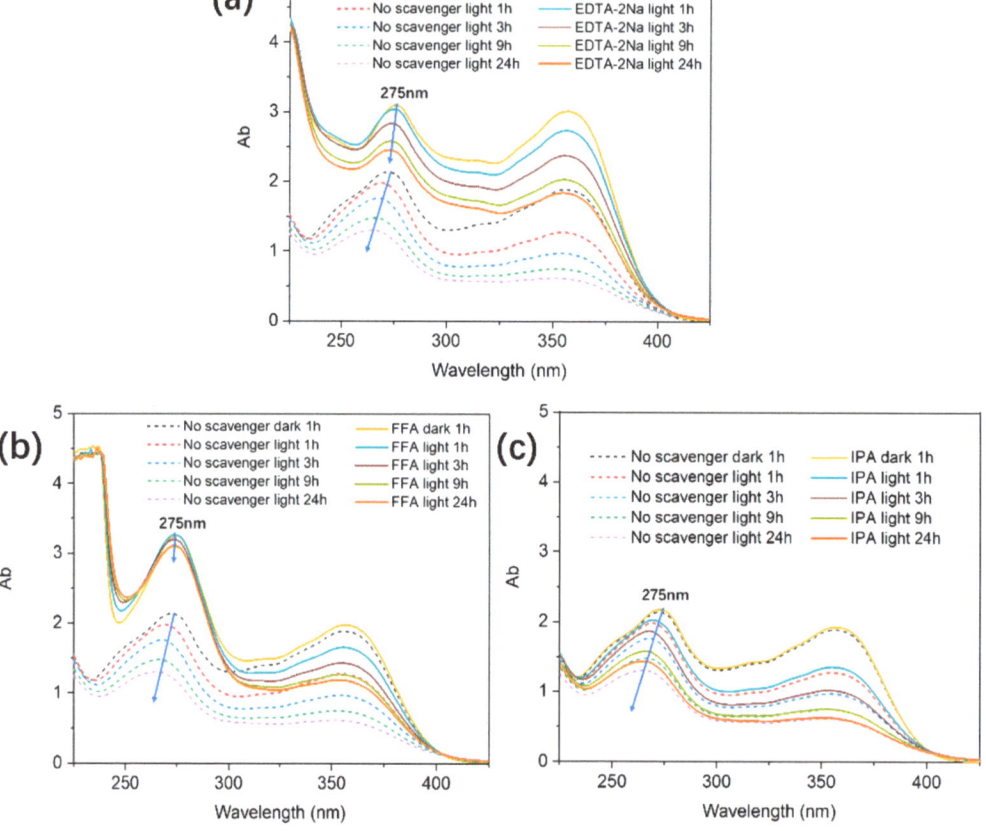

Figure 5. UV-Vis absorption spectra of TC solutions at different time intervals: (**a**) the effect of EDTA-2Na, (**b**) the effect of FFA, and (**c**) the effect of IPA.

To shed more light on the mechanism of TC degradation by the GO–light system, the intermediate products of TC during GO–light treatment were evaluated by liquid chromatography–electrospray ionization–tandem mass spectrometry (LC-ESIMS/MS) analysis. Figure 6a shows the total ion current LC-MS/MS chromatogram of TC treated by the GO–light system at different times. Based on the MS analysis, seven different kinds of products can be identified at m/z = 477 (retention time 6.4 min), 305 (retention time 7.8 min), 349 (retention time 8.3 min), 459 (retention time 8.9 min), 333 (retention time 10.4 min), and 435 (retention time 10.4 min), respectively. The detailed mass spectra corresponding to each chromatographic peak are given in Figure S4. The possible degradation products of TC are proposed in Table S2, where m/z = 445 (retention time 8.5 min) is taken as the parent TC.

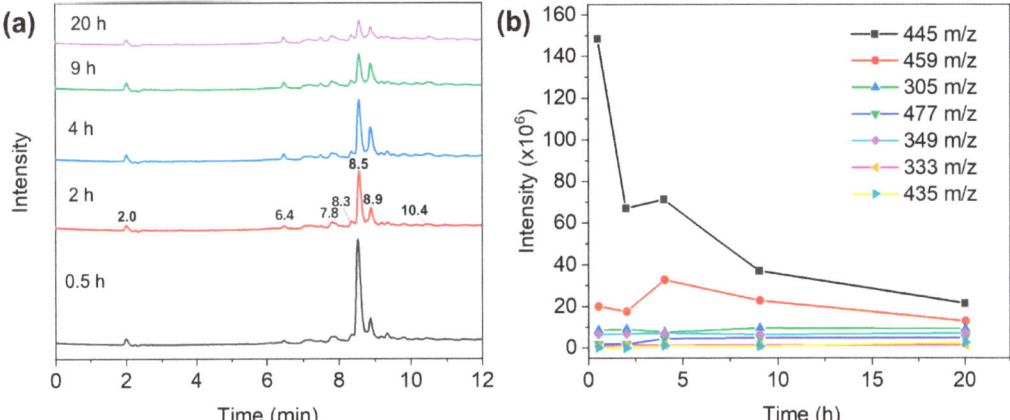

Figure 6. (**a**) Total ion current LC-MS/MS chromatogram of TC solution treated by GO irradiation at different time points. (**b**) Product evolution of TC during the removal of TC process by the GO–light system.

As shown in Figure 6a, the amount of TC gradually decreases with increasing GO–light treatment time. Among the TC photocatalytic degradation products, the abundance of m/z = 459 product is the most obvious, indicating that this intermediate is the main degradation product in the process of TC removal by the GO–light system. Product m/z = 459 can be obtained by introducing two carbonyl groups to the *para*-positions of the TC aromatic ring in the presence of singlet oxygen and superoxide radicals [57,58]. With increasing treatment time, the concentration of the intermediate shows a trend of first increasing and then decreasing (Figure 6b). This can be explained by that a large amount of the TC present in the early stage of GO–light treatment is degraded into m/z 459 by ROS produced in the system, and the intermediate may be further degraded through adsorption or remain on the GO surface as the reaction proceeds. The double bond at the C11a-C12 position of TC may cause C11a to be hydroxylated by •OH because the electron-withdrawing group is more vulnerable to radical attack. In addition, hydroxylation may occur at the CH$_3$-NR site, leading to the production of the m/z = 477 product [58,59].

The m/z = 435 degradation products can be formed by demethylation of dimethyl amine of TC under $^1O_2$ and •O_2^- attack and hydroxylation destruction under H_2O_2/H_2O attack [28,60–62]. The carbon–carbon double bond on m/z = 435 can be attacked by ROS, and ring A is subsequently cracked during photocatalytic oxidation to produce intermediate m/z = 349 [63]. A similar reaction mechanism can be introduced to form the intermediate m/z = 333 [64]. The product m/z = 349 can be further decarboxylated to form another product m/z = 305 [63]. Notably, there is also a distinct peak at the retention time of 2.0 min in the LC-MS chromatogram, which could be attributed to the partial dissolution of GO in water, as the same chromatogram peak and the same mass spectra (Figure S5) appear at the retention time of 2.0 min under dark conditions. Combining our experimental outcomes and literature results, we arrive at the possible reaction pathways and the degraded products of TC degradation by the GO–light system proposed in Figure 7.

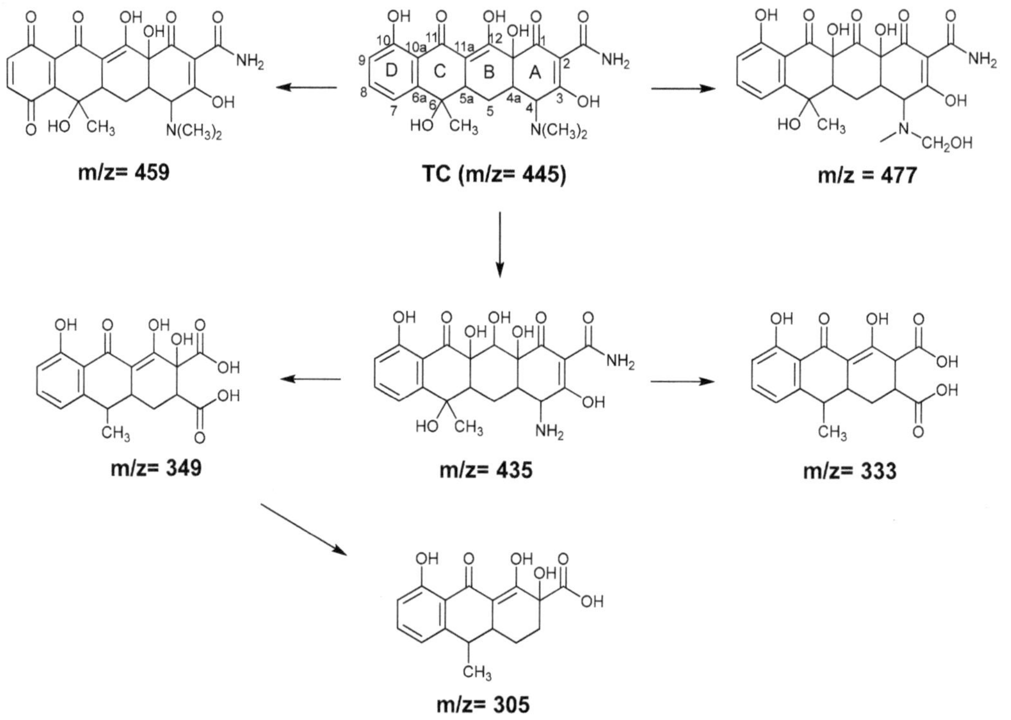

Figure 7. Proposed photodegradation pathways and the degraded products of TC by the GO–light system.

The DFT method was used to reveal the adsorption property of TC on GO under light irradiation (Figure S6). Because TC is a photosensitive molecule, excited-state TC was used as a model for the GO–light system. The binding energies of GO with the excited-state TC and ground-state TC were calculated to be −4.91 ev and −2.31 ev, respectively. The theoretical results indicated that TC can adsorb more easily on the GO surface under light irradiation compared to under dark conditions, which also contributed to the enhanced removal rate of TC by the GO–light system. The possible removal mechanism of TC by GO under irradiation is illustrated in Figure 8. As a semiconductor-like material, GO could generate oxidative (valence band holes, h^+) and reductive (conduction band electron, e^-) transient species when exposed to sunlight. In addition, sunlight irradiation should change GO from the ground state to the excited state (GO*), which in turn induces the formation of singlet oxygen ($^1O_2$) through the energy transfer between GO* and dissolved oxygen in water [65]. The photoinduced electrons could quickly migrate to the surface of GO. The abundant oxygen functional groups (OFGs) on the GO surface facilitate the generation of GO radical anions and subsequent formation of $·O_2^-$ [66]. The migration of electrons can improve the separation efficiency of photogenerated e^-–h^+ pairs and enhance the h^+-dominated direct oxidation on TC reaction [67]. It is also possible that hydroxy radicals (·OH) might be produced from $·O_2^-$ [68], but ·OH plays only a minor role in photo-enhanced TC removal in the presence of GO.

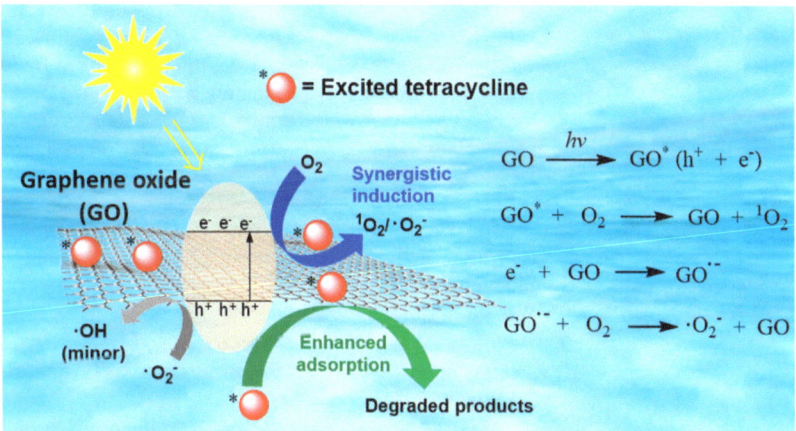

Figure 8. The proposed mechanism of TC degradation by a GO–light system (red circle with star symbol represents excited tetracycline).

From a fundamental perspective, the structural homogeneity of GO is an important factor in its photocatalytic effects on generating ROS and degrading organic substances on its surface. Gaining a deeper insight into this aspect, however, requires a more carefully controlled synthesis of GO and thorough characterizations of the structure and composition of GO. It is also worth noting that the molecular structures of tetracycline and many other antibiotics contain stereogenic centers and, therefore, show optical activity. The use of polarized light to induce selective photoexcitation and subsequent degradation on the surface of GO represents another intriguing direction for future work. Moreover, tuning the nonlinear optical effects of GO may create a new avenue for optimizing and enhancing the performance of GO in combination with other functional nanomaterials (e.g., metal and metal oxide nanoparticles) [69]. Studies along these directions are warranted for future work to further improve the performance of our GO-based photocatalytic systems.

3. Materials and Methods

3.1. Chemical Reagents

Detailed information on the chemical reagents used in this study is provided in Text S1.

3.2. Preparation of GO

GO was prepared from natural graphite powder using an improved Hummers method (see Text S2 for more details) [70]. The characterization methods of GO are presented in Text S3.

3.3. Removal of TC under Light Condition

A xenon lamp (300 W) was used as a simulated sunlight source, and the distance between TC solution and light source was kept at 10 cm. The conical flask containing TC solution and GO sample was placed in a water bath and was blown with a fan to maintain the sample solution at room temperature (25 °C) during the TC removal test. An experiment that was conducted under the same conditions without the presence of GO was used as a control. Further, an experiment in which a conical flask containing tetracycline solution and GO sample was directly irradiated by xenon light without temperature control was also conducted and the results were used to evaluate the thermal effect of the light irradiation. A typical TC removal experiment was carried out through the following steps: 10 mg of GO was added to a 50 mL solution of TC (100 mg·L^{-1}). The resulting suspension was stirred under irradiation or dark conditions for a certain period of time. After that, the sample was centrifuged and aliquots from the top of the solution were collected for analysis. In order to study the effect of pH on TC removal, the pH values of TC solutions were adjusted in the range of 3.0–10.0, using a small amount of 0.1 M hydrochloric acid or 0.1 M sodium hydroxide solution. Ethylenediaminetetraacetic acid disodium salt (EDTA-2Na), furfuryl alcohol (FFA), Superoxide dismutase (SOD), and isopropanol (IPA), were used as holes, $^1O_2$, $\bullet O_2^-$, and $\bullet OH$ scavengers, respectively. All experiments were performed in triplicate.

3.4. Analytical Methods

The concentration of TC in solution of each sample was determined by the UV-Vis absorption method. The TC removal rate (R) at a time (t) can be calculated using the following formula:

$$R = \frac{C_0 - C_t}{C_0} \quad (3)$$

where C_0 and C_t are the initial concentration of TC and the concentration of TC at time t, respectively.

Electron spin resonance (ESR) experiments were performed using a spectrometer (Brucker EMX, Germany) equipped with a 300 W xenon lamp. The test conditions for $\bullet OH$, $^1O_2$, $\bullet O_2^-$, and holes are given in Text S4. Photodegradation intermediates of TC were detected using an HPLC–MS system (Agilent 1290/6460, Triple Quad MS). Detailed information on the HPLC–MS system analysis is given in Text S5. Detailed information on the computational modeling is provided in Text S6.

4. Conclusions

The removal of TC from water by the GO–light system has been systematically studied. Our results show that light irradiation significantly enhances the removal of TC. More than 90% of TC was removed within 20 h (100 mg·L^{-1} TC, 200 mg·L^{-1} GO) under light irradiation, which is 50% more efficient than the action of GO in dark conditions. Radical scavenging experiments, ESR, and UV-Vis spectral analysis all point to the fact that $^1O_2$, $\bullet O_2^-$, and h$^+$ are responsible for the enhanced TC removal. The degradation pathway of TC is proposed based on the intermediates identified by the LC-ESIMS/MS technique. The studies provide experimental and theoretical support for the development of a new strategy for the removal of pollutants from water. At the same time, recycling or isolating GO after water treatment is still a challenge as GO is highly dispersible in water due to its abundant oxygen functional groups. This challenge is expected to be overcome by designing GO composites that can be readily isolated out of water and retain the performance of GO in terms of excellent absorptivity and photoactivity. Overall, we envision the concept of enhanced adsorption and synergistic induction of ROS generation will find extensive applications in sustainable materials and environmental technologies.

Supplementary Materials: The following supporting information can be downloaded at: https://www.mdpi.com/article/10.3390/molecules29163765/s1. Text S1. Chemical reagents; Text S2. Preparation and characterization of GO; Text S3–S6. Detailed information of analytic methods; TC removal model; ESR spectra; UV-Vis spectra; Total ion current LC-MS/MS chromatogram analysis during TC removal and corresponding mass spectra; Proposed intermediate structures; Computational modeling. Figure S1. (a) FTIR spectrum of prepared GO; (b) XRD spectrum and TEM image of GO. (c) UV-VIS absorption spectrum of GO suspended in water. Figure S2. The influence of various TC concentrations (30 to 200 mg·L^{-1}) on the removal effect of TC by the GO-Light system. Table S1. First order reaction kinetics of tetracycline removal by GO-Light system in the presence of various radical scavengers. Figure S3. UV–vis absorption spectra of TC solutions at different time intervals under light and dark conditions. Figure S4. Mass spectra corresponding to each chromatography peak in the total ion current LC-MS/MS chromatogram of tetracycline solution treated by GO under light. (2 h as a typical example). Table S2. The identified of TC and its possible transformation products during the photocatalysis. Figure S5. (a) Total ion current LC-MS/MS chromatogram of tetracycline solution treated by GO under dark and light conditions; GO-Light control is the pure water treated by GO under light. (b) Mass spectra collected at retention time of 2.1 min. Figure S6. Configuration for TC and GO structure interaction, references [71–76].

Author Contributions: K.N.: Conceptualization, Formal analysis, Investigation, Methodology, Supervision, Writing—original draft, Writing—review and editing. Y.C.: Data curation, Formal analysis. R.X.: Data curation; Formal analysis. Y.Z.: Writing—review and editing. M.G.: Supervision, Writing—review and editing. All authors have read and agreed to the published version of the manuscript.

Funding: This research is supported by the Zhejiang Provincial Natural Science Foundation of China under Grant No. LTGS24B070001.

Institutional Review Board Statement: Not applicable.

Informed Consent Statement: Not applicable.

Data Availability Statement: Data are contained within the article and Supplementary Materials.

Conflicts of Interest: The authors declare that they have no known competing financial interests or personal relationships that could have appeared to influence the work reported in this paper.

References

1. Olabi, A.G.; Abdelkareem, M.A.; Wilberforce, T.; Sayed, E.T. Application of graphene in energy storage device—A review. *Renew. Sustain. Energy Rev.* **2021**, *135*, 110026. [CrossRef]
2. Huang, H.; Shi, H.; Das, P.; Qin, J.; Li, Y.; Wang, X.; Su, F.; Wen, P.; Li, S.; Lu, P.; et al. The Chemistry and Promising Applications of Graphene and Porous Graphene Materials. *Adv. Funct. Mater.* **2020**, *30*, 1909035. [CrossRef]
3. Zhang, F.; Yang, K.; Liu, G.; Chen, Y.; Wang, M.; Li, S.; Li, R. Recent advances on graphene: Synthesis, properties and applications. *Compos. Part A Appl. Sci. Manuf.* **2022**, *160*, 107051. [CrossRef]
4. Wu, J.; Jia, L.; Zhang, Y.; Qu, Y.; Jia, B.; Moss, D.J. Graphene Oxide for Integrated Photonics and Flat Optics. *Adv. Mater.* **2021**, *33*, 2006415. [CrossRef] [PubMed]
5. Han, Y.; Ma, S.; Ma, J.; Guiraud, P.; Guo, X.; Zhang, Y.; Jiao, T. In-situ desorption of acetaminophen from the surface of graphene oxide driven by an electric field: A study by molecular dynamics simulation. *Chem. Eng. J.* **2021**, *418*, 129391. [CrossRef]
6. Loh, K.P.; Bao, Q.; Eda, G.; Chhowalla, M. Graphene oxide as a chemically tunable platform for optical applications. *Nat. Chem.* **2010**, *2*, 1015–1024. [CrossRef] [PubMed]
7. Valentini, C.; Montes-García, V.; Livio, P.A.; Chudziak, T.; Raya, J.; Ciesielski, A.; Samorì, P. Tuning the electrical properties of graphene oxide through low-temperature thermal annealing. *Nanoscale* **2023**, *15*, 5743–5755. [CrossRef] [PubMed]
8. Du, W.; Wu, H.; Chen, H.; Xu, G.; Li, C. Graphene oxide in aqueous and nonaqueous media: Dispersion behaviour and solution chemistry. *Carbon* **2020**, *158*, 568–579. [CrossRef]
9. Wang, H.; Hu, Y.H. Effect of Oxygen Content on Structures of Graphite Oxides. *Ind. Eng. Chem. Res.* **2011**, *50*, 6132–6137. [CrossRef]
10. Mousavi, S.M.; Hashemi, S.A.; Kalashgrani, M.Y.; Gholami, A.; Binazadeh, M.; Chiang, W.-H.; Rahman, M.M. Recent advances in energy storage with graphene oxide for supercapacitor technology. *Sustain. Energy Fuels* **2023**, *7*, 5176–5197. [CrossRef]
11. Ha, S.H.; Jeong, Y.S.; Lee, Y.J. Free Standing Reduced Graphene Oxide Film Cathodes for Lithium Ion Batteries. *ACS Appl. Mater. Interfaces* **2013**, *5*, 12295–12303. [CrossRef] [PubMed]
12. Zhang, K.; Fu, Q.; Pan, N.; Yu, X.; Liu, J.; Luo, Y.; Wang, X.; Yang, J.; Hou, J. Direct writing of electronic devices on graphene oxide by catalytic scanning probe lithography. *Nat. Commun.* **2012**, *3*, 1194. [CrossRef] [PubMed]
13. Chung, C.; Kim, Y.-K.; Shin, D.; Ryoo, S.-R.; Hong, B.H.; Min, D.-H. Biomedical Applications of Graphene and Graphene Oxide. *Acc. Chem. Res.* **2013**, *46*, 2211–2224. [CrossRef] [PubMed]
14. Putri, L.K.; Tan, L.-L.; Ong, W.-J.; Chang, W.S.; Chai, S.-P. Graphene oxide: Exploiting its unique properties toward visible-light-driven photocatalysis. *Appl. Mater. Today* **2016**, *4*, 9–16. [CrossRef]
15. Cruz, M.; Gomez, C.; Duran-Valle, C.J.; Pastrana-Martínez, L.M.; Faria, J.L.; Silva, A.M.T.; Faraldos, M.; Bahamonde, A. Bare TiO_2 and graphene oxide TiO_2 photocatalysts on the degradation of selected pesticides and influence of the water matrix. *Appl. Surf. Sci.* **2017**, *416*, 1013–1021. [CrossRef]
16. Pastrana-Martínez, L.M.; Morales-Torres, S.; Kontos, A.G.; Moustakas, N.G.; Faria, J.L.; Doña-Rodríguez, J.M.; Falaras, P.; Silva, A.M.T. TiO_2, surface modified TiO_2 and graphene oxide-TiO_2 photocatalysts for degradation of water pollutants under near-UV/Vis and visible light. *Chem. Eng. J.* **2013**, *224*, 17–23. [CrossRef]
17. Pastrana-Martínez, L.M.; Morales-Torres, S.; Likodimos, V.; Figueiredo, J.L.; Faria, J.L.; Falaras, P.; Silva, A.M.T. Advanced nanostructured photocatalysts based on reduced graphene oxide–TiO_2 composites for degradation of diphenhydramine pharmaceutical and methyl orange dye. *Appl. Catal. B Environ.* **2012**, *123–124*, 241–256. [CrossRef]
18. Li, B.; Liu, T.; Wang, Y.; Wang, Z. ZnO/graphene-oxide nanocomposite with remarkably enhanced visible-light-driven photocatalytic performance. *J. Colloid Interface Sci.* **2012**, *377*, 114–121. [CrossRef] [PubMed]

19. Pastrana-Martínez, L.M.; Morales-Torres, S.; Likodimos, V.; Falaras, P.; Figueiredo, J.L.; Faria, J.L.; Silva, A.M.T. Role of oxygen functionalities on the synthesis of photocatalytically active graphene–TiO$_2$ composites. *Appl. Catal. B Environ.* **2014**, *158–159*, 329–340. [CrossRef]
20. Linley, S.; Liu, Y.; Ptacek, C.J.; Blowes, D.W.; Gu, F.X. Recyclable Graphene Oxide-Supported Titanium Dioxide Photocatalysts with Tunable Properties. *ACS Appl. Mater. Interfaces* **2014**, *6*, 4658–4668. [CrossRef]
21. Liu, J.; Ke, J.; Li, D.; Sun, H.; Liang, P.; Duan, X.; Tian, W.; Tadé, M.O.; Liu, S.; Wang, S. Oxygen Vacancies in Shape Controlled Cu$_2$O/Reduced Graphene Oxide/In$_2$O$_3$ Hybrid for Promoted Photocatalytic Water Oxidation and Degradation of Environmental Pollutants. *ACS Appl. Mater. Interfaces* **2017**, *9*, 11678–11688. [CrossRef] [PubMed]
22. Jiang, X.; Wang, J. Enhanced photocatalytic activity of three-dimensional TiO$_2$/reduced graphene oxide aerogel by efficient interfacial charge transfer. *Appl. Surf. Sci.* **2023**, *612*, 155849. [CrossRef]
23. Tong, Z.; Yang, D.; Shi, J.; Nan, Y.; Sun, Y.; Jiang, Z. Three-Dimensional Porous Aerogel Constructed by g-C$_3$N$_4$ and Graphene Oxide Nanosheets with Excellent Visible-Light Photocatalytic Performance. *ACS Appl. Mater. Interfaces* **2015**, *7*, 25693–25701. [CrossRef] [PubMed]
24. Pedrosa, M.; Pastrana-Martínez, L.M.; Pereira, M.F.R.; Faria, J.L.; Figueiredo, J.L.; Silva, A.M.T. N/S-doped graphene derivatives and TiO$_2$ for catalytic ozonation and photocatalysis of water pollutants. *Chem. Eng. J.* **2018**, *348*, 888–897. [CrossRef]
25. Xing, M.; Fang, W.; Yang, X.; Tian, B.; Zhang, J. Highly-dispersed boron-doped graphene nanoribbons with enhanced conductibility and photocatalysis. *Chem. Commun.* **2014**, *50*, 6637–6640. [CrossRef] [PubMed]
26. Tang, Z.-R.; Zhang, Y.; Zhang, N.; Xu, Y.-J. New insight into the enhanced visible light photocatalytic activity over boron-doped reduced graphene oxide. *Nanoscale* **2015**, *7*, 7030–7034. [CrossRef] [PubMed]
27. Peng, W.; Li, X. Synthesis of a sulfur-graphene composite as an enhanced metal-free photocatalyst. *Nano Res.* **2013**, *6*, 286–292. [CrossRef]
28. Zhang, Q.; Jiang, L.; Wang, J.; Zhu, Y.; Pu, Y.; Dai, W. Photocatalytic degradation of tetracycline antibiotics using three-dimensional network structure perylene diimide supramolecular organic photocatalyst under visible-light irradiation. *Appl. Catal. B Environ.* **2020**, *277*, 119122. [CrossRef]
29. Adeleye, A.S.; Wang, X.; Wang, F.; Hao, R.; Song, W.; Li, Y. Photoreactivity of graphene oxide in aqueous system: Reactive oxygen species formation and bisphenol A degradation. *Chemosphere* **2018**, *195*, 344–350. [CrossRef]
30. Oh, J.; Chang, Y.H.; Kim, Y.-H.; Park, S. Thickness-dependent photocatalytic performance of graphite oxide for degrading organic pollutants under visible light. *Phys. Chem. Chem. Phys.* **2016**, *18*, 10882–10886. [CrossRef]
31. Li, C.; Xu, Q.; Xu, S.; Zhang, X.; Hou, X.; Wu, P.J.R.a. Synergy of adsorption and photosensitization of graphene oxide for improved removal of organic pollutants. *RSC Adv.* **2017**, *7*, 16204–16209. [CrossRef]
32. Bustos-Ramírez, K.; Barrera-Díaz, C.E.; De Icaza-Herrera, M.; Martínez-Hernández, A.L.; Natividad-Rangel, R.; Velasco-Santos, C. 4-chlorophenol removal from water using graphite and graphene oxides as photocatalysts. *J. Environ. Health Sci. Eng.* **2015**, *13*, 33. [CrossRef] [PubMed]
33. Hou, W.-C.; Chowdhury, I.; Goodwin, D.G., Jr.; Henderson, W.M.; Fairbrother, D.H.; Bouchard, D.; Zepp, R.G. Photochemical Transformation of Graphene Oxide in Sunlight. *Environ. Sci. Technol.* **2015**, *49*, 3435–3443. [CrossRef] [PubMed]
34. Shams, M.; Guiney, L.M.; Huang, L.; Ramesh, M.; Yang, X.; Hersam, M.C.; Chowdhury, I. Influence of functional groups on the degradation of graphene oxide nanomaterials. *Environ. Sci. Nano* **2019**, *6*, 2203–2214. [CrossRef]
35. Pedrosa, M.; Da Silva, E.S.; Pastrana-Martínez, L.M.; Drazic, G.; Falaras, P.; Faria, J.L.; Figueiredo, J.L.; Silva, A.M.T. Hummers' and Brodie's graphene oxides as photocatalysts for phenol degradation. *J. Colloid Interface Sci.* **2020**, *567*, 243–255. [CrossRef] [PubMed]
36. Zou, Y.; Wang, W.; Wang, H.; Pan, C.; Xu, J.; Pozdnyakov, I.P.; Wu, F.; Li, J. Interaction between graphene oxide and acetaminophen in water under simulated sunlight: Implications for environmental photochemistry of PPCPs. *Water Res.* **2023**, *228*, 119364. [CrossRef] [PubMed]
37. Du, L.; Ahmad, S.; Liu, L.; Wang, L.; Tang, J. A review of antibiotics and antibiotic resistance genes (ARGs) adsorption by biochar and modified biochar in water. *Sci. Total Environ.* **2023**, *858*, 159815. [CrossRef]
38. Yan, L.; Liu, Y.; Zhang, Y.; Liu, S.; Wang, C.; Chen, W.; Liu, C.; Chen, Z.; Zhang, Y. ZnCl$_2$ modified biochar derived from aerobic granular sludge for developed microporosity and enhanced adsorption to tetracycline. *Bioresour. Technol.* **2020**, *297*, 122381. [CrossRef]
39. Song, Z.; Ma, Y.-L.; Li, C.-E. The residual tetracycline in pharmaceutical wastewater was effectively removed by using MnO$_2$/graphene nanocomposite. *Sci. Total Environ.* **2019**, *651*, 580–590. [CrossRef]
40. Gao, Y.; Li, Y.; Zhang, L.; Huang, H.; Hu, J.; Shah, S.M.; Su, X. Adsorption and removal of tetracycline antibiotics from aqueous solution by graphene oxide. *J. Colloid Interface Sci.* **2012**, *368*, 540–546. [CrossRef]
41. Minale, M.; Gu, Z.; Guadie, A.; Kabtamu, D.M.; Li, Y.; Wang, X. Application of graphene-based materials for removal of tetracyclines using adsorption and photocatalytic-degradation: A review. *J. Environ. Manag.* **2020**, *276*, 111310. [CrossRef] [PubMed]
42. Fathy, M.; Gomaa, A.; Taher, F.A.; El-Fass, M.M.; Kashyout, A.E.-H.B. Optimizing the preparation parameters of GO and rGO for large-scale production. *J. Mater. Sci.* **2016**, *51*, 5664–5675. [CrossRef]
43. Sharma, N.; Arif, M.; Monga, S.; Shkir, M.; Mishra, Y.K.; Singh, A. Investigation of bandgap alteration in graphene oxide with different reduction routes. *Appl. Surf. Sci.* **2020**, *513*, 145396. [CrossRef]

44. Rauf, M.A.; Ashraf, S.S. Fundamental principles and application of heterogeneous photocatalytic degradation of dyes in solution. *Chem. Eng. J.* **2009**, *151*, 10–18. [CrossRef]
45. Rhoden, C.R.B.; Bruckmann, F.d.S.; Salles, T.d.R.; Kaufmann Junior, C.G.; Mortari, S.R. Study from the influence of magnetite onto removal of hydrochlorothiazide from aqueous solutions applying magnetic graphene oxide. *J. Water Process Eng.* **2021**, *43*, 102262. [CrossRef]
46. Yuan, J.; Li, H.; Wang, G.; Zhang, C.; Wang, Y.; Yang, L.; Li, M.; Lu, J. Adsorption, isolated electron/hole transport, and confined catalysis coupling to enhance the photocatalytic degradation performance. *Appl. Catal. B Environ.* **2022**, *303*, 120892. [CrossRef]
47. Gottfried, V.; Kimel, S. Temperature effects on photosensitized processes. *J. Photochem. Photobiol. B Biol.* **1991**, *8*, 419–430. [CrossRef] [PubMed]
48. Bertini, I.; Banci, L.; Luchinat, C.; Bielski, B.H.J.; Cabelli, D.E.; Mullenbach, G.T.; Hallewell, R.A. An investigation of a human erythrocyte SOD modified at position 137. *J. Am. Chem. Soc.* **1989**, *111*, 714–719. [CrossRef]
49. Palominos, R.A.; Mondaca, M.A.; Giraldo, A.; Peñuela, G.; Pérez-Moya, M.; Mansilla, H.D. Photocatalytic oxidation of the antibiotic tetracycline on TiO_2 and ZnO suspensions. *Catal. Today* **2009**, *144*, 100–105. [CrossRef]
50. Yang, Y.; Bian, Z. Oxygen doping through oxidation causes the main active substance in g-C_3N_4 photocatalysis to change from holes to singlet oxygen. *Sci. Total Environ.* **2021**, *753*, 141908. [CrossRef]
51. Li, L.; Niu, C.-G.; Guo, H.; Wang, J.; Ruan, M.; Zhang, L.; Liang, C.; Liu, H.-Y.; Yang, Y.-Y. Efficient degradation of Levofloxacin with magnetically separable $ZnFe_2O_4$/NCDs/Ag_2CO_3 Z-scheme heterojunction photocatalyst: Vis-NIR light response ability and mechanism insight. *Chem. Eng. J.* **2020**, *383*, 123192. [CrossRef]
52. He, W.; Kim, H.-K.; Wamer, W.G.; Melka, D.; Callahan, J.H.; Yin, J.-J. Photogenerated Charge Carriers and Reactive Oxygen Species in ZnO/Au Hybrid Nanostructures with Enhanced Photocatalytic and Antibacterial Activity. *J. Am. Chem. Soc.* **2014**, *136*, 750–757. [CrossRef]
53. Beliakova, M.M.; Bessonov, S.I.; Sergeyev, B.M.; Smirnova, I.G.; Dobrov, E.N.; Kopylov, A.M. Rate of Tetracycline Photolysis during Irradiation at 365 nm. *Biochemistry* **2003**, *68*, 182–187. [CrossRef] [PubMed]
54. Verma, B.; Headley, J.V.; Robarts, R.D. Behaviour and fate of tetracycline in river and wetland waters on the Canadian Northern Great Plains. *J. Environ. Sci. Health Part A* **2007**, *42*, 109–117. [CrossRef] [PubMed]
55. Wu, S.; Hu, H.; Lin, Y.; Zhang, J.; Hu, Y.H. Visible light photocatalytic degradation of tetracycline over TiO_2. *Chem. Eng. J.* **2020**, *382*, 122842. [CrossRef]
56. Gao, B.; Iftekhar, S.; Srivastava, V.; Doshi, B.; Sillanpää, M. Insights into the generation of reactive oxygen species (ROS) over polythiophene/ZnIn2S4 based on different modification processing. *Catal. Sci. Technol.* **2018**, *8*, 2186–2194. [CrossRef]
57. Nguyen, H.V.-M.; Lee, D.-H.; Lee, H.-S.; Shin, H.-S. Investigating the different transformations of tetracycline using birnessite under different reaction conditions and various humic acids. *Environ. Pollut.* **2023**, *339*, 122763. [CrossRef] [PubMed]
58. Shen, Q.; Wang, Z.; Yu, Q.; Cheng, Y.; Liu, Z.; Zhang, T.; Zhou, S. Removal of tetracycline from an aqueous solution using manganese dioxide modified biochar derived from Chinese herbal medicine residues. *Environ. Res.* **2020**, *183*, 109195. [CrossRef] [PubMed]
59. Dong, G.; Huang, L.; Wu, X.; Wang, C.; Liu, Y.; Liu, G.; Wang, L.; Liu, X.; Xia, H. Effect and mechanism analysis of MnO_2 on permeable reactive barrier (PRB) system for the removal of tetracycline. *Chemosphere* **2018**, *193*, 702–710. [CrossRef]
60. Xie, Z.; Feng, Y.; Wang, F.; Chen, D.; Zhang, Q.; Zeng, Y.; Lv, W.; Liu, G. Construction of carbon dots modified MoO_3/g-C_3N_4 Z-scheme photocatalyst with enhanced visible-light photocatalytic activity for the degradation of tetracycline. *Appl. Catal. B Environ.* **2018**, *229*, 96–104. [CrossRef]
61. Chen, Y.; Yin, R.; Zeng, L.; Guo, W.; Zhu, M. Insight into the effects of hydroxyl groups on the rates and pathways of tetracycline antibiotics degradation in the carbon black activated peroxydisulfate oxidation process. *J. Hazard. Mater.* **2021**, *412*, 125256. [CrossRef] [PubMed]
62. Luo, Y.; Zheng, A.; Li, J.; Han, Y.; Xue, M.; Zhang, L.; Yin, Z.; Xie, C.; Chen, Z.; Ji, L.; et al. Integrated adsorption and photodegradation of tetracycline by bismuth oxycarbonate/biochar nanocomposites. *Chem. Eng. J.* **2023**, *457*, 141228. [CrossRef]
63. Guo, J.; Jiang, L.; Liang, J.; Xu, W.; Yu, H.; Zhang, J.; Ye, S.; Xing, W.; Yuan, X. Photocatalytic degradation of tetracycline antibiotics using delafossite silver ferrite-based Z-scheme photocatalyst: Pathways and mechanism insight. *Chemosphere* **2021**, *270*, 128651. [CrossRef] [PubMed]
64. Chen, Y.-Y.; Ma, Y.-L.; Yang, J.; Wang, L.-Q.; Lv, J.-M.; Ren, C.-J. Aqueous tetracycline degradation by H_2O_2 alone: Removal and transformation pathway. *Chem. Eng. J.* **2017**, *307*, 15–23. [CrossRef]
65. Chong, Y.; Ge, C.; Fang, G.; Wu, R.; Zhang, H.; Chai, Z.; Chen, C.; Yin, J.-J. Light-Enhanced Antibacterial Activity of Graphene Oxide, Mainly via Accelerated Electron Transfer. *Environ. Sci. Technol.* **2017**, *51*, 10154–10161. [CrossRef] [PubMed]
66. Zhao, F.-F.; Wang, S.-C.; Zhu, Z.-L.; Wang, S.-G.; Liu, F.-F.; Liu, G.-Z. Effects of oxidation degree on photo-transformation and the resulting toxicity of graphene oxide in aqueous environment. *Environ. Pollut.* **2019**, *249*, 1106–1114. [CrossRef] [PubMed]
67. Qutob, M.; Rafatullah, M.; Qamar, M.; Alorfi, H.S.; Al-Romaizan, A.N.; Hussein, M.A. A review on heterogeneous oxidation of acetaminophen based on micro and nanoparticles catalyzed by different activators. *Nanotechnol. Rev.* **2022**, *11*, 497–525. [CrossRef]
68. Hou, W.-C.; BeigzadehMilani, S.; Jafvert, C.T.; Zepp, R.G. Photoreactivity of Unfunctionalized Single-Wall Carbon Nanotubes Involving Hydroxyl Radical: Chiral Dependency and Surface Coating Effect. *Environ. Sci. Technol.* **2014**, *48*, 3875–3882. [CrossRef]

69. Jiménez-Marín, E.; Moreno-Valenzuela, J.; Trejo-Valdez, M.; Martinez-Rivas, A.; Vargas-García, J.R.; Torres-Torres, C. Laser-induced electrical signal filtering by multilayer reduced graphene oxide decorated with Au nanoparticles. *Opt. Express* **2019**, *27*, 7330–7343. [CrossRef]
70. Lavin-Lopez, M.d.P.; Romero, A.; Garrido, J.; Sanchez-Silva, L.; Valverde, J.L. Influence of Different Improved Hummers Method Modifications on the Characteristics of Graphite Oxide in Order to Make a More Easily Scalable Method. *Ind. Eng. Chem. Res.* **2016**, *55*, 12836–12847. [CrossRef]
71. Adamo, C.; Barone, V. Toward reliable density functional methods without adjustable parameters: The PBE0 model. *J. Chem. Phys.* **1999**, *110*, 6158–6170. [CrossRef]
72. Weigend, F.; Ahlrichs, R. Balanced basis sets of split valence, triple zeta valence and quadruple zeta valence quality for H to Rn: Design and assessment of accuracy. *Phys. Chem. Chem. Phys.* **2005**, *7*, 3297–3305. [CrossRef] [PubMed]
73. Tian Lu, Molclus Program, Version 1.9.9.2. Available online: http://www.keinsci.com/research/molclus.html (accessed on 5 August 2024).
74. Bannwarth, C.; Caldeweyher, E.; Ehlert, S.; Hansen, A.; Pracht, P.; Seibert, J.; Spicher, S.; Grimme, S. Extended tight-binding quantum chemistry methods. *WIREs Comput. Mol. Sci.* **2021**, *11*, e1493. [CrossRef]
75. Grimme, S.; Bannwarth, C.; Shushkov, P. A Robust and Accurate tight-binding quantum chemical method for structures, vibrational frequencies, and noncovalent interactions of large molecular systems parametrized for all spd-block elements (Z = 1–86). *J. Chem. Theory Comput.* **2017**, *13*, 1989–2009. [CrossRef]
76. Bannwarth, C.; Ehlert, S.; Grimme, S. GFN2-xTB—An accurate and broadly parametrized self-consistent tight-binding quantum chemical method with multipole electrostatics and density-dependent dispersion contributions. *J. Chem. Theory Comput.* **2019**, *15*, 1652–1671. [CrossRef]

Disclaimer/Publisher's Note: The statements, opinions and data contained in all publications are solely those of the individual author(s) and contributor(s) and not of MDPI and/or the editor(s). MDPI and/or the editor(s) disclaim responsibility for any injury to people or property resulting from any ideas, methods, instructions or products referred to in the content.

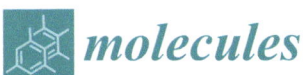

Review

Carbon Dots Derived from Non-Biomass Waste: Methods, Applications, and Future Perspectives

Wenjing Chen [1], Hong Yin [2,*], Ivan Cole [2], Shadi Houshyar [2] and Lijing Wang [1]

[1] School of Fashion and Textiles, RMIT University, Brunswick, VIC 3056, Australia; s3981322@student.rmit.edu.au (W.C.); lijing.wang@rmit.edu.au (L.W.)

[2] School of Engineering, STEM College, RMIT University, Melbourne, VIC 3000, Australia; ivan.cole@rmit.edu.au (I.C.); shadi.houshyar@rmit.edu.au (S.H.)

* Correspondence: hong.yin@rmit.edu.au

Abstract: Carbon dots (CDs) are luminescent carbon nanoparticles with significant potential in analytical sensing, biomedicine, and energy regeneration due to their remarkable optical, physical, biological, and catalytic properties. In light of the enduring ecological impact of non-biomass waste that persists in the environment, efforts have been made toward converting non-biomass waste, such as ash, waste plastics, textiles, and papers into CDs. This review introduces non-biomass waste carbon sources and classifies them in accordance with the 2022 Australian National Waste Report. The synthesis approaches, including pre-treatment methods, and the properties of the CDs derived from non-biomass waste are comprehensively discussed. Subsequently, we summarize the diverse applications of CDs from non-biomass waste in sensing, information encryption, LEDs, solar cells, and plant growth promotion. In the final section, we delve into the future challenges and perspectives of CDs derived from non-biomass waste, shedding light on the exciting possibilities in this emerging area of research.

Keywords: carbon dots; non-biomass waste; environment management; textiles; sustainability

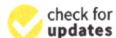

Citation: Chen, W.; Yin, H.; Cole, I.; Houshyar, S.; Wang, L. Carbon Dots Derived from Non-Biomass Waste: Methods, Applications, and Future Perspectives. *Molecules* **2024**, *29*, 2441. https://doi.org/10.3390/molecules 29112441

Academic Editor: Giuseppe Cirillo

Received: 11 April 2024
Revised: 17 May 2024
Accepted: 20 May 2024
Published: 22 May 2024

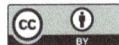

Copyright: © 2024 by the authors. Licensee MDPI, Basel, Switzerland. This article is an open access article distributed under the terms and conditions of the Creative Commons Attribution (CC BY) license (https:// creativecommons.org/licenses/by/ 4.0/).

1. Introduction

Escalating global greenhouse gas emissions pose a threat to the sustainability of our planet [1]. Waste management practices, including collection and landfill operations, account for approximately 5% of atmospheric greenhouse gas emissions [2,3]. The growing volume of waste generation presents a significant challenge in terms of responsible disposal and environmental protection. In this context, various strategies, including reducing, reusing, recycling, and recovery, have been implemented to promote resource efficiency and environmental friendliness and develop a competitive low-carbon economy [4,5]. However, a considerable portion of waste still ends up in landfills. Non-biomass wastes, such as plastics and textiles, when consigned to landfills, can cause long-term ecological impacts on the planet, as they could persist in the environment for centuries or even millennia [6–9]. The issue is further exacerbated by the bans on the export of waste materials like plastic, paper, glass, and tyres to countries where value may be added to the waste materials. Figure 1 shows waste generation and management methods categorized by material types. Notably, the highest recovery rate is for metals at 87%, closely followed by building and demolition materials at 81%. In contrast, plastics and textiles exhibit the lowest recovery rates, standing at 13% and 21%, respectively, underscoring the critical need for more effective approaches to address these persistent waste management challenges [10,11].

Carbon dots (CDs) represent a relatively recent entrant in the domain of "zero-dimensional" carbon nanoparticles, characterized by their small sizes from 1 to 10 nm. Due to their excellent optical, physical, biological, and catalytic properties, CDs have been linked to widespread interest and have found diverse applications in fields such as environmental treatment and protection, sensing, drug delivery, bioimaging, fluorescent inks, catalysis, heavy metal ion detection, and more [12–16]. CDs can be synthesized from various precursors, including waste materials. A literature search on the synthesis, properties, and applications of waste-derived CDs was conducted using keywords including waste, rubbish, trash, carbon dots, CDs, carbon quantum dots, and carbon nanodots. As shown in Table 1, there has been a predominant focus in the literature on CDs derived from natural waste, especially biomass residues [14,17–30]. Limited attention has been granted to CDs derived from non-biomass waste materials, such as plastics, sludge, wastepaper, waste kitchen chimney oil, and waste soot (e.g., kerosene fuel soot and candle soot) [14,18,20]. Considering the increasing generation of non-biomass wastes and their non-biodegradable nature, there is a need for a comprehensive review that addresses the conversion of non-biomass waste into valuable CDs. In this review, we first classify non-biomass waste sources according to the 2022 Australian *National Waste Report* (https://www.dcceew.gov.au/sites/default/files/documents/national-waste-report-2022.pdf (accessed on 23 November 2023)) and subsequently summarize the synthesis methods, characterizations, and properties of the CDs prepared from these non-biomass waste materials. This review further provides a survey of the applications of non-biomass-waste-derived CDs, such as sensing, information encryption, LEDs, solar cells, and plant growth promotion. Finally, we outline the challenges ahead and suggest avenues for future work to foster the advancement and commercialization of CDs derived from non-biomass waste.

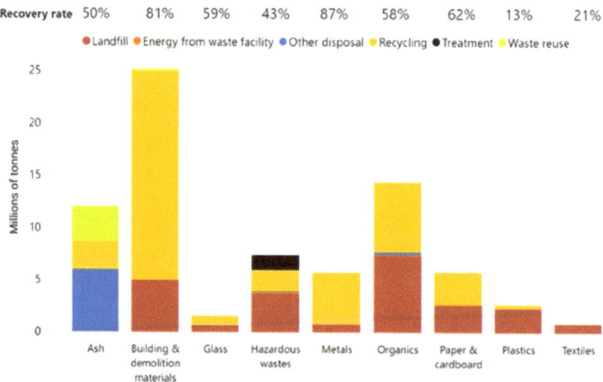

Figure 1. Waste generation and management methods categorized by material type, Australia 2020–2021 [11].

Table 1. Summary of the foci of past reviews on waste-derived CDs.

Title	Foci	Ref.
A Review of Carbon Dots Produced from Biomass Wastes	• Methods and applications of CDs from biomass waste. • Advantages and disadvantages of CDs from biomass waste. • Major influencing factors on photoluminescence characteristics.	[17]
Recent Trends in the use of Green Sources for Carbon Dot Synthesis—A short review	Synthesis of CDs from green sources including biomass waste and non-biomass waste.	[18]
A Review on Multifunctional Carbon-Dots Synthesized from Biomass Waste: Design/Fabrication, Characterization and Applications	• Methods and applications of CDs from biomass waste. • Structure analysis, physical, and chemical properties of CDs. • The factors affecting the bandgap formation mechanisms of the CDs produced by hydrothermal methods.	[19]
Carbon Quantum Dots Synthesis from Waste and By-Products: Perspectives and Challenges	Potentials, advantages, and challenges in synthesizing CDs from waste after comparing the quantum yield.	[20]

Table 1. *Cont.*

Title	Foci	Ref.
Food Waste as a Carbon Source in Carbon Quantum Dots Technology and their Applications in Food Safety Detection	• Approaches, characterizations, and applications of CDs from food wastes. • Applications on food quality and safety detection, especially on sensing food additives and heavy metal ions.	[21]
Green Carbon Dots with Multifaceted Applications—Waste to Wealth Strategy	Synthesis routes, fluorescent properties and mechanisms, and applications of CDs from wastes with a focus on hydrothermal approach.	[14]
Recent Advances of Biomass Carbon Dots on Syntheses, Characterization, Luminescence Mechanism, and Sensing Applications	• Synthesis and properties improvement methods for CDs from biomass. • Characterization of the structure, composition of biomass-derived CDs, and the regulation of fluorescence color. • Luminescence mechanism and sensing applications.	[22]
Sustainable Synthesis of Multifunctional Carbon Dots using Biomass and their Applications: A mini review	• Synthesis methods, especially hydrothermal methods, applications, and characterizations of CDs from plant sources. • Separation technologies.	[23]
Carbon Dots based on Natural Resources: Synthesis and Applications in Sensors	Synthesis of CDs from biomass resources and their sensing applications.	[24]
Biomass-Based Carbon Dots: Current Development and Future Perspectives	Advantages and disadvantages on synthesis, properties, and applications of CDs from biomass waste and chemicals.	[25]
New Insight into the Engineering of Green Carbon Dots: Possible Applications in Emerging Cancer Theragnostic	Synthesis, physicochemical properties, and possible applications of CDs from natural sources.	[26]
Green Synthesis of Carbon Quantum Dots and their Environmental Applications	• Synthesis and physicochemical properties and stability of CDs. • Applications in wastewater treatment and biomedical fields.	[27]
Sustainable Development of Carbon Nanodots Technology: Natural Products as a Carbon Source and Applications to Food Safety	• Synthesis of CDs from food and food waste. • Application of photoluminescent CDs in food safety.	[28]
Biomass-Derived Carbon Dots and Their Applications	• Simple synthesis routes and specific optical properties of CDs from biomass. • Applications in biosensing, bioimaging, optoelectronics, and catalysis.	[29]
Plastic Waste-Derived Carbon Dots: Insights of Recycling Valuable Materials Towards Environmental Sustainability	Synthesis routes, characterizations, and potential applications of CDs from plastic waste.	[30]
The Role of Fluorescent Carbon Dots in the Fate of Plastic Waste	• Approaches, properties, and applications of CDs from plastic waste. • The role of CDs in the fate of plastic waste.	[31]

2. Waste Precursors

Non-biomass waste materials include a broad spectrum, such as ash, building and demolition materials, glass, metals, organics, paper and carboard, plastics, textiles, leather, rubber, and various composite materials. Developing innovative methodologies for converting non-biomass waste to CDs has attracted increasing attention from both industry and academy [11].

In the realm of CDs, particle size and quantum yield (QY) are important factors that dictate their properties. Generally, a high fluorescent emission efficiency is associated with small particles and a narrow size distribution [32]. Fluorescence QY is a quantitative indicator of the substance's ability to emit fluorescence, defined as the ratio of emitted photons to absorbed photons [33]. The prevailing opinions attribute the emission of CDs to their surface state, carbon core state, molecule state, and their synergistic effect [34–37]. Unlike semiconductor quantum dots, the emission wavelength of CDs cannot be tuned by controlling their particle size alone. In contrast, various factors, such as heteroatom doping, solvatochromic effect, concentration-dependent effect, and surface functionalization, all contribute to the optical properties of CDs [38]. A wide range of waste precursors and different synthetic procedures (e.g., hydrothermal, microwave, refluxing, and pyrolysis) result in a wide size distribution in the CD product. Due to the unknown composition of the waste precursors, the prepared CDs are also accompanied by unreacted impurities or by-products that interfere with their pristine emission properties. Therefore, conventional CDs derived from waste normally show a wide emission wavelength with a full width at half-maximum of more than 100 nm [39–42]. In this literature review, a systematic search method was employed to gather existing research on CDs derived from non-biomass waste, focusing on their precursor materials (including ash [32,39,42–55], waste plastics [40,56–78], wastepaper [79–83], waste textiles [84–89], cigarette filters [90], sewage sludge [41,91], and engine oil) [92]. As shown in Figure 2, 55 relevant articles met our rigorous inclusion criteria. There are 24 and 16 articles on waste plastic- and ash-derived CDs, accounting for 44% and 29% of the total publications, respectively. Additionally, the numbers of research articles on CDs from waste textiles and wastepaper are six and five, respectively.

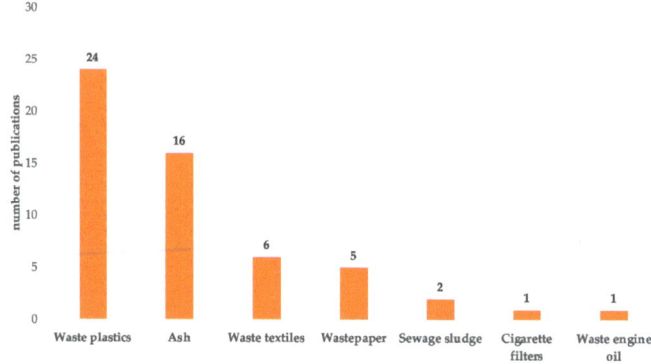

Figure 2. Published papers (up to the end of 2023) on the CDs derived from non-biomass waste based on their precursor materials.

2.1. Ash

Ash is a residual by-product of coal-fired power generation [11], and ash waste has surged due to population growth and economic development. Traditional methods of managing coal ash waste are dry storage and wet disposal. Recently, resource recovery has offered a more sustainable alternative with significant environmental, social, and economic benefits, thus attracting considerable attention [93]. The composition of ash waste depends on the source material being burned, such as coal and plants, while the main chemical constituent in ash is carbon [94]. Various types of CDs have been extensively reported, including those derived from candle soot, cigarettes, oil fly ash, diesel soot, and toner powder, from 2011 to 2023 [32,39,42–55]. Table 2 lists the comprehensive details of the CDs derived from ash waste, including the methods utilized, particle sizes, and QY.

The ball milling technique is a typical top-down method to fabricate nanomaterials and has been widely used to generate carbon nanoparticles (CNPs) from ash waste. CNPs produced via ball milling generally exhibit large sizes. CNPs with cluster sizes ranging from 22.3 nm to 35 nm were successfully synthesized from oil fly ash by ball milling in a dry medium, followed by sonication in liquid media containing deionized water and nitric acid. In another instance, CNPs with sizes less than 100 nm were synthesized from oil fly ash, using high-energy ball milling in an acetic acid medium [43,44]. In contrast, certain direct burning methods have produced significantly smaller CDs. For example, CDs within a size range of 4.5 to 7.0 nm were derived from cigarette smoke, while even smaller-sized CDs with narrower size distribution (2.0–4.0 nm) were obtained from burning of flammable organic materials, such as ethanol, n-butanol, domestic candle, and benzene [32,50].

Table 2. CDs prepared from waste ash and coal and their corresponding properties.

Method	Carbon Precursor	Conditions	Size (nm)	QY (%)	Ref.
Ball Milling	Oil fly ash	25 Hz and 400 rpm for 45 h in the air	<35	NA	[43]
	Oil fly ash	25 Hz for 45 h in acetic acid	<100	NA	[44]
Burn	Cigarette Smoking	In the air	4.5–7.0	NA	[50]
	Ethanol, n-Butanol, Domestic candle, and Benzene	In the air	2.0–4.0	NA	[32]
Chemical Oxidation	Pollutant diesel soot	10 h	20–50	1.9	[42]
	Vehicle exhaust waste soot	100 °C for 12 h	2.2–4.6	3	[51]
	Candle soot	140 °C for 12 h	112	0.5	[53]
	Waste candle soot	110 °C for 6 h	2.0–5.0	NA	[46]
	Fullerene carbon soot	80–120 °C for 12–36 h	2.0–3.0	3–5	[54]
	Kerosene fuel soot	100 °C for 12 h	1.0–7.0	NA	[52]
	Candle soot	80 °C for 6 h	2.0–5.0	NA	[49]
	Candles	20 h	10–45	NA	[48]
	Coal-T20	Ice-cold condition for 6 h	2.0–5.0	3	[95]
	Coal-NK	Ice-cold condition for 6 h	10–30	4	[95]
	Coal-T60	Ice-cold condition for 6 h	1.0–6.0	8	[95]
	Coal-NG	Ice-cold condition for 6 h	1.0–4.0	14	[95]
	Gondwana coal, Damodar Coal, Tertiary Indian coal	2 h	4.8–14.0	NA	[96]
	Pennsylvania anthracite, and Kentucky bituminous coals	Ice-cold condition for 5–6 h	2.0–12.0	4–53	[97]
Soxhlet-Purification	Diesel soot	In acetone	20–30	~8	[39]
Hydrothermal Method	Bike Pollutant Soot	160 °C for 10 h	1–10	NA	[45]
Microwave pyrolysis	Red toner powder	350 W for 30 s	1–4	9.2 for internal and 8.4 for external efficiency	[55]

Chemical oxidation is another method to prepare CDs from ash. CDs with a size of 2–3 nm and a high QY of 3–5% were synthesized using fullerene carbon soot through a nitric acid refluxing approach [54]. Coals from the northeastern coalfield (Cenozoic age) in India, including Coal-NK, Coal-NG, Coal-T60, and Coal-T20, were used in a wet-chemical ultrasonic stimulation process to produce CDs with different sizes (1–4 nm, 1–6 nm, 2–5 nm, and 10–30 nm) and QY values ranging from 3 to 14%. This method stands out for its environmental friendliness and cost-effective coal feedstocks [95].

Microwave pyrolysis has emerged as a predominant method for CDs synthesis owing to its high efficiency, energy conservation, and straightforward equipment operation [98–100]. In a recent publication, CDs with an average size of 2.1 nm were derived from waste toner powder via microwave pyrolysis in an ethanol solvent. These CDs demonstrated a yellow emission at 557 nm upon excitation at 300 nm, holding promises for potential LED applications [55].

Emissions from vehicles have a detrimental impact on the global environment and accelerate climate change [101–103]. To address these issues, numerous policies, legislation, and enforcement strategies were developed to control exhaust emissions from vehicles [104,105]. Recent research by Chaudhary et al. (2022) showed that CDs with just 2 nm in size could be prepared using bike pollutant soot and distilled water through a hydrothermal process [45]. Additionally, Soxhlet-purification was effectively employed to transform harmful diesel soot into larger CDs with an average size of 20–30 nm and a QY of ~8% [39].

2.2. Waste Plastics

Plastics play a critical role in the global economy but create increasing environmental concerns due to non-biodegradability and recycling difficulties [106–108]. It is estimated that a staggering 87% of plastic waste ends up in landfills [11]. Since polymers generally contain abundant carbon chains, repurposing plastics into CDs presents an efficient strategy to transform waste into a valuable resource. The plastic resources used for CD synthesis from 2018 to 2023 are summarized in Figure 3a [40,56–78]. Table 3 lists the main approaches for synthesizing CDs from waste plastics, including the hydrothermal and pyrolysis method. The pyrolysis approach is a common chemical method to convert plastic waste into carbon materials at elevated temperatures. In contrast, the hydrothermal approach is the most widely used method for CD synthesis from plastics due to its lower operating temperature, high yield, ability to obtain CDs with a small size, and narrow size distribution [109,110].

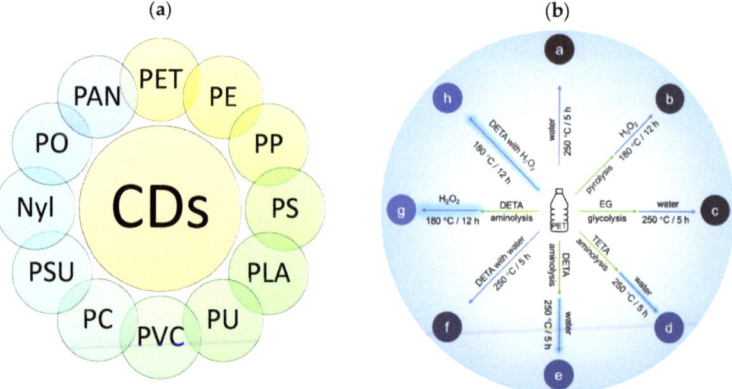

Figure 3. (a) Resources to fabricate CDs from plastics during 2018–2023 [40,56–78], Note: PET: polyester, PE: polyethylene, PP: polypropylene, PS: polystyrene, PLA: polylactide, PU: polyurethane, PVC: polyvinylchloride, PC: polycarbonate, PSU: polysulfone, Nyl: nylon, PO: polyolefins, and PAN: polyacrylonitrile. (b) CDs from PET via Various Conversion Routes [56]. Reproduced with permission from Elsevier.

Compared with ashes, waste plastics tend to generate CDs with higher QYs. The main composition of ashes is carbon, with multiple elements, including calcium, magnesium, aluminum, and silicon in their oxide forms [111]. These materials have been subjected to a high temperature calcination and remained stable in these conditions. In contrast, the carbonaceous backbones in plastic wastes are more susceptible to hydrolysis, ring opening, and crosslinking reactions involved in CD synthesis. As a result, various compounds with different types of polar functional groups are produced, leading to a high QY [37,112]. Kumari et al. (2020) fabricated CDs from single-use plastic waste, including plastic bags, cups, and bottles made up of polyethylene, polypropylene, and PET based polymers, respectively [67]. The waste was first heated at 300 °C for 2 h. Afterwards, the calcinated samples were added into 15 mL of deionized water and subjected to hydrothermal treatment at 200 °C for 5 h. The fluorescence QY values for CDs ranged from 60% to 69%, and the CDs prepared from PET-based waste bottles demonstrated the highest QY [67]. As shown in Table 3, most high QY values were obtained from waste PET bottles. It could be related to its carbonaceous backbone with abundant oxygen-containing functional groups that facilitate hydrolysis, condensation, and later carbonization [113]. Research conducted by Wang et al. (2023) converted PET waste bottles into CDs using a direct hydrothermal ammonolysis approach, resulting in CDs with an average size of 2 nm and an impressive QY of 87.36% [54]. In this process, ammonium hydroxide and pyromellitic acid were used as precursors together with PET. The as-prepared PET-CDs were not only successfully doped with nitrogen in the form of pyrrole N structures but also covered with -NH_2 and -COOH groups on the surface [54]. All these factors act collectively, contributing to their extremely high QY.

Table 3. CDs prepared from waste plastics and their corresponding properties.

Method	Carbon Precursor	Conditions	QY (%)	Size (nm)	Ref.
Hydrothermal approach	Waste PET bottles	180 °C for 12 h in diethylenetriamine (DETA) with H_2O_2	9.1	3.9–12.9	[56]
	Waste PET bottles	260 °C for 12 h in ammonia water	87.36	1.1–3.1	[57]
	Waste PET bottles	260 °C for 36 h	48.16	1.6–2.9	[58]
	PLA polymeric waste	240 °C for 4 h in ultrapure water	NA	2.99 ± 0.57	[59]
	PS plastics	180 °C for 8 h with HNO_3 and ethylenediamine	NA	2.66–5.18	[61]
	Waste PET bottles	110 °C for 15 h in H_2O_2	NA	1.3–4.0	[62]
	PE plastic bags PP surgical masks	180 °C for 12 h in HNO_3	14 16	1.0–8.0	[63]
	Waste PET bottles	200 °C for 8 h in deionized water	31.81	3.0–10.0	[65]
	Plastic polybags Cups Bottles	300 °C for 2 h of thermal calcination and 200 °C for 5 h of hydrothermal treatment in deionized water	60–69	NA	[67]
	Waste PET bottles	350 °C for 2 h in air and hydrothermal treatment at 180 °C for 12 h in H_2O_2 solution.	5.2	3.0–10.0	[68]
	Waste expanded PS Foam	200 °C for 5 h in HNO_3	W-CDs *: 5.2, Y-CDs *: 3.4% O-CDs *: 3.1%	W-CDs *: 4.5, Y-CDs *: 3.5, O-CDs *: 2.3	[69]
	Waste medical masks	200 °C for 10 h in deionized water	NA	1.0–6.0	[71]
	Waste polyolefins	120 °C for 12 h in HNO_3 and H_2SO_4	4.84	1.5–3.5	[72]
	Waste PET bottles	180 °C for 12 h in H_2O_2	5.2	3.0–10.0	[76]
	Waste PET bottles	260 °C for 24 h	14.2	1.8–4.6	[77]
Pyrolysis method	Waste plastic cups	350 °C for 2 h	59	<10	[66]
	Waste PET bottles	800 °C for 1h	NA	2000–8000	[40]
	PU foam	200, 250, and 300 °C for 2, 4, and 6 h	33	5.0–8.0	[74]
	HDPE/LDPE, PET, PS, PVC, PP	800 °C for 1 h	NA	NA	[75]

* Note: W-CD: white CDs; Y-CD: yellow CDs; O-CD: orange CDs; PET: polyester; PLA: polylactide; PS: polystyrene; PE: polyethylene; PP: polypropylene; PU: polyurethane; HDPE: High-Density Polyethylene; LDPE: Low-Density Polyethylene; PVC: polyvinylchloride; NA: not available.

Unlike ash waste, which naturally exists in a powdered form to be used for CD synthesis, plastic wastes generally need additional pre-treatment processes to convert their different morphologies into powders suitable for the subsequent reactions. The pre-treatment methods include grinding, alcoholysis, hydrolytic degradation, aminolysis, pyrolysis, thermal treatment, and more [56,58,59]. Some studies have reported the pyrolysis of plastics at a high temperature of 300–400 °C for about 2 h, either in an oven or a microwave, before a hydrothermal process [60,62,65,67,68,72,76]. Chan et al. (2022) used various pre-treatment routes for PET, including pyrolysis, glycolysis, and aminolysis with or without an oxidizing agent (Figure 3b) [56]. The fluorescence properties of CDs derived from waste PET showed that direct hydrothermal synthesis of PET or a combination of pyrolysis or glycolysis pre-treatment resulted in non-fluorescent or weak fluorescent products. Whereas the aminolysis of PET bottle plastics followed by hydrothermal synthesis led to a dramatic increase in fluorescence (ten to one hundred times higher than the original). Adding a small amount of oxidant (H_2O_2) to the hydrothermal mixture achieved a conversion yield of 25.3% and a QY of 9.1%.

2.3. Waste Textiles and Wastepaper

As shown in Figure 4, the primary sources of fibers in global textile production include synthetic fibers (polyester, polyamide, and PP), manmade cellulose fibers (like viscose and acetate), plant-based fibers (including cotton), and animal fibers (such as wool and silk) [114]. Wastepaper comes from newsprint, magazine, printing and writing papers, and packaging papers. Cellulose is the main chemical component of cotton and paper for synthesizing CDs. Table 4 summarizes the methods, sizes, and QY of CDs prepared from waste textiles, wastepaper, and cellulose.

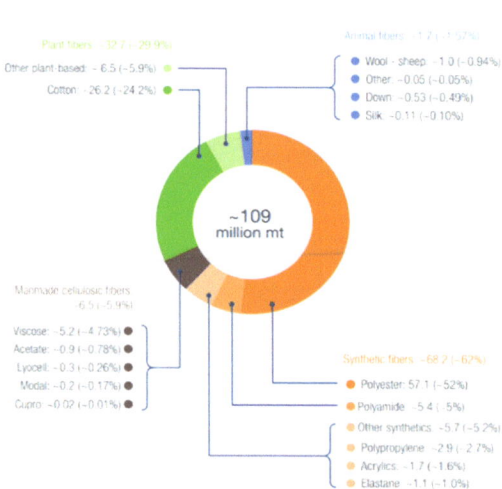

Figure 4. Global fiber productions in 2020 [114].

Among synthetic fibers, PET is a prominent waste material and has been widely used for CD synthesis. Using a pre-treatment step combined with a hydrothermal process, CDs with smaller size and higher QY were obtained from waste PET. CDs derived from terylene waste were successfully generated using a hydrothermal method (at 260 °C for 18 h), resulting in particles with sizes of 2.5–7.0 nm and a QY of 49.36% [87]. Wang et al. (2022) synthesized CDs with sizes ranging from 1.6 to 4.6 nm and a high QY of 97.30% from PET textiles [85]. The method involves the initial synthesis of PET oligomer from PET fibers in a microwave reactor, followed by a hydrothermal reaction (at 260 °C for 24 h) of PET oligomer.

Silk, a natural biomaterial with rich nitrogen, is widely used to produce carbon materials [115,116]. CDs with nitrogen doping attracted attention because of their improved optical and electrical properties [117]. Waste silk cloth has been utilized as a carbon source to prepare CDs in an acid solution using a hydrothermal method (at 250 °C for 5 h), resulting in CDs with sizes ranging from 2.2 to 6.1 nm and a QY of 19.1% [88].

Table 4 illustrates that the hydrothermal method is the most widely reported to prepare CDs from waste cotton and wastepaper. The CDs derived from wastepaper (4.5 nm) had similar particle sizes to those derived from cellulose (4.2 nm) via a hydrothermal process at 180 °C. However, their QY shows a significant difference, standing at 10.8% and 21.7%, respectively. Burning is another method of making CDs from wastepaper. Water-soluble fluorescent CDs with a QY of 9.3% and a size distribution of 2–5 nm were obtained by simply incinerating wastepaper [80].

Table 4. CDs prepared from waste textiles and wastepaper and their corresponding properties.

Method	Carbon Precursor	Conditions	QY (%)	Size (nm)	Ref.
Hydrothermal method	Wastepaper	150–200 °C for 10 h	10.80	150 °C: 4.0–12.0 180 °C: 3.0–7.0 200 °C: 2.0–5.0	[79]
	Kraft softwood pulp	240 °C for 4 h	NA	Diameter: 2–6 Length: 40–60	[118]
	Carbon paper	180 °C for 8 h	~5.1	4.8	[81]
	Wastepaper	210 °C for 12 h	10–27	2.6 to 4.4	[82]
	Wastepaper	220 °C for 15 h	20	2–4	[83]
	Degrease cotton (Human waste)	200 °C for 13 h	10.20	2–4	[84]
	Waste PET textiles	260 °C for 24 h	97.30	1.6–4.6	[85]
	Absorbent cotton	200 °C for 15 h	NA	1.4–5.6	[86]
	Terylene waste	260 °C for 18 h	49.36	2.5–7.0	[87]
	Waste silk cloth	250 °C for 5 h	19.10	2.2 ± 6.1	[88]
	Eucalyptus fibers	120 °C, 140 °C, 160 °C, and 180 °C for 24 h	NA	1.5–4.0	[89]
	Cellulose	180 °C for 72 h	21.7	4.2	[119]
	Cellulose	210 °C for 14 h	32.3	5.45	[120]
	Cellulose	200 °C for 12 h	2.9–18.3	2.11–8.72	[121]
	Microcrystalline Cellulose	240 °C for 12 h	54	0.5–6.5	[122]
Burn	Wastepaper	Burn	9.3	2–5	[80]

Note: NCC/CDs: nanocrystalline cellulose/carbon dots.

Similar to waste plastics, textiles and paper are solid waste materials and require pre-treatment prior to the preparation of CDs. Chemical pre-treatments can remove impurities from waste textiles. For example, waste PET fibers were converted to PET oligomers through glycolysis pre-treatment using ethylene glycol and zinc acetate dehydrates and subsequent microwave reactions. The resulting CDs have high QYs of 49.36% and 97.30%, with relatively small average sizes of 4.3 nm and 2.8 nm, respectively [85,87]. Various chemical methods have been reported to remove lignin from eucalyptus fibers, obtaining a refined cellulose fraction. This process often involves four sequential heat treatments with acetic acid and sodium chloride to remove lignin, followed by heating in the presence of potassium oxychloride to eliminate hemicellulose. The obtained N-CDs had an average size of 2.46 nm [89]. The high QY generated from PET-based waste was also confirmed in Table 4, where PET textiles were used as the precursor, and the QY could reach 97.3%. PET-CDs were prepared using a hydrothermal method with urea and homophthalic acid as co-precursors. The obtained CDs were not only successfully doped with nitrogen in the form of pyrrole N structures but also covered with -NH$_2$ and abundant oxygen-containing functional groups [85].

Doping heteroatoms into CDs is an effective way to enhance QY. The most common doping element is nitrogen, which is generally introduced using N-containing small molecules, such as p-phenylenediamine, urea, ethylenediamine, and ammonia water as co-precursors [112,123–125]. Sulphur and phosphorus have also been co-doped with nitrogen by adding concentrated phosphoric and sulphuric acids, respectively [126–129]. These non-waste precursors help promote the hydrolysis and carbonization reactions and introduce heteroatom doping and surface functional groups, aiming to enhance the QY and induce specific interactions with analytes for sensing applications.

2.4. Other Wastes

Recently, sewage sludge [41], cigarette filters [90], and waste engine oil [92] have emerged as novel CD precursors. The pre-treatment approaches for converting these wastes into CDs depend on the composition of the materials. As urbanization continues, the volume of urban sludge composed of carbon-based substances increases rapidly. The untreated and inadequately treated sewage poses a significant threat to human life [130–132]. Sewage management technologies include various methods, such as landfill disposal, land spreading, anaerobic digestion, thermochemical processes, and integration into building materials [91,133]. Hu et al. reported the conversion of sewage sludge into useful CDs. This process involves pre-treatment through drying and grounding, followed by microwave irradiation. The resulting CDs had an average size of 4.0 nm with a high QY of 21.7% and could be used for fluorescent sensing applications, particularly for para-nitrophenol detection [41]. Waste engine oil was transformed into CDs using a direct hydrothermal method (220 °C for 12 h). The CDs showed a high QY of 11.4% and a size distribution of 2–10 nm with excellent detection selectivity and sensitivity towards Fe^{3+} (Figure 5) [92].

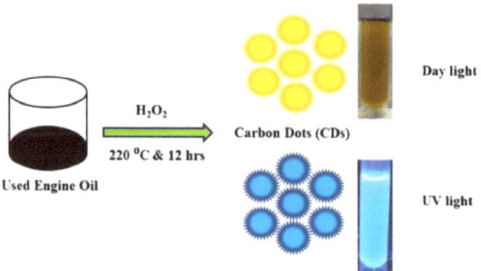

Figure 5. Waste-engine-oil-derived CDs. Reused with permission [92]. Copyright 2022 Elsevier.

3. Applications of CDs Derived from Non-Biomass Waste

CDs derived from non-biomass waste have similar favorable properties, such as low toxicity, biocompatibility, high photostability, and fluorescence. These waste-derived CDs find applications in sensing, information encryption, LEDs, solar cells, and growth promotion.

3.1. Sensing

Table 5 summarizes the pre-treatment methods, synthesis techniques, and the corresponding sensing performance of reported CDs derived from non-biomass waste sources. The most common method to prepare CDs for sensing applications is the hydrothermal method, conducted at temperatures from 120 °C to 260 °C. Prior to this, the waste was subjected to various pre-treatment processes, such as purifying, grinding, sieving, drying, nitration, pyrolysis, oxidation, and microwave alcoholysis. CDs derived from non-biomass waste have been primarily utilized for the detection of heavy metal ions, followed by small molecules, pH, and bacteria. In Table 5, the fluorescence properties of CDs were used for almost all sensors, and one exception is that the impedance response of CDs derived from bike pollutant soot was used to detect relative humidity [41]. The fluorescence sensing behavior is dominated by turn-off detection, which involves the intensity quenching upon interacting with the analytes. The quenching mechanisms include static or dynamic quenching. In static quenching, a non-emissive complex is formed between the CDs and the analyte, causing a previously emissive state to return to the ground state without an emission. Dynamic quenching, often referred to as collisional quenching, occurs because of the collisions or close contact between the analyte and the excited CDs, which result in an energy transfer without an emission. Dynamic quenching includes several mechanisms, such as photo-induced electron transfer, Förster resonance energy transfer, surface energy transfer, and inner filter effect (IFE) [134].

Table 5. Sensing applications of CDs derived from non-biomass waste.

Carbon Precursor	Pre-Treatment	Method	Analyte	Limits of Detection (LOD)	Linear Range	Ref.
Harmful diesel soot	Magnetically purified	Soxhlet-purification with acetone	Fe^{3+} and Hg^{2+}	Fe^{3+}: ~352 nM Hg^{2+}: ~898 nM	NA	[39]
Candle soot	HNO_3 and ethanol treatment	Stirring at 80 °C for 6 h with ethylene diamine and sodium lauryl sulphate (SDS)	Hg^{2+} and Fe^{3+}	Fe^{3+}: 10 nM Hg^{2+}: 50 nM	Fe^{3+}: 20–50 μM Hg^{2+}: 20–50 μM	[49]
PS plastics	Nitration	Solvothermal treatment at 180 °C for 8 h	Hg^{2+}, Fe^{3+}, and GSH	NA	Fe^{3+}: 0.25–10 μM Hg^{2+}: 0.5–20 μM GSH: 1–50 μM	[61]
Waste medical masks	NA	Hydrothermal treatment at 200 °C for 10 h	$Na_2S_2O_4$ and Fe^{3+}	$Na_2S_2O_4$: 19.44 μM Fe^{3+}: 0.11 μM	$Na_2S_2O_4$: 0.1–5 mM Fe^{3+}: 1–300 μM	[71]
Waste engine oil	Filtration process by filter paper	Hydrothermal treatment at 200 °C for 12 h	Fe^{3+}	0.055 μM	0.6–3.3 μM	[92]
Waste PET bottles	Pyrolysis at 350 °C for 2 h in air	Hydrothermal treatment at 180 °C for 12 h	Fe^{3+} and pyrophosphate ions	Fe^{3+}: 0.21 μM pyrophosphate: 0.86 μM	Fe^{3+}: 0.5–400 μM pyrophosphate: 2–600 μM	[76]
Waste PET bottles	Shredding and air oxidation at 350 °C for 2 h.	Hydrothermal treatment at 170 °C for 8 h	Pb^{2+}	21 nM	0–2 μM	[68]
Waste expanded PS	NA	One-step solvothermal method at 150 °C for 8 h	Au^{3+}	53 nM	0–18 μM	[70]
White PU foam	Crushed	Pyrolysis at 200, 250, and 300 °C for 2, 4, and 6 h in H_2SO_4	Ag^+	2.8 μM	NA	[74]
Waste PO	Pyrolysis by ultrasonic and chemical oxidation approach at 700 W for 2 h.	Hydrothermal method at 120 °C for 12 h	Cu^{2+}	6.33 nM	1–8.0 μM	[72]
Degrease cotton	NA	One-pot hydrothermal method at 200 °C for 13 h	Cr^{4+}	0.12 μg/mL	1–6 mmol/L	[84]
Waste plastic cups	NA	Simple thermal calcination at 350 °C for 2 h	Sulphite anion	0.34 μM	0.001–50 μm	[66]
Sewage sludge	Dried and grounded into fine powder	Microwave-assisted heating with 700 W for 30 min.	Para-Nitrophenol	0.069 μM	0.2–20 μM	[41]
Cigarette filters	Cut and dried in an oven at 80 °C for 1 h	One-pot hydrothermal method at 240 °C for 15 h	Tetracycline	0.06 μM	0–80 μM	[90]

Table 5. *Cont.*

Carbon Precursor	Pre-Treatment	Method	Analyte	Limits of Detection (LOD)	Linear Range	Ref.
Carbon paper	Burn	Hydrothermal route at 180 °C for 8 h	Trinitrotoluene	32.7 nM	4.4 nM–26.4 μM	[81]
Vehicle exhaust waste soot	NA	One-pot acid reflexion method with nitric acid at 100 °C for 12 h	Tartrazine	26 nM	0.1 to 0.5 μM	[51]
Wastepaper	NA	Hydrothermal method at 220 °C for 15 h	Organophosphorus pesticides	3 ng/mL	0.01–1.0 μg/mL	[83]
PET waste bottles	Microwave alcoholysis with 540 W for 20 min followed by crushing into powder	Solvothermal method at 260 °C for 36 h	Water in organic solvent	0.00001%	NA	[58]
Pollutant diesel soot	Purified via Soxhlet extraction method with different organic solvents	Chemical oxidation method refluxed 10 h	Cholesterol and *E. coli*	NA	NA	[42]
Single-use plastic waste such as plastic polybags, cups, and bottles	Calcination at 300 °C for 2 h.	Hydrothermal treatment at 200 °C for 5 h,	*E. coli*	108 CFU/mL	NA	[67]
Waste PET bottles	Microwave alcoholysis with 540 W for 20 min followed by crashing into powder	Solvothermal method at 260 °C for 24 h	pH	NA	NA	[77]
Bike pollutant soot	Ground for 1 h and sieved using 15 mm sieving paper	Hydrothermal treatment at 160 °C for 10 h	Humidity	NA	NA	[45]

Note: NA: not available.

Heavy metals, such as Fe^{3+}, Hg^{2+}, Cu^{2+}, Cr^{4+}, and Au^{3+}, can accumulate in the ecosystems, causing harmful effects on the environment and living organisms [135]. CDs derived from various non-biomass waste categories using the hydrothermal method have been reported for highly selective and sensitive heavy metal sensing. For example, CDs prepared from medical masks, waste engine oil, and waste PET were utilized for Fe^{3+} quantitation with linear ranges of 1–300 μM, 0.5–400 μM, and 0.6–3.3 μM and limits of detections (LODs) of 0.11 μM, 0.21 μM, and 0.055 μM, respectively. The average size of CDs ranged from 3.7 nm to 6 nm. CDs with average sizes from 2.5 nm to 6 nm, derived from PET, polyolefin, and cotton using the hydrothermal approach, have enabled sensitive and selective detections of Pb^{2+}, Cu^{2+}, and Cr^{4+} with LODs of 21 nM, 6.33 nM, and 0.12 μg/mL, respectively. The hydroxyl and carboxyl groups on the surface of the CDs interact with heavy metal ions, resulting in static or IFE fluorescence quenching [71,75,83,92]. Doping with nitrogen is a common strategy to enhance the fluorescent properties and increase quenching probabilities of CDs because of the presence of functional groups such as amine, hydroxyl, carbonyl, nitryl, and alkene [49,117]. Additionally, N-CDs derived from candle soot have an average size between 2 nm to 5 nm and have been used for quantifying Fe^{3+} and Hg^{2+} in water with a similar linear range of 20–50 μM. The LODs for Fe^{3+} and Hg^{2+} are 10 nM and 50 nM, respectively. The fluorescence generated by electron transfer of N-CDs is captured by empty 'd' orbital of Fe^{3+} and Hg^{2+}, leading to a PET quenching mechanism [49]. N-CDs with a QY of 20% and an average size of 4.0 ± 1.2 nm were synthesized from waste-expanded polystyrene (EPS) using the one-step solvothermal method, exhibiting selectivity for Au^{3+} quantitation with an LOD of 53 nM [70]. PU, rich in nitrogen atoms, is an ideal candidate for synthesizing highly photoluminescent CDs with enhanced QYs. N-CDs derived from waste white PU foam had diameters ranging from

5 nm to 8 nm and a relatively high QY of 33%. The CDs could detect Ag^+ with an LOD of 2.8 µM. The quenching effect is attributed to static quenching due to a strong interaction between the S-doped surface of CDs and Ag^+ [73].

In addition to heavy metals, CDs from non-biomass sources have been employed to detect small molecules, such as para-nitrophenol [41], tetracycline [90], trinitrotoluene [81], tartrazine [51], pesticides [83], water in organic solvent [45,58], and cholesterol [42]. The CDs prepared from PET waste showed a highly selective and sensitive detection of ferric ion (Fe^{3+}) through a quenching effect, and the fluorescence could be restored specifically with pyrophosphate anion (PPi), rendering the CDs/Fe^{3+} sensor promising for PPi detection [75]. The static quenching mechanism of CDs was caused by Fe^{3+} due to the formation of nonfluorescent CD-Fe^{3+} complexes. Compared with CDs, PPi possessed a stronger affinity toward Fe^{3+} to generate PPi-Fe^{3+} complexes, thus releasing CDs and recovering the fluorescence. Similarly, the burning ash of the wastepaper was used as a carbon source to synthesize CDs. The fluorescence of obtained CDs could be turned off by Fe^{3+}, which was derived from Fe^{2+} oxidized by H_2O_2. Organophosphorus pesticides effectively inhibited the production of H_2O_2 by destroying the acetylcholinesterase activity, so the fluorescence of CDs was turned on in the presence of organophosphorus pesticides [82]. N-CDs synthesized from carbon paper and waste PET derived using solvothermal methods have small average sizes of 4.8 nm and 1.93 nm, respectively. They have been used for the quantitation of tetracycline and trinitrotoluene in both water and in organic solvents. Furthermore, CDs were prepared from single-use plastic waste, such as plastic polybags, cups, and bottles, via a hydrothermal method (at 200 °C for 5 h) with high QY of 60%, 65%, and 69%, respectively. They demonstrated the ability to effectively sense *E. coli* with an LOD of 108 CFU/mL [67]. Empty PET bottles were pre-treated using a microwave reactor, followed by crushing into powder using a pulverizer. Nitrogen- and phosphorus-doped CDs with spherical structures and an average particle size of 2.8 nm have been applied for pH sensing in the range of 2.3 to 12.3 [77].

3.2. Information Encryption

CDs are considered one of the most promising candidates for information encryption due to their polychromatic emission, a wide array of luminous categories, and stable physicochemical properties [136]. These versatile materials have been successfully synthetized from wastepaper using various solvents, such as deionized water, ethanol, and 2-propanol, using a hydrothermal method at 210 °C. The obtained CDs with average sizes from 2.6 nm to 4.4 nm and QYs of 12%, 27%, and 10% showed emission colors spanning from blue to yellow and have found applications as anti-counterfeiting ink for fluorescent flexible films [82].

3.3. LEDs

LEDs, as solid-state devices, have a crucial role in relieving the energy crisis. CDs have made significant contributions to recent advancements in LEDs because of their excellent photoluminescence and high stability [137]. Table 6 summarizes the LED applications of CDs derived from non-biomass wastes. CDs prepared from waste PET, non-degradable products and waste EPS prepared using solvothermal approaches could have multiple colors with particle sizes from 2.0 nm to 4.5 nm. Waste-PET-derived CDs also exhibited a range of colors, including colorless, white, yellow, blue–green, and brown [57,58,69,77,85]. Biohazardous products, such as PPE plastic waste, used disposable gloves, face shields, syringes, and food storage containers and bottles, were utilized to prepare CDs using a pyrolytic method. The resulting N-CDs emitted white light and possessed a high QY of 41% [73]. Furthermore, CDs with an average size of 2.1 nm were derived from waste toner powder via microwave irradiation. These CDs emitted yellow light at 557 nm under 300 nm excitation and had been used in LEDs [55].

Table 6. LED applications of CDs derived from non-biomass waste.

Carbon Precursor	Method	Emission Peak (nm)	Light Color	Size (nm)	QY (%)	Ref.
Waste PET bottles	Hydrothermal	485	Colorless to brown	2.0	87.36	[57]
Waste PET bottles	Solvothermal	360 470	Yellow light warm light	2.3	48.16	[58]
Waste expanded PS	Solvothermal	470 530 630	White Yellow Orange	4.5 3.5 2.3	5.2 3.4 3.1	[69]
PPE plastic waste, used disposable gloves, face shields, syringes, and food storage containers and bottles	Pyrolytic	436 495	White light	NA	41	[73]
Waste PET bottles	Solvothermal	460	White light	2.8	14.2	[77]
Waste PET textiles	Hydrothermal	485	Blue-green light	2.8	97.3	[85]
Wasted toner powder	Microwave irradiation	557	Yellow light	2.1	9.2 for internal and 8.4 for external efficiency	[55]

3.4. Solar Cells

Solar energy conversion is pivotal in addressing climate change [138]. The transformation of non-biomass waste into CDs can reduce pollution, and their subsequent utilization in solar energy conversion holds the potential to yield substantial societal, economic, and environmental benefits. A series of CDs have been successfully synthesized from absorbent cotton using a one-pot hydrothermal method. By introducing different dopants, such as carbamide, thiourea, and 1,3-diaminopropane, the average particle sizes were significantly reduced from 24.2 nm to 1.7 nm, 5.6 nm, and 1.4 nm, respectively. The 1,3-diaminopropane-doped CDs showed the highest power conversion efficiency (PCE) of 0.527%, which was 299% higher than that achieved without dopant (0.176%) [86].

3.5. Plant Growth Promotion

CDs, as a new type of carbon material have demonstrated their potential to boost plant growth [139,140]. For instance, PET was thermally treated at 400 °C for 2 h and crushed into a fine powder using ball milling, followed by a subsequent hydrothermal process (110 °C for 15 h) in the presence of H_2O_2 solution. When applied at concentrations of 0.25 mg/mL to 2 mg/mL, these CDs with an average size of 2.5 ± 0.5 nm could enhance the development of shoots and roots during germination and growth of pea (*Pisum sativum*). It is believed that the interaction between CDs and pea seeds promotes growth [62]. Similarly, CDs prepared from various plastic products via direct thermal treatment at high temperatures (800 °C for 1 h) promoted the growth of C. arietinum seeds within the concentration range of 0.1 mg/mL to 0.5 mg/mL [40]. However, the specific mechanism remains unclear. Furthermore, carbon nanomaterials with sizes ranging from 20 nm to 100 nm were synthesized from oil fly ash using a high-energy ball milling method. These CDs had been used in the treatment of *Phaseolus vulgaris* L. and *Cicer arietinum* L. plants [43].

4. Conclusions

The rising concerns about air and water pollution, land degradation, and the economic cost associated with increasing waste have garnered significant social concerns. An effective approach to address these issues is to convert waste into CDs for high-end applications. Considering that CDs derived from biomass waste have been widely reported, this review focuses on non-biomass waste, especially the related preparation methods, properties, and applications. Selecting the most suitable methods for synthesizing CDs from non-biomass waste requires careful consideration of the properties of the waste materials. Compared to CDs derived from chemicals, the complexity of the raw material composition presents a significant challenge. Pre-treatments, which may involve physical and chemical methods, are often essential to remove impurities and convert solid waste into powder forms suitable for CDs synthesis. However, the complexity of these procedures, the use of highly toxic chemicals, and the requirement for high temperatures and pressure may limit the applicability of these methods. CDs obtained from non-biomass waste have found applications in sensing, information encryption, LEDs, solar cells, and plant growth promotion.

The conversion of non-biomass waste into CDs is still in the early stages. The mechanism for enhancing QYs remains unclear. Industrial-scale production of CDs from non-biomass waste materials represents an efficient way of value-adding and reducing environmental impact. Challenges in this research field include:

(1) Expanding the range of non-biomass waste materials as carbon precursors for CDs synthesis.
(2) Simplifying pre-treatment procedures by reducing the use of toxic chemicals, lowering temperatures, and decreasing pressure.
(3) Exploring methods to enhance the properties of CDs, especially QY.
(4) Developing techniques to synthesize CDs from mixed non-biomass waste sources.
(5) Broadening the scope of CD applications from non-biomass waste.

Combining waste management strategies with CD synthesis technology offers an effective approach to addressing these technical challenges. Analyzing the components within the non-biomass waste and referencing methods used for precursors with similar chemical structures can be highly beneficial in developing a new route to convert non-biomass waste into CDs. Various synthetic approaches for CDs from chemicals encompass top-down methods, such as ball milling, laser ablation, arc discharge, chemical oxidation, electrochemical methods, micro-fluidization, and plasma approaches, as well as bottom-up approaches, such as pyrolytic methods, template, microwave-assisted, ultrasonic, hydrothermal/solvothermal, and chemical oxidation. Some of these methods have been used to convert non-bio waste to CDs, including reflux, hydrothermal, ball milling, ultrasonic irradiation, pyrolysis, and microwave-assisted methods. The applicability of the other methods warrants further study. In the experimental design, the selection of non-toxic, cost-effective, and environmentally friendly chemicals and methods is crucial to minimize any potential environmental pollution. The guiding principle should be followed when designing CDs from non-biomass waste. Surface functionalization and the doping of chemical heteroatoms have been designed to enhance the optical, electrical, and chemical properties of CDs, thereby expanding their potential applications.

Author Contributions: W.C.: Formal analysis, investigation, resources, and original draft writing; H.Y.: Conceptualization, methodology, and review and editing; I.C.: Supervision and review and editing; S.H.: Supervision, resources, investigation, and review and editing; L.W.: Supervision, resources, project administration, and review and editing. All authors have read and agreed to the published version of the manuscript.

Funding: This research received no external funding.

Acknowledgments: The study has been supported by the Australian Government Research Training Program (RTP) scholarship. The authors acknowledge the scholarship support of this research by the Australian Research Council (ARC) through the Linkage Project LP190101294.

Conflicts of Interest: The authors declare no conflicts of interest.

References

1. Parmesan, C.; Morecroft, M.D.; Trisurat, Y. Climate Change 2022: Impacts, Adaptation and Vulnerability. Ph.D. Thesis, GIEC, Geneva, Switzerland, 2022.

2. Gautam, M.; Agrawal, M. Greenhouse gas emissions from municipal solid waste management: A review of global scenario. In *Carbon Footprint Case Studies: Municipal Solid Waste Management, Sustainable Road Transport and Carbon Sequestration*; Springer: Berlin/Heidelberg, Germany, 2021; pp. 123–160.
3. Maria, C.; Góis, J.; Leitão, A. Challenges and perspectives of greenhouse gases emissions from municipal solid waste management in Angola. *Energy Rep.* **2020**, *6*, 364–369. [CrossRef]
4. Yu, K.H.; Zhang, Y.; Li, D.; Montenegro-Marin, C.E.; Kumar, P.M. Environmental planning based on reduce, reuse, recycle and recover using artificial intelligence. *Environ. Impact Assess. Rev.* **2021**, *86*, 106492. [CrossRef]
5. Zorpas, A.A. Strategy development in the framework of waste management. *Sci. Total Environ.* **2020**, *716*, 137088. [CrossRef] [PubMed]
6. Kumar, R.; Verma, A.; Shome, A.; Sinha, R.; Sinha, S.; Jha, P.K.; Kumar, R.; Kumar, P.; Shubham; Das, S. Impacts of plastic pollution on ecosystem services, sustainable development goals, and need to focus on circular economy and policy interventions. *Sustainability* **2021**, *13*, 9963. [CrossRef]
7. Shams, M.; Alam, I.; Mahbub, M.S. Plastic pollution during COVID-19: Plastic waste directives and its long-term impact on the environment. *Environ. Adv.* **2021**, *5*, 100119. [CrossRef] [PubMed]
8. Moazzem, S.; Wang, L.; Daver, F.; Crossin, E. Environmental impact of discarded apparel landfilling and recycling. *Resour. Conserv. Recycl.* **2021**, *166*, 105338. [CrossRef]
9. Moazzem, S.; Crossin, E.; Daver, F.; Wang, L. Environmental impact of apparel supply chain and textile products. *Environ. Dev. Sustain.* **2021**, *24*, 9757–9775. [CrossRef]
10. Tomaras, J. Waste Management and Recycling. 2021. Available online: https://www.aph.gov.au/About_Parliament/Parliamentary_Departments/Parliamentary_Library/pubs/rp/BudgetReview202021/WasteManagementRecycling (accessed on 25 November 2023).
11. Joe Pickin, C.W.; O'Farrell, K.; Stovell, L.; Nyunt, P.; Guazzo, S.; Lin, Y.; Caggiati-Shortell, G.; Chakma, P.; Edwards, C.; Lindley, B.; et al. *National Waste Report 2022*; The Department of Climate Change, Energy, the Environment and Water: Docklands, VIC, Australia, 2022.
12. Tu, L.; Li, Q.; Qiu, S.; Li, M.; Shin, J.; Wu, P.; Singh, N.; Li, J.; Ding, Q.; Hu, C.; et al. Recent developments in carbon dots: A biomedical application perspective. *R. Soc. Chem. J.* **2023**, *11*, 338–353. [CrossRef] [PubMed]
13. Tran, N.-A.; Hien, N.T.; Hoang, N.M.; Dang, H.-L.T.; Van Quy, T.; Hanh, N.T.; Vu, N.H.; Dao, V.-D. Carbon dots in environmental treatment and protection applications. *Desalination* **2023**, *548*, 116285. [CrossRef]
14. Shahraki, H.S.; Ahmad, A.; Bushra, R. Green carbon dots with multifaceted applications—Waste to wealth strategy. *FlatChem* **2022**, *31*, 100310. [CrossRef]
15. Truskewycz, A.; Yin, H.; Halberg, N.; Lai, D.T.; Ball, A.S.; Truong, V.K.; Rybicka, A.M.; Cole, I. Carbon dot therapeutic platforms: Administration, distribution, metabolism, excretion, toxicity, and therapeutic potential. *Small* **2022**, *18*, 2106342. [CrossRef] [PubMed]
16. Houshyar, S.; Yin, H.; Pope, L.; Zizhou, R.; Dekiwadia, C.; Hill-Yardin, E.L.; Yeung, J.M.; John, S.; Fox, K.; Tran, N. Smart suture with iodine contrasting nanoparticles for computed tomography. *OpenNano* **2023**, *9*, 100120. [CrossRef]
17. Kang, C.; Huang, Y.; Yang, H.; Yan, X.F.; Chen, Z.P. A review of carbon dots produced from biomass wastes. *Nanomaterials* **2020**, *10*, 2316. [CrossRef] [PubMed]
18. Kurian, M.; Paul, A. Recent trends in the use of green sources for carbon dot synthesis—A short review. *Carbon Trends* **2021**, *3*, 100032. [CrossRef]
19. Khairol Anuar, N.K.; Tan, H.L.; Lim, Y.P.; So'aib, M.S.; Abu Bakar, N.F. A review on multifunctional carbon-dots synthesized from biomass waste: Design/fabrication, characterization and applications. *Front. Energy Res.* **2021**, *9*, 67. [CrossRef]
20. de Oliveira, B.P.; da Silva Abreu, F.O.M. Carbon quantum dots synthesis from waste and by-products: Perspectives and challenges. *Mater. Lett.* **2021**, *282*, 128764. [CrossRef]
21. Fan, H.; Zhang, M.; Bhandari, B.; Yang, C.-h. Food waste as a carbon source in carbon quantum dots technology and their applications in food safety detection. *Trends Food Sci. Technol.* **2020**, *95*, 86–96. [CrossRef]
22. Lou, Y.; Hao, X.; Liao, L.; Zhang, K.; Chen, S.; Li, Z.; Ou, J.; Qin, A.; Li, Z. Recent advances of biomass carbon dots on syntheses, characterization, luminescence mechanism, and sensing applications. *Nano Sel.* **2021**, *2*, 1117–1145. [CrossRef]
23. Perumal, S.; Atchudan, R.; Edison, T.N.J.I.; Lee, Y.R. Sustainable synthesis of multifunctional carbon dots using biomass and their applications: A mini-review. *J. Environ. Chem. Eng.* **2021**, *9*, 105802. [CrossRef]
24. Lin, X.; Xiong, M.; Zhang, J.; He, C.; Ma, X.; Zhang, H.; Kuang, Y.; Yang, M.; Huang, Q. Carbon dots based on natural resources: Synthesis and applications in sensors. *Microchem. J.* **2021**, *160*, 105604. [CrossRef]
25. Wareing, T.C.; Gentile, P.; Phan, A.N. Biomass-based carbon dots: Current development and future perspectives. *ACS Nano* **2021**, *15*, 15471–15501. [CrossRef] [PubMed]
26. Radnia, F.; Mohajeri, N.; Zarghami, N. New insight into the engineering of green carbon dots: Possible applications in emerging cancer theranostics. *Talanta* **2020**, *209*, 120547. [CrossRef] [PubMed]
27. Manikandan, V.; Lee, N.Y. Green synthesis of carbon quantum dots and their environmental applications. *Environ. Res.* **2022**, *212*, 113283. [CrossRef] [PubMed]
28. Huang, C.-C.; Hung, Y.-S.; Weng, Y.-M.; Chen, W.; Lai, Y.-S. Sustainable development of carbon nanodots technology: Natural products as a carbon source and applications to food safety. *Trends Food Sci. Technol.* **2019**, *86*, 144–152. [CrossRef]

29. Meng, W.; Bai, X.; Wang, B.; Liu, Z.; Lu, S.; Yang, B. Biomass-derived carbon dots and their applications. *Energy Environ. Mater.* **2019**, *2*, 172–192. [CrossRef]
30. Arpita; Kumar, P.; Kataria, N.; Narwal, N.; Kumar, S.; Kumar, R.; Khoo, K.S.; Show, P.L. Plastic Waste-Derived Carbon Dots: Insights of Recycling Valuable Materials Towards Environmental Sustainability. *Curr. Pollut. Rep.* **2023**, *9*, 433–453. [CrossRef] [PubMed]
31. Hallaji, Z.; Bagheri, Z.; Ranjbar, B. The role of fluorescent carbon dots in the fate of plastic waste. *J. Environ. Chem. Eng.* **2023**, *11*, 110322. [CrossRef]
32. Zhang, S.; Zhang, L.; Huang, L.; Zheng, G.; Zhang, P.; Jin, Y.; Jiao, Z.; Sun, X. Study on the fluorescence properties of carbon dots prepared via combustion process. *J. Lumin.* **2019**, *206*, 608–612. [CrossRef]
33. Chahal, S.; Macairan, J.-R.; Yousefi, N.; Tufenkji, N.; Naccache, R. Green synthesis of carbon dots and their applications. *RSC Adv.* **2021**, *11*, 25354–25363. [CrossRef]
34. Hu, S.; Trinchi, A.; Atkin, P.; Cole, I. Tunable photoluminescence across the entire visible spectrum from carbon dots excited by white light. *Angew. Chem. Int. Ed.* **2015**, *54*, 2970–2974. [CrossRef]
35. Kolanowska, A.; Dzido, G.; Krzywiecki, M.; Tomczyk, M.M.; Łukowiec, D.; Ruczka, S.; Boncel, S. Carbon quantum dots from amino acids revisited: Survey of renewable precursors toward high quantum-yield blue and green fluorescence. *ACS Omega* **2022**, *7*, 41165–41176. [CrossRef]
36. Zhu, S.; Tang, S.; Zhang, J.; Yang, B. Control the size and surface chemistry of graphene for the rising fluorescent materials. *Chem. Commun.* **2012**, *48*, 4527–4539. [CrossRef] [PubMed]
37. Yan, F.; Sun, Z.; Zhang, H.; Sun, X.; Jiang, Y.; Bai, Z. The fluorescence mechanism of carbon dots, and methods for tuning their emission color: A review. *Microchim. Acta* **2019**, *186*, 583. [CrossRef] [PubMed]
38. Sk, M.A.; Ananthanarayanan, A.; Huang, L.; Lim, K.H.; Chen, P. Revealing the tunable photoluminescence properties of graphene quantum dots. *J. Mater. Chem. C* **2014**, *2*, 6954–6960. [CrossRef]
39. Kaushik, J.; Saini, D.; Singh, R.; Dubey, P.; Sonkar, S.K. Surface adhered fluorescent carbon dots extracted from the harmful diesel soot for sensing Fe (III) and Hg (II) ions. *New J. Chem.* **2021**, *45*, 20164–20172.
40. Mondal, N.K.; Singha, P.; Sen, K.; Mondal, A.; Debnath, P.; Mondal, A.; Mishra, D. Waste plastics acts as a good growth promoter: A laboratory-based study. *Res. Sq.* **2023**. [CrossRef]
41. Hu, Y.; Gao, Z. Sewage sludge in microwave oven: A sustainable synthetic approach toward carbon dots for fluorescent sensing of para-Nitrophenol. *J. Hazard. Mater.* **2020**, *382*, 121048. [CrossRef] [PubMed]
42. Tripathi, K.M.; Sonker, A.K.; Sonkar, S.K.; Sarkar, S. Pollutant soot of diesel engine exhaust transformed to carbon dots for multicoloured imaging of E. coli and sensing cholesterol. *RSC Adv.* **2014**, *4*, 30100–30107. [CrossRef]
43. Alluqmani, S.M.; Alabdallah, N.M. Preparation and application of nanostructured carbon from oil fly ash for growth promotion and improvement of agricultural crops with different doses. *Sci. Rep.* **2022**, *12*, 17033. [CrossRef]
44. Alluqmani, S.M.; Loulou, M.; Ouerfelli, J.; Alshahrie, A.; Salah, N. Annealing effect on structural and optical properties of nanostructured carbon of oil fly ash modified titania thin-film. *Results Phys.* **2021**, *25*, 104335. [CrossRef]
45. Chaudhary, P.; Verma, A.; Mishra, A.; Yadav, D.; Pal, K.; Yadav, B.; Kumar, E.R.; Thapa, K.B.; Mishra, S.; Dwivedi, D. Preparation of carbon quantum dots using bike pollutant soot: Evaluation of structural, optical and moisture sensing properties. *Phys. E Low-Dimens. Syst. Nanostructures* **2022**, *139*, 115174. [CrossRef]
46. Ganesan, K.; Hayagreevan, C.; Jeevagan, A.J.; Adinaveen, T.; Sophie, P.L.; Amalraj, M.; Bhuvaneshwari, D. Candle soot derived carbon dots as potential corrosion inhibitor for stainless steel in HCl medium. *J. Appl. Electrochem.* **2023**, *54*, 89–102. [CrossRef]
47. Huang, H.; Cui, Y.; Liu, M.; Chen, J.; Wan, Q.; Wen, Y.; Deng, F.; Zhou, N.; Zhang, X.; Wei, Y. A one-step ultrasonic irradiation assisted strategy for the preparation of polymer-functionalized carbon quantum dots and their biological imaging. *J. Colloid Interface Sci.* **2018**, *532*, 767–773. [CrossRef] [PubMed]
48. Li, Y.; Chen, T.; Ma, Y. Nanosized carbon dots from organic matter and biomass. *J. Wuhan Univ. Technol. Mater. Sci. Ed.* **2016**, *31*, 823–826. [CrossRef]
49. Pankaj, A.; Tewari, K.; Singh, S.; Singh, S.P. Waste candle soot derived nitrogen doped carbon dots based fluorescent sensor probe: An efficient and inexpensive route to determine Hg (II) and Fe (III) from water. *J. Environ. Chem. Eng.* **2018**, *6*, 5561–5569. [CrossRef]
50. Song, Y.; Lu, F.; Li, H.; Wang, H.; Zhang, M.; Liu, Y.; Kang, Z. Degradable carbon dots from cigarette smoking with broad-spectrum antimicrobial activities against drug-resistant bacteria. *ACS Appl. Bio Mater.* **2018**, *1*, 1871–1879. [CrossRef] [PubMed]
51. Thulasi, S.; Kathiravan, A.; Asha Jhonsi, M. Fluorescent carbon dots derived from vehicle exhaust soot and sensing of tartrazine in soft drinks. *ACS Omega* **2020**, *5*, 7025–7031. [CrossRef] [PubMed]
52. Venkatesan, S.; Mariadoss, A.J.; Arunkumar, K.; Muthupandian, A. Fuel waste to fluorescent carbon dots and its multifarious applications. *Sens. Actuators B Chem.* **2019**, *282*, 972–983. [CrossRef]
53. Wang, Q.; Zheng, H.; Long, Y.; Zhang, L.; Gao, M.; Bai, W. Microwave–hydrothermal synthesis of fluorescent carbon dots from graphite oxide. *Carbon* **2011**, *49*, 3134–3140. [CrossRef]
54. Zhang, Q.; Sun, X.; Ruan, H.; Yin, K.; Li, H. Production of yellow-emitting carbon quantum dots from fullerene carbon soot. *Sci. China Mater.* **2017**, *60*, 141–150. [CrossRef]
55. Hong, W.T.; Moon, B.K.; Yang, H.K. Microwave irradiation and color converting film application of carbon dots originated from wasted toner powder. *Mater. Res. Bull.* **2022**, *156*, 111999. [CrossRef]

56. Chan, K.; Zinchenko, A. Aminolysis-assisted hydrothermal conversion of waste PET plastic to N-doped carbon dots with markedly enhanced fluorescence. *J. Environ. Chem. Eng.* **2022**, *10*, 107749. [CrossRef]
57. Wang, R.; Li, S.; Huang, H.; Liu, B.; Gao, L.; Qu, M.; Wei, Y.; Wei, J. Preparation of carbon dots from PET waste by one-step hydrothermal method and its application in light blocking films and LEDs. *J. Fluoresc.* **2023**, *33*, 1305–1315. [CrossRef] [PubMed]
58. Ma, G.; Wang, R.; Zhang, M.; Dong, Z.; Zhang, A.; Qu, M.; Gao, L.; Wei, Y.; Wei, J. Solvothermal preparation of nitrogen-doped carbon dots with PET waste as precursor and their application in LEDs and water detection. *Spectrochim. Acta Part A Mol. Biomol. Spectrosc.* **2023**, *289*, 122178. [CrossRef] [PubMed]
59. Lauria, A.; Lizundia, E. Luminescent carbon dots obtained from polymeric waste. *J. Clean. Prod.* **2020**, *262*, 121288. [CrossRef]
60. Hu, Y.; Li, M.; Gao, Z.; Wang, L.; Zhang, J. Waste polyethylene terephthalate derived carbon dots for separable production of 5-hydroxymethylfurfural at low temperature. *Catal. Lett.* **2021**, *151*, 2436–2444. [CrossRef]
61. Li, H.; Li, Y.; Xu, Y. Nitrogen-doped carbon dots from polystyrene for three analytes sensing and their logic recognition. *Inorg. Chem. Commun.* **2023**, *148*, 110369. [CrossRef]
62. Liang, L.; Wong, S.C.; Lisak, G. Effects of plastic-derived carbon dots on germination and growth of pea (*Pisum sativum*) via seed nano-priming. *Chemosphere* **2023**, *316*, 137868. [CrossRef] [PubMed]
63. Abdelhameed, M.; Elbeh, M.; Baban, N.S.; Pereira, L.; Matula, J.; Song, Y.-A.; Ramadi, K.B. High-yield, one-pot upcycling of polyethylene and polypropylene waste into blue-emissive carbon dots. *Green Chem.* **2023**, *25*, 1925–1937. [CrossRef]
64. Kommula, B.; Banoo, M.; Roy, R.S.; Sil, S.; Sah, A.K.; Rawat, B.; Chakraborty, S.; Meena, P.; Kailasam, K.; Gautam, U.K. Landscaping sustainable conversion of waste plastics to carbon dots and enormous diversity in O_2 harvesting, hypoxia, autophagy. *Carbon* **2023**, *213*, 118304. [CrossRef]
65. Muro-Hidalgo, J.M.; Bazany-Rodríguez, I.J.; Hernández, J.G.; Pabello, V.M.L.; Thangarasu, P. Histamine Recognition by Carbon Dots from Plastic Waste and Development of Cellular Imaging: Experimental and Theoretical Studies. *J. Fluoresc.* **2023**, *33*, 2041–2059. [CrossRef] [PubMed]
66. Kumari, M.; Chaudhary, G.R.; Chaudhary, S.; Umar, A. Rapid analysis of trace sulphite ion using fluorescent carbon dots produced from single use plastic cups. *Eng. Sci.* **2021**, *17*, 101–112. [CrossRef]
67. Kumari, M.; Chaudhary, S. Modulating the physicochemical and biological properties of carbon dots synthesised from plastic waste for effective sensing of E. coli. *Colloids Surf. B Biointerfaces* **2020**, *196*, 111333. [CrossRef] [PubMed]
68. Ghosh, A.; Das, G. Environmentally benign synthesis of fluorescent carbon nanodots using waste PET bottles: Highly selective and sensitive detection of Pb^{2+} ions in aqueous medium. *New J. Chem.* **2021**, *45*, 8747–8754. [CrossRef]
69. Song, H.; Liu, X.; Wang, B.; Tang, Z.; Lu, S. High production-yield solid-state carbon dots with tunable photoluminescence for white/multi-color light-emitting diodes. *Sci. Bull.* **2019**, *64*, 1788–1794. [CrossRef] [PubMed]
70. Ramanan, V.; Siddaiah, B.; Raji, K.; Ramamurthy, P. Green synthesis of multifunctionalized, nitrogen-doped, highly fluorescent carbon dots from waste expanded polystyrene and its application in the fluorimetric detection of Au^{3+} ions in aqueous media. *ACS Sustain. Chem. Eng.* **2018**, *6*, 1627–1638. [CrossRef]
71. Li, S.; Hu, J.; Aryee, A.A.; Sun, Y.; Li, Z. Three birds, one stone: Disinfecting and turning waste medical masks into valuable carbon dots for sodium hydrosulfite and Fe^{3+} detection enabled by a simple hydrothermal treatment. *Spectrochim. Acta Part A Mol. Biomol. Spectrosc.* **2023**, *296*, 122659. [CrossRef]
72. Kumari, A.; Kumar, A.; Sahu, S.K.; Kumar, S. Synthesis of green fluorescent carbon quantum dots using waste polyolefins residue for Cu^{2+} ion sensing and live cell imaging. *Sens. Actuators B Chem.* **2018**, *254*, 197–205. [CrossRef]
73. Perikala, M.; Bhardwaj, A. Waste to white light: A sustainable method for converting biohazardous waste to broadband white LEDs. *RSC Adv.* **2022**, *12*, 11443–11453. [CrossRef]
74. Cruz, M.I.S.D.; Thongsai, N.; de Luna, M.D.G.; In, I.; Paoprasert, P. Preparation of highly photoluminescent carbon dots from polyurethane: Optimization using response surface methodology and selective detection of silver (I) ion. *Colloids Surf. A Physicochem. Eng. Asp.* **2019**, *568*, 184–194. [CrossRef]
75. Shaw, V.; Mondal, A.; Mondal, A.; Koley, R.; Mondal, N.K. Effective utilization of waste plastics towards sustainable control of mosquito. *J. Clean. Prod.* **2023**, *386*, 135826. [CrossRef]
76. Hu, Y.; Gao, Z.; Yang, J.; Chen, H.; Han, L. Environmentally benign conversion of waste polyethylene terephthalate to fluorescent carbon dots for "on-off-on" sensing of ferric and pyrophosphate ions. *J. Colloid Interface Sci.* **2019**, *538*, 481–488. [CrossRef] [PubMed]
77. Wang, R.; Chen, X.; Li, Q.; Zhang, A.; Ma, G.; Wei, Y.; Qu, M.; Gao, L.; Wei, J. Solvothermal preparation of nitrogen and phosphorus-doped carbon dots with PET waste as precursor and its application. *Mater. Today Commun.* **2023**, *34*, 104918. [CrossRef]
78. Gu, W.; Dong, Z.; Zhang, A.; Ma, T.; Hu, Q.; Wei, J.; Wang, R. Functionalization of PET with carbon dots as copolymerizable flame retardants for the excellent smoke suppressants and mechanical properties. *Polym. Degrad. Stab.* **2022**, *195*, 109766. [CrossRef]
79. Wei, J.; Zhang, X.; Sheng, Y.; Shen, J.; Huang, P.; Guo, S.; Pan, J.; Liu, B.; Feng, B. Simple one-step synthesis of water-soluble fluorescent carbon dots from waste paper. *New J. Chem.* **2014**, *38*, 906–909. [CrossRef]
80. Wei, J.; Shen, J.; Zhang, X.; Guo, S.; Pan, J.; Hou, X.; Zhang, H.; Wang, L.; Feng, B. Simple one-step synthesis of water-soluble fluorescent carbon dots derived from paper ash. *RSC Adv.* **2013**, *3*, 13119–13122. [CrossRef]
81. Devi, S.; Gupta, R.K.; Paul, A.K.; Tyagi, S. Waste carbon paper derivatized Carbon Quantum Dots/(3-Aminopropyl) triethoxysilane based fluorescent probe for trinitrotoluene detection. *Mater. Res. Express* **2018**, *6*, 025605. [CrossRef]

82. Park, S.J.; Park, J.Y.; Chung, J.W.; Yang, H.K.; Moon, B.K.; Yi, S.S. Color tunable carbon quantum dots from wasted paper by different solvents for anti-counterfeiting and fluorescent flexible film. *Chem. Eng. J.* **2020**, *383*, 123200. [CrossRef]
83. Lin, B.; Yan, Y.; Guo, M.; Cao, Y.; Yu, Y.; Zhang, T.; Huang, Y.; Wu, D. Modification-free carbon dots as turn-on fluorescence probe for detection of organophosphorus pesticides. *Food Chem.* **2018**, *245*, 1176–1182. [CrossRef]
84. Wang, J.; Qiu, F.; Li, X.; Wu, H.; Xu, J.; Niu, X.; Pan, J.; Zhang, T.; Yang, D. A facile one-pot synthesis of fluorescent carbon dots from degrease cotton for the selective determination of chromium ions in water and soil samples. *J. Lumin.* **2017**, *188*, 230–237. [CrossRef]
85. Wu, Y.; Ma, G.; Zhang, A.; Gu, W.; Wei, J.; Wang, R. Preparation of carbon dots with ultrahigh fluorescence quantum yield based on PET waste. *ACS Omega* **2022**, *7*, 38037–38044. [CrossRef] [PubMed]
86. Huang, P.; Xu, S.; Zhang, M.; Zhong, W.; Xiao, Z.; Luo, Y. Modulation doping of absorbent cotton derived carbon dots for quantum dot-sensitized solar cells. *Phys. Chem. Chem. Phys.* **2019**, *21*, 26133–26145. [CrossRef] [PubMed]
87. Wu, Y.; Wang, R.; Xie, W.; Ma, G.; Zhang, A.; Liu, B.; Huang, H.; Gao, L.; Qu, M.; Wei, Y. Solvent-thermal preparation of sulfur and nitrogen-doped carbon dots with PET waste as precursor and application in light-blocking film. *J. Nanoparticle Res.* **2023**, *25*, 18. [CrossRef]
88. Vadivel, R.; Nirmala, M.; Raji, K.; Siddaiah, B.; Ramamurthy, P. Synthesis of highly luminescent carbon dots from postconsumer waste silk cloth and investigation of its electron transfer dynamics with methyl viologen dichloride. *J. Indian Chem. Soc.* **2021**, *98*, 100181. [CrossRef]
89. Chen, X.; Song, Z.; Li, S.; Thang, N.T.; Gao, X.; Gong, X.; Guo, M. Facile one-pot synthesis of self-assembled nitrogen-doped carbon dots/cellulose nanofibril hydrogel with enhanced fluorescence and mechanical properties. *Green Chem.* **2020**, *22*, 3296–3308. [CrossRef]
90. Zhao, Z.; Guo, Y.; Zhang, T.; Ma, J.; Li, H.; Zhou, J.; Wang, Z.; Sun, R. Preparation of carbon dots from waste cellulose diacetate as a sensor for tetracycline detection and fluorescence ink. *Int. J. Biol. Macromol.* **2020**, *164*, 4289–4298. [CrossRef] [PubMed]
91. Zhao, Y.; Yang, Z.; Niu, J.; Du, Z.; Federica, C.; Zhu, Z.; Yang, K.; Li, Y.; Zhao, B.; Pedersen, T.H. Systematical analysis of sludge treatment and disposal technologies for carbon footprint reduction. *J. Environ. Sci.* **2023**, *128*, 224–249. [CrossRef]
92. Kalanidhi, K.; Nagaraaj, P. A green approach for synthesis of highly fluorescent carbon dots from waste engine oil: A strategy for waste to value added products. *Diam. Relat. Mater.* **2022**, *121*, 108724. [CrossRef]
93. Zhang, Y.; Wang, L.; Chen, L.; Ma, B.; Zhang, Y.; Ni, W.; Tsang, D.C. Treatment of municipal solid waste incineration fly ash: State-of-the-art technologies and future perspectives. *J. Hazard. Mater.* **2021**, *411*, 125132. [CrossRef]
94. Zhang, Y.; Li, H.; Gao, S.; Geng, Y.; Wu, C. A study on the chemical state of carbon present in fine ash from gasification. *Asia-Pac. J. Chem. Eng.* **2019**, *14*, e2336. [CrossRef]
95. Das, T.; Saikia, B.K.; Dekaboruah, H.; Bordoloi, M.; Neog, D.; Bora, J.J.; Lahkar, J.; Narzary, B.; Roy, S.; Ramaiah, D. Blue-fluorescent and biocompatible carbon dots derived from abundant low-quality coals. *J. Photochem. Photobiol. B Biol.* **2019**, *195*, 1–11. [CrossRef] [PubMed]
96. Raj, A.M.; Chirayil, G.T. Facile synthesis of preformed mixed nano-carbon structure from low rank coal. *Manag. Syst. Prod. Eng.* **2018**, *36*, 14–20.
97. Saikia, M.; Hower, J.C.; Das, T.; Dutta, T.; Saikia, B.K. Feasibility study of preparation of carbon quantum dots from Pennsylvania anthracite and Kentucky bituminous coals. *Fuel* **2019**, *243*, 433–440. [CrossRef]
98. Jiang, Y.; Wang, J.C.; Meng, F.; Wang, B.; Cheng, Y.; Zhu, C. N-doped carbon dots synthesized by rapid microwave irradiation as highly fluorescent probes for Pb^{2+} detection. *New J. Chem.* **2015**, *39*, 3357–3360. [CrossRef]
99. Jiang, K.; Wang, Y.; Gao, X.; Cai, C.; Lin, H. Facile, quick, and gram-scale synthesis of ultralong-lifetime room-temperature-phosphorescent carbon dots by microwave irradiation. *Angew. Chem. Int. Ed.* **2018**, *57*, 6216–6220. [CrossRef] [PubMed]
100. de Medeiros, T.V.; Manioudakis, J.; Noun, F.; Macairan, J.-R.; Victoria, F.; Naccache, R. Microwave-assisted synthesis of carbon dots and their applications. *J. Mater. Chem. C* **2019**, *7*, 7175–7195. [CrossRef]
101. Marinello, S.; Lolli, F.; Gamberini, R. Roadway tunnels: A critical review of air pollutant concentrations and vehicular emissions. *Transp. Res. Part D Transp. Environ.* **2020**, *86*, 102478. [CrossRef]
102. Kumar, P.G.; Lekhana, P.; Tejaswi, M.; Chandrakala, S. Effects of vehicular emissions on the urban environment-a state of the art. *Mater. Today Proc.* **2021**, *45*, 6314–6320. [CrossRef]
103. Gu, M.; Pan, Y.; Walters, W.W.; Sun, Q.; Song, L.; Wang, Y.; Xue, Y.; Fang, Y. Vehicular emissions enhanced ammonia concentrations in winter mornings: Insights from diurnal nitrogen isotopic signatures. *Environ. Sci. Technol.* **2022**, *56*, 1578–1585. [CrossRef]
104. Milku Augustine, K.; Attiogbe, F.; Derkyi, N.; Atepor, L. A Review of Policies and Legislations of Vehicular Exhaust Emissions in Ghana and Their Enforcement. *Aerosol Sci. Eng.* **2023**, *7*, 169–181. [CrossRef]
105. Gulia, S.; Tiwari, R.; Mendiratta, S.; Kaur, S.; Goyal, S.; Kumar, R. Review of scientific technology-based solutions for vehicular pollution control. *Clean Technol. Environ. Policy* **2020**, *22*, 1955–1966. [CrossRef]
106. Li, Z.; Wang, L.; Li, Y.; Feng, Y.; Feng, W. Frontiers in carbon dots: Design, properties and applications. *Mater. Chem. Front.* **2019**, *3*, 2571–2601. [CrossRef]
107. Evode, N.; Qamar, S.A.; Bilal, M.; Barceló, D.; Iqbal, H.M. Plastic waste and its management strategies for environmental sustainability. *Case Stud. Chem. Environ. Eng.* **2021**, *4*, 100142. [CrossRef]
108. Gu, J.-D. Biodegradability of plastics: The issues, recent advances, and future perspectives. *Environ. Sci. Pollut. Res.* **2021**, *28*, 1278–1282. [CrossRef] [PubMed]

109. Sharuddin, S.D.A.; Abnisa, F.; Daud, W.M.A.W.; Aroua, M.K. A review on pyrolysis of plastic wastes. *Energy Convers. Manag.* **2016**, *115*, 308–326. [CrossRef]
110. Maqsood, T.; Dai, J.; Zhang, Y.; Guang, M.; Li, B. Pyrolysis of plastic species: A review of resources and products. *J. Anal. Appl. Pyrolysis* **2021**, *159*, 105295. [CrossRef]
111. Vassilev, S.V.; Kitano, K.; Takeda, S.; Tsurue, T. Influence of mineral and chemical composition of coal ashes on their fusibility. *Fuel Process. Technol.* **1995**, *45*, 27–51. [CrossRef]
112. Naik, V.M.; Bhosale, S.V.; Kolekar, G.B. A brief review on the synthesis, characterisation and analytical applications of nitrogen doped carbon dots. *Anal. Methods* **2022**, *14*, 877–891. [CrossRef] [PubMed]
113. Dhenadhayalan, N.; Lin, K.C.; Saleh, T.A. Recent advances in functionalized carbon dots toward the design of efficient materials for sensing and catalysis applications. *Small* **2020**, *16*, 1905767. [CrossRef]
114. National Clothing Product Stewardship Schemes. Available online: https://ausfashioncouncil.com/wp-content/uploads/2023/05/AFC-NCPSS-Data-Report.pdf (accessed on 30 November 2023).
115. Wang, C.; Xia, K.; Zhang, Y.; Kaplan, D.L. Silk-based advanced materials for soft electronics. *Acc. Chem. Res.* **2019**, *52*, 2916–2927. [CrossRef]
116. He, H.; Zhang, Y.; Wang, P.; Hu, D. Preparation of sponge-cake-like N-doped porous carbon materials derived from silk fibroin by chemical activation. *Microporous Mesoporous Mater.* **2021**, *317*, 110998. [CrossRef]
117. Munusamy, S.; Mandlimath, T.R.; Swetha, P.; Al-Sehemi, A.G.; Pannipara, M.; Koppala, S.; Shanmugam, P.; Boonyuen, S.; Pothu, R.; Boddula, R. Nitrogen-doped carbon dots: Recent developments in its fluorescent sensor applications. *Environ. Res.* **2023**, *231*, 116046. [CrossRef]
118. Li, W.; Wang, S.; Li, Y.; Ma, C.; Huang, Z.; Wang, C.; Li, J.; Chen, Z.; Liu, S. One-step hydrothermal synthesis of fluorescent nanocrystalline cellulose/carbon dot hydrogels. *Carbohydr. Polym.* **2017**, *175*, 7–17. [CrossRef]
119. Shen, P.; Gao, J.; Cong, J.; Liu, Z.; Li, C.; Yao, J. Synthesis of cellulose-based carbon dots for bioimaging. *ChemistrySelect* **2016**, *1*, 1314–1317. [CrossRef]
120. Liao, X.; Chen, C.; Zhou, R.; Huang, Q.; Liang, Q.; Huang, Z.; Zhang, Y.; Hu, H.; Liang, Y. Comparison of N-doped carbon dots synthesized from the main components of plants including cellulose, lignin, and xylose: Characterized, fluorescence mechanism, and potential applications. *Dye Pigment.* **2020**, *183*, 108725. [CrossRef]
121. Huang, H.; Ge, H.; Ren, Z.; Huang, Z.; Xu, M.; Wang, X. Controllable synthesis of biocompatible fluorescent carbon dots from cellulose hydrogel for the specific detection of Hg^{2+}. *Front. Bioeng. Biotechnol.* **2021**, *9*, 617097. [CrossRef]
122. Wu, P.; Li, W.; Wu, Q.; Liu, Y.; Liu, S. Hydrothermal synthesis of nitrogen-doped carbon quantum dots from microcrystalline cellulose for the detection of Fe^{3+} ions in an acidic environment. *RSC Adv.* **2017**, *7*, 44144–44153. [CrossRef]
123. Zhang, W.; Li, L.; Yan, M.; Ma, J.; Wang, J.; Liu, C.; Bao, Y.; Jin, H.; Fan, Q. Turning waste into treasure: Multicolor carbon dots synthesized from waste leather scrap and their application in anti-counterfeiting. *ACS Sustain. Chem. Eng.* **2023**, *11*, 5082–5092. [CrossRef]
124. Craciun, A.; Diac, A.; Focsan, M.; Socaci, C.; Magyari, K.; Maniu, D.; Mihalache, I.; Veca, L.; Astilean, S.; Terec, A. Surface passivation of carbon nanoparticles with p-phenylenediamine towards photoluminescent carbon dots. *RSC Adv.* **2016**, *6*, 56944–56951. [CrossRef]
125. Kaur, M.; Kaur, M.; Sharma, V.K. Nitrogen-doped graphene and graphene quantum dots: A review onsynthesis and applications in energy, sensors and environment. *Adv. Colloid Interface Sci.* **2018**, *259*, 44–64. [CrossRef]
126. Xu, Y.; Wang, C.; Sui, L.; Ran, G.; Song, Q. Phosphoric acid densified red emissive carbon dots with a well-defined structure and narrow band fluorescence for intracellular reactive oxygen species detection and scavenging. *J. Mater. Chem. C* **2023**, *11*, 2984–2994. [CrossRef]
127. Goswami, J.; Rohman, S.S.; Guha, A.K.; Basyach, P.; Sonowal, K.; Borah, S.P.; Saikia, L.; Hazarika, P. Phosphoric acid assisted synthesis of fluorescent carbon dots from waste biomass for detection of Cr (VI) in aqueous media. *Mater. Chem. Phys.* **2022**, *286*, 126133. [CrossRef]
128. Zhang, Y.; Tan, B.; Zhang, X.; Guo, L.; Zhang, S. Synthesized carbon dots with high N and S content as excellent corrosion inhibitors for copper in sulfuric acid solution. *J. Mol. Liq.* **2021**, *338*, 116702. [CrossRef]
129. Zhang, Y.; Zhang, S.; Tan, B.; Guo, L.; Li, H. Solvothermal synthesis of functionalized carbon dots from amino acid as an eco-friendly corrosion inhibitor for copper in sulfuric acid solution. *J. Colloid Interface Sci.* **2021**, *604*, 1–14. [CrossRef]
130. Liang, Y.; Xu, D.; Feng, P.; Hao, B.; Guo, Y.; Wang, S. Municipal sewage sludge incineration and its air pollution control. *J. Clean. Prod.* **2021**, *295*, 126456. [CrossRef]
131. Rangabhashiyam, S.; dos Santos Lins, P.V.; de Magalhães Oliveira, L.M.; Sepulveda, P.; Ighalo, J.O.; Rajapaksha, A.U.; Meili, L. Sewage sludge-derived biochar for the adsorptive removal of wastewater pollutants: A critical review. *Environ. Pollut.* **2022**, *293*, 118581. [CrossRef]
132. Chen, X.; Jeyaseelan, S.; Graham, N. Physical and chemical properties study of the activated carbon made from sewage sludge. *Waste Manag.* **2002**, *22*, 755–760. [CrossRef]
133. Ding, A.; Zhang, R.; Ngo, H.H.; He, X.; Ma, J.; Nan, J.; Li, G. Life cycle assessment of sewage sludge treatment and disposal based on nutrient and energy recovery: A review. *Sci. Total Environ.* **2021**, *769*, 144451. [CrossRef]
134. Zu, F.; Yan, F.; Bai, Z.; Xu, J.; Wang, Y.; Huang, Y.; Zhou, X. The quenching of the fluorescence of carbon dots: A review on mechanisms and applications. *Microchim. Acta* **2017**, *184*, 1899–1914. [CrossRef]

135. Bhat, S.A.; Hassan, T.; Majid, S. Heavy metal toxicity and their harmful effects on living organisms–a review. *Int. J. Med. Sci. Diagn. Res.* **2019**, *3*, 106–122.
136. Wu, Y.; Chen, X.; Wu, W. Multiple Stimuli-Response Polychromatic Carbon Dots for Advanced Information Encryption and Safety. *Small* **2023**, *19*, 2206709. [CrossRef]
137. Ji, C.; Xu, W.; Han, Q.; Zhao, T.; Deng, J.; Peng, Z. Light of Carbon: Recent Advancements of Carbon Dots for LEDs. *Nano Energy* **2023**, *114*, 108623. [CrossRef]
138. Olabi, A.; Abdelkareem, M.A. Renewable energy and climate change. *Renew. Sustain. Energy Rev.* **2022**, *158*, 112111. [CrossRef]
139. Hu, J.; Jia, W.; Wu, X.; Zhang, H.; Wang, Y.; Liu, J.; Yang, Y.; Tao, S.; Wang, X. Carbon dots can strongly promote photosynthesis in lettuce (*Lactuca sativa* L.). *Environ. Sci. Nano* **2022**, *9*, 1530–1540. [CrossRef]
140. Guo, B.; Liu, G.; Wei, H.; Qiu, J.; Zhuang, J.; Zhang, X.; Zheng, M.; Li, W.; Zhang, H.; Hu, C. The role of fluorescent carbon dots in crops: Mechanism and applications. *SmartMat* **2022**, *3*, 208–225. [CrossRef]

Disclaimer/Publisher's Note: The statements, opinions and data contained in all publications are solely those of the individual author(s) and contributor(s) and not of MDPI and/or the editor(s). MDPI and/or the editor(s) disclaim responsibility for any injury to people or property resulting from any ideas, methods, instructions or products referred to in the content.

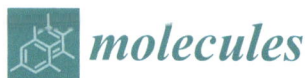

Article

Sequestration of an Azo Dye by a Potential Biosorbent: Characterization of Biosorbent, Adsorption Isotherm and Adsorption Kinetic Studies

Bharti Gaur [1], Jyoti Mittal [1], Syed Ansar Ali Shah [2], Alok Mittal [1,*] and Richard T. Baker [2,*]

[1] Department of Chemistry, Maulana Azad National Institute of Technology, Bhopal 462 003, India; jyalmittal@yahoo.co.in (J.M.)
[2] Department of Chemistry, University of St. Andrews, Fife, St. Andrews KY16 9ST, UK; saas1@st-andrews.ac.uk
* Correspondence: aljymittal@gmail.com (A.M.); rtb5@st-andrews.ac.uk (R.T.B.)

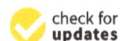

Citation: Gaur, B.; Mittal, J.; Shah, S.A.A.; Mittal, A.; Baker, R.T. Sequestration of an Azo Dye by a Potential Biosorbent: Characterization of Biosorbent, Adsorption Isotherm and Adsorption Kinetic Studies. *Molecules* 2024, 29, 2387. https://doi.org/10.3390/molecules29102387

Academic Editor: Fabio Ganazzoli

Received: 27 April 2024
Revised: 15 May 2024
Accepted: 17 May 2024
Published: 19 May 2024

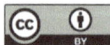

Copyright: © 2024 by the authors. Licensee MDPI, Basel, Switzerland. This article is an open access article distributed under the terms and conditions of the Creative Commons Attribution (CC BY) license (https://creativecommons.org/licenses/by/4.0/).

Abstract: This study explores the detailed characterization of a biosorbent (Hen Feather) and its efficient use in eradicating the azo dye Metanil Yellow (MY) from its aqueous solutions. Effects of a range of experimental parameters, including pH, initial dye concentration, biosorbent dosage and contact time on the adsorption, were studied. A detailed physical and chemical characterization of the biosorbent was made using SEM, XRD, XPS and FTIR. During the optimization of adsorption parameters, the highest dye uptake of almost 99% was recorded at pH 2, dye concentration 2×10^{-5} M, 0.05 g of biosorbent and a contact period of 75 min. Various adsorption isotherm models were studied to gather different adsorption and thermodynamic parameters. The linearity of the Langmuir, Freundlich and D-R adsorption isotherms indicate homogeneous, multilayer chemisorption with high adsorption affinity between the dye and biosorbent. Values of the changes in the Gibbs free energy ($\Delta G°$) and the enthalpy ($\Delta H°$) of the adsorption process have been calculated, these values indicate that it is a spontaneous and endothermic process. Kinetics of the adsorption were also measured, and it was established that the adsorption of MY over Hen Feather follows a pseudo-second-order kinetic model at temperatures 30, 40 and 50 °C. The findings of this investigation clearly indicate that the studied biosorbent exhibits a high affinity towards the dye (MY), and it can be effectively, economically and efficiently used to sequestrate and eradicate MY from its aqueous solutions.

Keywords: hen feather; metanil yellow; adsorption isotherm; adsorption kinetics; thermodynamics

1. Introduction

Water contamination is a severe threat to humanity. Rapid population increase leading to speedy industrialization is the main cause of water pollution. Industrial effluents contain a variety of chemical impurities in dissolved and suspended forms, of which dissolved nonbiodegradable materials such as bulky organic dyes are considered to be highly toxic to living beings and the most difficult to remove. These organic dyes also obstruct sunlight, which impairs photosynthesis in water resources and harms aquatic life [1,2]. The removal of dyes from water via a safe method is essential, and adsorption is an established economic, effective and operationally practicable technique [3]. In adsorption operations, the selection of an adsorbent determines the efficacy and cost-effectiveness of the procedure [4]. Hence, a cheap and easily available waste material with extraordinarily high adsorption abilities can be an excellent choice as an adsorbent [5].

Previous studies claim that, of the available variety of dyes, dyes belonging to the azo group pose severe toxicity due to their carcinogenic and mutagenic behaviour [6]. The azo dye studied in this work, Metanil Yellow (MY), contains diazotized metanilic acid and diphenylamine. It is widely applied to stain paper, nylon, silk, wool and other materials and effluents of these industries contain large amounts of this toxic dye. Due to the resemblance in colour, adulterators replace costly turmeric with MY in many edible products, and this is one of the menaces of the usage of this dye [7]. Indeed, its use as a food additive has been banned due to its established severely toxic nature [8]. Many studies have confirmed that MY can lead to cardiovascular disease, damage the central venous region of liver tissue and cause histopathological abnormalities in the kidneys of goats [9]. Exposure of fish to MY results in collapsed cytoplasm, nucleus pyknosis and cardiotoxicity [10].

Based on several observations, it has been discovered that MY harms the testicles and reproductive systems of rats and guinea pigs [11,12]. It also causes inflammatory irritation when it comes into contact with the skin. It is now well established that the presence of harmful methemoglobinemia and cyanosis caused by MY adversely affects humans. Hence, when MY is ingested orally, all crucial human organs (heart, liver, kidneys, intestines, reproductive systems, neurological system, gastric tissues, etc.) can be harmed [10,13]. Therefore, keeping the toxicity of MY in view, the eradication of MY from its aqueous solution using a safe method like adsorption is highly desirable.

In the present work for the removal of MY, a bio-waste material, Hen Feather (HF), has been employed as the adsorbent since no attempt has so far been made to adsorb MY using HF. It contains a highly flexible and porous structure in the soft and the hard parts and is distinct from any other natural or artificial fibres. The shaft of the feather called the rachis is the hard part, while barbs, which originate from the rachis, and barbules, which emerge as branches from barbs, are both considered soft parts [14,15]. Chemically, Hen Feathers possess organic materials, especially protein (approximately 84%) [16]. It is pertinent to note that the soft parts of Hen Feathers (barbs/barbules) have a special cross-section that is not found in other protein fibres like wool and silk. The porous nature and high surface area of Hen Feather make it a potent biosorbent for the eradication of bulky organic dyes.

The present paper is an attempt to first explore the physical and chemical structure of the Hen Feather using a variety of analytical techniques, including scanning electron microscopy (SEM), X-ray diffraction (XRD), X-ray photoelectron spectroscopy (XPS) and Fourier transform infra-red (FTIR) spectroscopy, and then to carry out detailed and systematic studies on the adsorption of MY over Hen Feathers in aqueous solution.

2. Results and Discussions

2.1. Characterization of Biosorbent

The SEM images presented in Figure 1 show the microstructure of the Hen Feather sample. Figure 1a,c exhibit the branch-like ramus, which supports the barbules sprouting from it. Both distal and proximal barbules can be seen, and a series of hooks that connect these together are also visible at the top of each of these images. Bamboo-like structures are seen in Figure 1c, and the material of a single barbule is viewed at a higher magnification in Figure 1d. Figure 2 presents SEM images of the Hen Feather sample after treatment with MY solution and drying. The presence of particles and plate-like structures, which may be aggregations of MY dye molecules, indicates that MY covers both flighted and bamboo-like feathers.

The XRD pattern presented in Figure 3 is very similar to patterns given for Hen Feathers and for pure keratin in the literature [17]. According to literature reports, the broad peak at ~19° results from the overlap of a peak at 17.8° and 19°, which correspond, respectively, to the α-helix and β-sheet structures [18]. A further peak at ~10°, which can be seen in Figure 3, also corresponds to the α-helix structure [19]. Since both broad peaks are intense, it is clear that both these structural conformations are common in this sample.

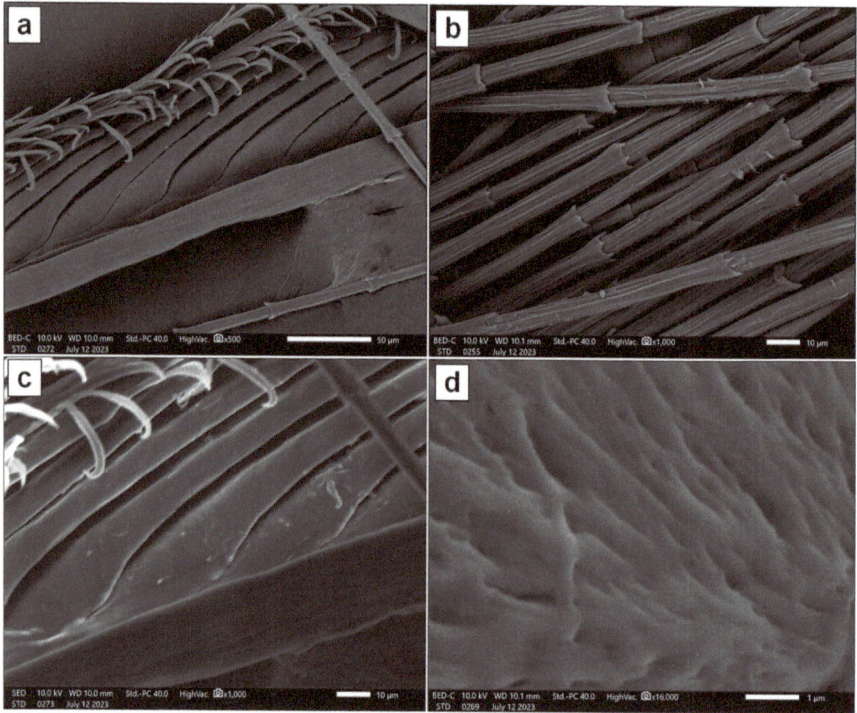

Figure 1. SEM images of Hen Feather taken at increasing magnifications and in both backscattered (**a,b,d**) and secondary (**c**) electron modes.

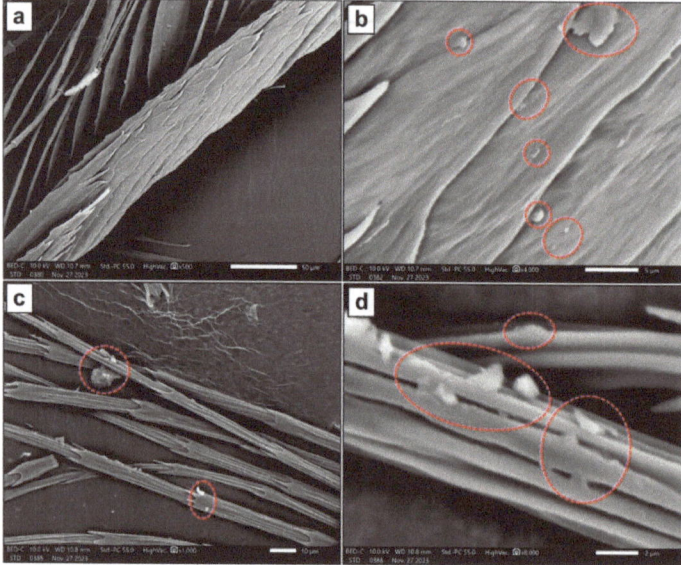

Figure 2. SEM images of Hen Feather treated with Metanil Yellow taken at a range of magnifications and in backscattered electron mode. Both flighted feather (**a,b**) and bamboo-like structures (**c,d**) are shown. (Examples of extraneous material, which may be aggregations of the dye, are circled in red).

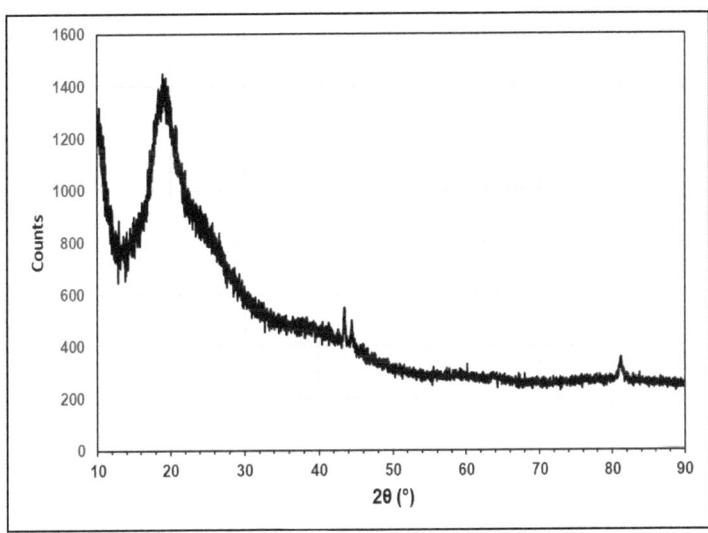

Figure 3. XRD pattern of pressed Hen Feather.

The FTIR spectrum of the Hen Feather is presented in Figure 4a. Previous studies [17] have shown that the FTIR spectra of Hen Feather and of pure keratin are very similar, indicating a high content of the latter in the former. The spectrum presented here is consistent with this. The main peaks are reported to relate to the peptide bonds in the keratin (-CONH) and have been labelled according to the convention as Amides A, I, II and III. The band at ~3270 cm^{-1} can be due to stretching vibrations of O–H and N–H and is known as Amide A. The band is at 1630 cm^{-1} (labelled as Amide I) and relates to a C=O stretch. The band at 1520 cm^{-1} (Amide II) is due to a C–H stretch and N–H bend, while the band at ~1230 cm^{-1} is a combination of several vibrations (C=O bend, C–C stretch, N–H bend and C–N stretch) and is labelled Amide III. Amide A is reported to relate to the α-helix structure of keratin; Amide II to the β-sheet structure; and Amide III to the combination of both of these structures. On this basis, both structures must be present in this Hen Feather sample. The spectra of Hen Feather after treatment with MY, and of pure crystalline MY are present in Figure 4b,c, respectively. The major vibrational bands assigned for MY by Dhakal et al. [7] are labelled on Figure 4c. Notable among these are the N-H stretch (3412, 3294 cm^{-1}), aromatic C-H stretch (~3020 cm^{-1}), stretching modes of the azo group, N=N, (1595, 1435 cm^{-1}), the stretch of the neighbouring C-N$_{azo}$ bonds (1045 cm^{-1}) and the S=O stretch (1339 cm^{-1}) of the sulfonic acid group on MY. In the MY-treated Hen Feather material, the Amide bands for the O-H/N-H, C=O and C-O bonds appear at the same frequencies as for the untreated sample. This suggests that the extensive hydrogen bonding present between carbonyl and the N atom in the keratin, which is a major component of Hen Feather, is not significantly changed by the addition of the dye. However, it should be noted that the relative intensity of the C-O peak at 1066 cm^{-1} does increase significantly. The dye was added to the Hen Feather by soaking it in an acidic solution of MY (pH 2), followed by drying. This may cause protonation of a proportion of the amide carbonyl species, giving a larger concentration in the enol form [20], resulting in a higher concentration of singly bonded C-O than before treatment with the MY solution.

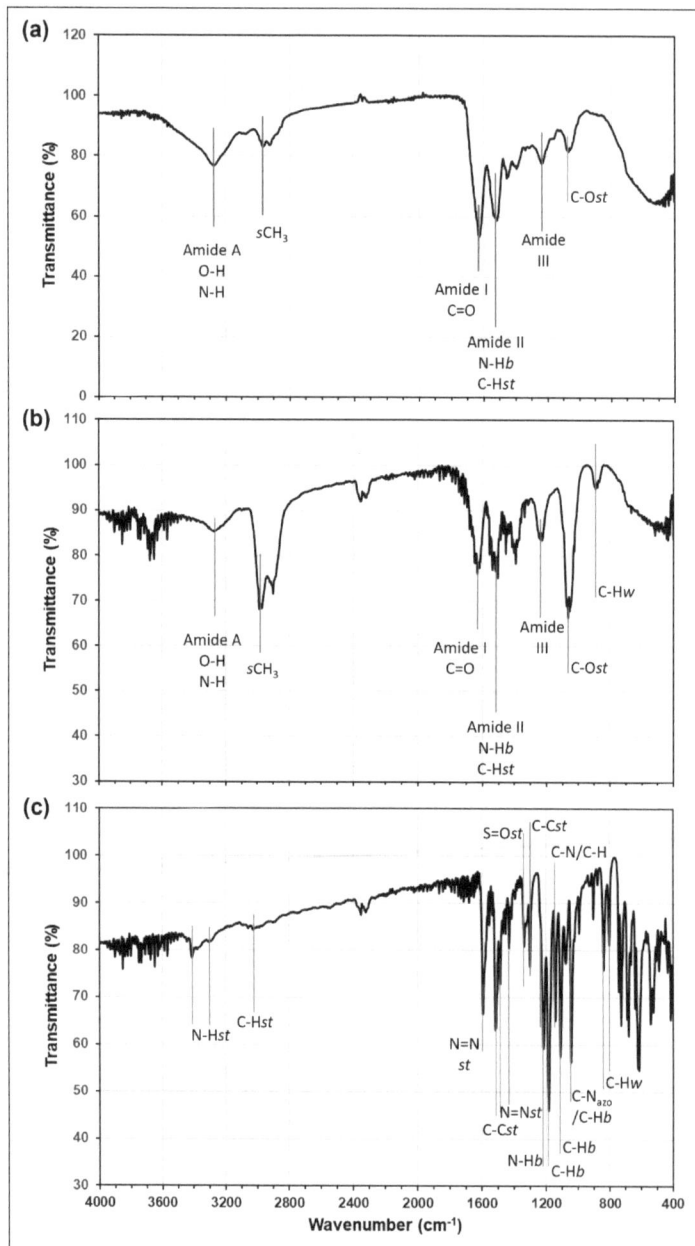

Figure 4. Fourier transform infra-red spectrum of (**a**) Hen Feather. (**b**) Hen Feather treated with MY solution (pH 2.0) and dried and (**c**) pure crystalline MY (sCH$_3$: symmetric mode of CH$_3$ Ion, *b*: bend and *st*: stretch).

XPS spectra of the Hen Feather sample are presented in Figure 5. The atomic surface composition of the sample was determined to be 85.4% C, 11.1% O, 2.9% N and 0.72% S. This is consistent with Hen Feather consisting predominantly of the polypeptide; keratin, which contains –CONH– linkages between amino acid units; and –S–S cross-linking. No charging of the sample was evident. The main C 1s peak at 284.5 eV is consistent with C–C and C–H environments. The small peak at 287.6 eV would match C in C=O groups, while another small peak at low binding energy—281.8 eV—is an artifact due to the use of charge compensation in the XPS instrument and can be ignored. The single peak for N 1s at 399.6 eV can be confidently attributed to N in amide groups, –N(C=O)–C–, which are very common in keratin. The main O 1s peak is consistent with C=O groups, while the smaller peak at 529.5 eV matches the C-O environment, which is present in some amino acids. In the S 2p region, the single peak seen should be attributed to electron-rich S environments such as S^{2-} or S_2^{2-} groups. This agrees with the known presence of –S–S– cross-linkages in keratin and Hen Feather.

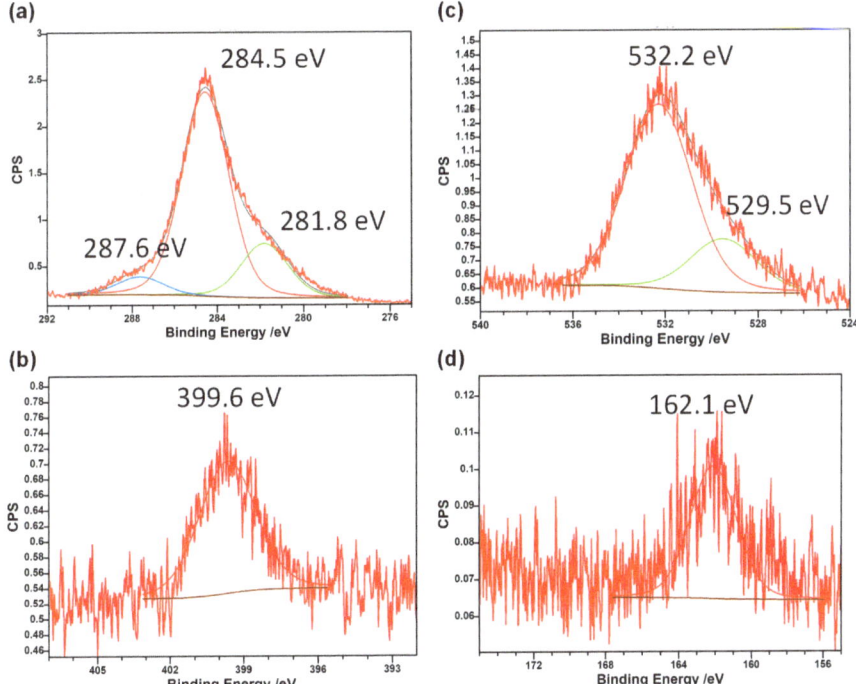

Figure 5. X-ray photoelectron spectra of Hen Feather at (**a**) C 1s, (**b**) N 1s, (**c**) O 1s and (**d**) S 2p regions.

Standard chemical methods [21] were applied to analyze the Hen Feather, and the sample was found to contain a maximum of about 82% of protein, while other components like fat, ash, crude fibre, available Lysine, Methionine and Cysteine each were almost less than 2%. The approximate results of the ultimate analysis of Hen Feathers are carbon (64.5%), nitrogen (10.5%), oxygen (22%) and sulphur (3%). The porosity (74%) density (0.3834 g·m^{-3}) and surface area (1170.6 cm^2·g^{-1}) of the Hen Feathers were determined by standard methods.

2.2. Preliminary Adsorption Studies

2.2.1. Influence of pH

To measure the effect of pH on the dye removal, 2×10^{-5} M MY was taken in 10 different flasks. The pH of each flask was maintained from 1.0 to 11.0. Figure 6 indicates that the highest dye uptake of about 99% was obtained at pH 2.0, and with increasing pH dye uptake, decreases almost linearly to about 45% at pH 11.0. Since the highest adsorption is achieved at pH 2.0, this pH was selected to carry out all subsequent studies.

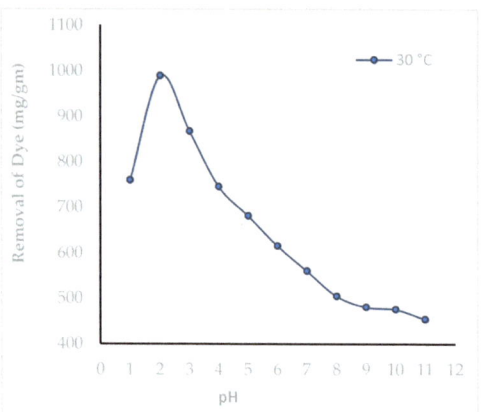

Figure 6. Influence of pH on the adsorptive removal of the dye Metanil Yellow over Hen Feathers (initial dye concentration: 2×10^{-5} M, adsorbent dosage: 0.05 g/20 mL, contact time: 75 min).

In the strong acidic medium at pH 2.0, electrostatic attraction of deprotonated MY and protonated HF results in the strong adsorption of MY over HF. With increasing pH, weaker electrostatic attraction force develops, which reduces the dye removal [22,23].

In order to determine the nature of the Hen Feathers, its weighed quantities (0.05, 0.10, 0.20, 0.30, 0.40 and 0.50 g) were dipped in 25 mL of distilled water (pH = 7.0), and the mixtures were taken in six 100 mL airtight measuring flasks. After almost 24 h, each mixture was filtered, and the pHs of the filtrates were recorded. It is interesting to note that each sample exhibited an increase in pH, thereby indicating the basic nature of Hen Feathers.

2.2.2. Influence of Biosorbent Dosage

Adsorption studies were performed by adding 0.01 to 0.15 g of Hen Feathers to a dye solution of concentration 2×10^{-5} M and pH 2. After agitating the solution for 75 min, the uptake of MY was monitored, and the results obtained are presented in Figure 7. It is found that initially, the percentage removal of MY increases with increasing amounts of Hen Feathers in the solution, and the highest dye uptake was recorded at a biosorbent amount of 0.05 g. Beyond this value, the dye uptake was constant. An increase in the dye adsorption is due to the availability of large numbers of binding sites; 0.05 g HF may be the reason for the increased adsorption of MY.

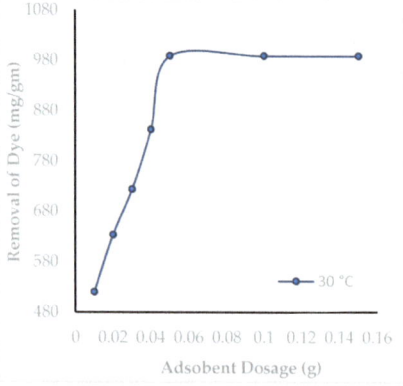

Figure 7. Influence of Hen Feather dosage on the adsorptive removal of Metanil Yellow (pH: 2, initial dye concentration: 2×10^{-5} M, contact time: 75 min).

2.2.3. Influence of Adsorbate Concentration

The effect of MY concentration on its removal at different temperatures was observed at pH 2.0 and by adding 0.05 g of Hen Feathers. At each temperature, the percentage removal increased linearly and attained a plateau at 2×10^{-5} M dye concentration. The increase in the amount of the MY with an increase in concentration may be due to large numbers of available binding sites of the biosorbent, but at dye concentrations around 2×10^{-5} M and above, the binding sites become almost saturated. Thus, the percentage removal of the dye attains almost a fixed value at each temperature.

2.2.4. Influence of Contact Time

To measure the effect of time of contact of MY and Hen Feather, their solutions were thoroughly agitated at different time periods (Figure 8). Figure 8 shows that 75 min are sufficient to attain equilibrium of adsorption of the MY–Hen Feather. Figure 8 clearly indicates that the proportion of MY adsorption increases steadily from a contact time of 15 to 75 min and then starts stabilizing due to coverage of the Hen Feather by MY.

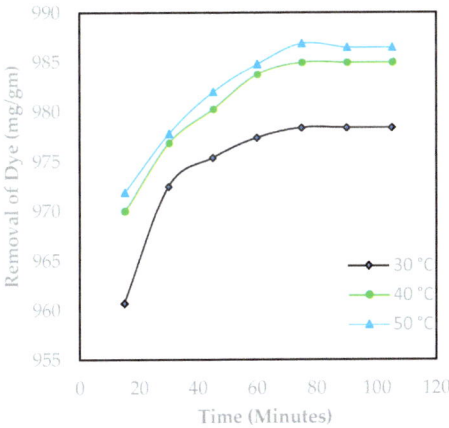

Figure 8. Influence of contact time on the adsorptive removal of Metanil Yellow over Hen Feathers (pH: 2.0, initial dye concentration: 2×10^{-5} M, adsorbent dosage: 0.05 g/20 mL).

2.3. Adsorption Isotherm Studies

Adsorption isotherms provide a great deal of information on the interaction in the adsorbate–adsorbent system, particularly adsorption behaviour, binding energy, thermodynamic parameters and nature of adsorption. Here, Langmuir, Freundlich, Temkin and Dubinin–Radushkevtich adsorption isotherms were all examined. The theory and other details regarding each adsorption isotherm are well documented in the literature [24,25]. In each case, experiments were performed by varying dye concentration and temperature and keeping the optimum values of other parameters as determined in the previous section.

2.3.1. Langmuir Adsorption Isotherm

It is well known that in the year 1916, Irving Langmuir postulated an experimental isotherm model. The model is helpful in establishing monolayer adsorption over homogeneous surfaces and in providing values of different thermodynamic parameters like change in Gibb's free energy ($\Delta G°$), enthalpy ($\Delta H°$), entropy ($\Delta S°$), etc., during the adsorption process. The linear form of the Langmuir adsorption isotherm model can be expressed as

$$\frac{1}{q_e} = \frac{1}{q_o} + \frac{1}{bq_o c_e} \qquad (1)$$

The amount of adsorbate adsorbed at equilibrium (mg·g^{-1}) is denoted by q_e, C_e denotes the dye's equilibrium molar concentration (mg·L^{-1}), q_o is the adsorbent's maximum adsorption capacity per unit mass (mg·g^{-1}) and b is the Langmuir constant (L·mg^{-1}). Graphs of $1/C_e$ versus $1/q_e$, plotted for different temperatures, give straight lines with regression coefficients close to unity (Figure 9). This indicates that the data obtained follow the Langmuir isotherm model, and the monolayer adsorption of the dye, MY, takes place over the homogeneous surface of Hen Feathers at all temperatures studied. The values of Langmuir adsorption constant 'b' are given in Table 1 and decreases with increase in temperature. High values of 'b' indicate strong interaction between MY and Hen Feather. However, with increasing temperatures, the value of 'b' decreases, thereby indicating weaker adsorption at higher temperatures.

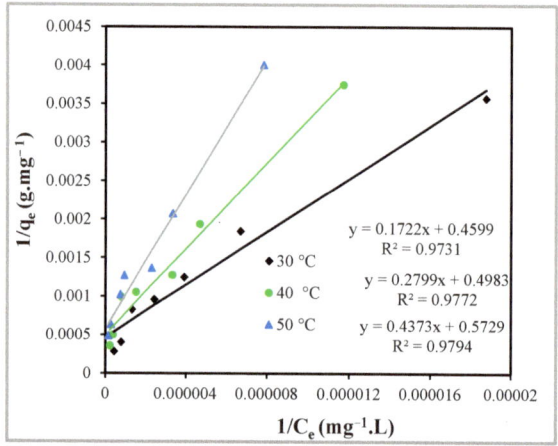

Figure 9. Langmuir adsorption isotherms at the temperatures indicated for the adsorption of Metanil Yellow over Hen Feathers at pH = 2.

Table 1. Values of various isotherm constants for the uptake of Metanil Yellow by Hen Feathers at the indicated temperatures.

Parameter	Langmuir Adsorption Isotherm		
	Temperature (°C)		
	30	40	50
$q_o \times 10^3$ (mg·g^{-1})	2.17	2.01	1.75
b (L·mg^{-1})	2.67	1.78	1.31
R^2	0.9731	0.9772	0.9794
Freundlich Adsorption Isotherm			
K_f (mol·g^{-1})	0.10	0.70	0.62
n	1.51	1.81	1.95
R^2	0.9809	0.9563	0.9364
Dubinin–Radushkevtich Adsorption Isotherm			
$X_m \times 10^{-2}$ (mol·g^{-1})	9.74	3.74	2.19
$b \times 10^{-9}$ (L·mol^{-1})	4.00	3.00	3.00
E (kJ mol^{-1})	11.18	12.91	12.91
R^2	0.9748	0.9564	0.9639

The values of 'b' were applied to evaluate a dimensionless separation factor (r), which is helpful in establishing the favourability of the ongoing adsorption process. The values of 'r' can be evaluated using the following equation:

$$r = \frac{1}{1 + bC_o} \quad (2)$$

Here, b and C_o have the same meanings as described above. At temperatures 30, 40 and 50 °C, the values of 'r' are found to be 0.047, 0.069 and 0.092. Since these values all fall between 0 and 1, the adsorption of MY over Hen Feathers can be considered a favourable process.

2.3.2. Freundlich Adsorption Isotherm

The Freundlich adsorption isotherm is related to multilayer formation over a heterogeneous surface and is mathematically expressed by the following expression:

$$\log q_e = \log k_f + \left(\frac{1}{n}\right) \log C_e \quad (3)$$

Here, k_f and n are the Freundlich constants, determined by the intercept and slope, respectively, C_e (mol·L^{-1}) is the equilibrium concentration and q_e (mol·g^{-1}) is the equilibrium capacity of the adsorbent.

To verify the applicability of the Freundlich adsorption isotherm model, graphs of log C_e versus log q_e were plotted (Figure 10). Figure 10 exhibits that straight lines with negative intercepts and regression coefficients close to unity were obtained at all temperatures. This indicates the adsorption of the dye MY over Hen Feathers can follow a multilayer formation even at low concentrations. Table 1 presents the values of various Freundlich constants.

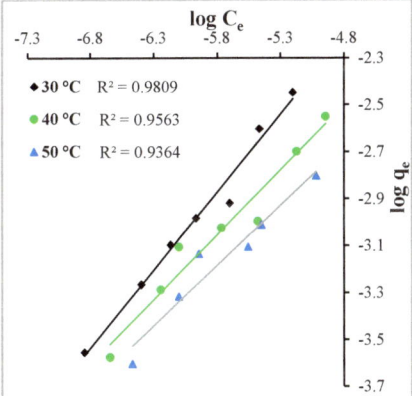

Figure 10. Freundlich adsorption isotherms at the temperatures indicated for the adsorption of Metanil Yellow over Hen Feather at pH = 2.

2.3.3. Dubinin–Radushkevtich Adsorption Isotherm

The Dubinin–Radushkevtich (DR) adsorption isotherm model is helpful in diagnosing adsorption behaviour, specifically whether the adsorbing molecules are undergoing chemisorption or physisorption. The following is the linear form of the DR adsorption isotherm model:

$$\ln C_{ads} = \ln X_m - \beta \in^2 \quad (4)$$

where C_{ads} (mol·g^{-1}), X_m (mol·g^{-1}) and β (mol^2·J^{-2}) are the amount of MY adsorbed per unit weight of Hen Feathers, the maximum adsorption capacity of Hen Feathers and the activity coefficient related to the mean adsorption energy, respectively. The Polanyi potential ($\in$) is given as

$$\epsilon = RT \cdot \ln\left(1 + \frac{1}{C_e}\right) \quad (5)$$

where T is the Kelvin temperature, and R (8.314 J·mol^{-1}K^{-1}) is the Gas Constant. The graph of ϵ^2 vs. lnC$_{ads}$ is presented in Figure 11. The straight lines depict regression coefficient values of near unity at all temperatures, indicating that the DR adsorption model can be applied in the ongoing adsorption process (Table 1). To ascertain whether the process is physisorption or chemisorption, mean sorption energy (E) was calculated using the following relationship:

$$E = \frac{1}{\sqrt{-2\beta}} \quad (6)$$

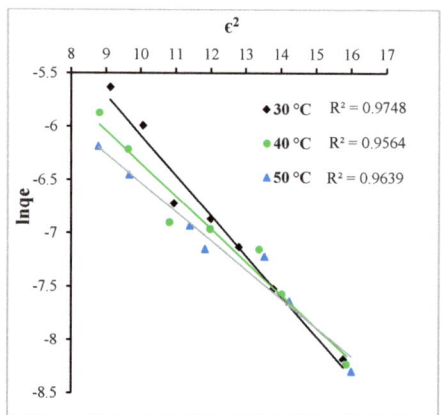

Figure 11. Dubinin–Radushkevitch adsorption isotherms at the temperatures indicated for the adsorption of Metanil Yellow over Hen Feathers at pH = 2.

Hutson and Yang [26] determined that for any adsorbate–adsorbent system, if the value of 'E' is less than 8 kJ·mol^{-1}, physisorption dominates, while a value between 8 and 16 kJ·mol^{-1} ascertains the chemisorption process. Due to values of more than 8 kJ/mol at all temperatures, it can be safely interpreted that the ongoing adsorption is chemisorption only.

2.3.4. Thermodynamic Parameters

The measurement of thermodynamic parameters is crucial for determining the process's viability and feasibility as well as for understanding the effect of temperature on MY adsorption. Using Equations (7) to (9), values of $\Delta G°$, $\Delta H°$ and $\Delta S°$ associated with the ongoing adsorption process were calculated (Table 2).

$$\Delta G° = -RT\ln b \quad (7)$$

$$\Delta H° = -R\left(\frac{T_2 T_1}{T_2 - T_1}\right) \times \ln\left(\frac{b_2}{b_1}\right) \quad (8)$$

$$\Delta S° = \frac{\Delta H° - \Delta G°}{T} \quad (9)$$

The negative values of $\Delta G°$ indicate that the process of adsorption of MY on Hen Feathers is feasible, while the positive values of ΔH confirm the endothermic nature of the adsorption. Similarly, by using Equation (9), it is ascertained that entropy ($\Delta S°$) is positive, thereby indicating an increased randomness at the MY–Hen Feather interface with minor structural changes in the Hen Feather.

Table 2. Values of various thermodynamic parameters for the uptake of the dye Metanil Yellow by Hen Feathers at the indicated temperatures.

Parameter	Temperature (°C)		
	30	40	50
$-\Delta G°$ (kJ·mol^{-1})	2.47	1.50	0.73
$\Delta H°$ (kJ·mol^{-1})	31.98	25.78	12.48
$\Delta S°$ (J·K^{-1}mol^{-1})	113.71	90.03	43.57

2.4. Kinetic Studies

In the kinetic studies, the rate and order of the adsorption process are calculated by monitoring the effect of contact time on the percentage removal of the dye. An amount of 0.05 g of Hen Feathers was added to a dye solution of 2×10^{-5} mole·L^{-1} concentration and pH 2.0 at fixed temperatures (30, 40 and 50 °C), and the flask was agitated on a mechanical shaker for a predetermined amount of time. To calculate the order of reaction, two well-established rate equations, namely Legergren's rate equation (Equation (10)) and the Ho–McKay rate equation (Equation (11)) for pseudo-first-order and pseudo-second-order reactions, respectively, were applied [27,28].

$$\log(q_e - q_t) = \log q_e - \frac{k_1}{2.303} \times t \qquad (10)$$

$$\frac{t}{q_t} = \frac{1}{k_2 q_e^2} + \frac{t}{q_e} \qquad (11)$$

Here, q_e (mol·g^{-1}), q_t (mol·g^{-1}), k_1 (min^{-1}) and k_2 (g·mol^{-1}·min^{-1}) are the amount adsorbed at equilibrium, amount adsorbed at time 't', pseudo-first-order rate constant and pseudo-second-order rate constant, respectively.

To establish an order of ongoing adsorption, using Equation (10), a plot of time vs. log($q_e - q_t$) and using Equation (11), a graph of time versus t/q_t was plotted (Figures 12 and 13). It is clear from Figure 13 that the values of the regression coefficients of the straight lines obtained at all three temperatures are close to unity, while in Figure 12, the lines obtained have low regression coefficient values. Thus, it can be safely interpreted that pseudo-second-order rate kinetics are operative in the MY adsorption over Hen Feather, and the rate constants of the reaction (k_2) are 2.933×10^4, 1.40×10^3 and 2.41×10^3 (L·mol^{-1} s^{-1}) at 30, 40 and 50 °C, respectively.

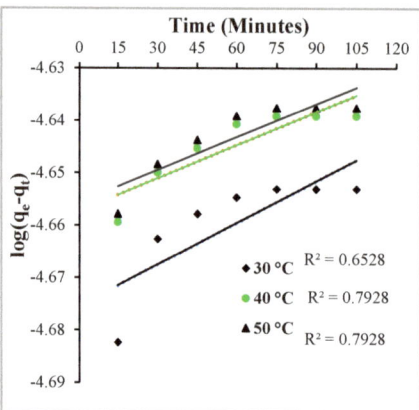

Figure 12. Legergren's plot for the adsorption of Metanil Yellow over Hen Feathers at the indicated temperatures.

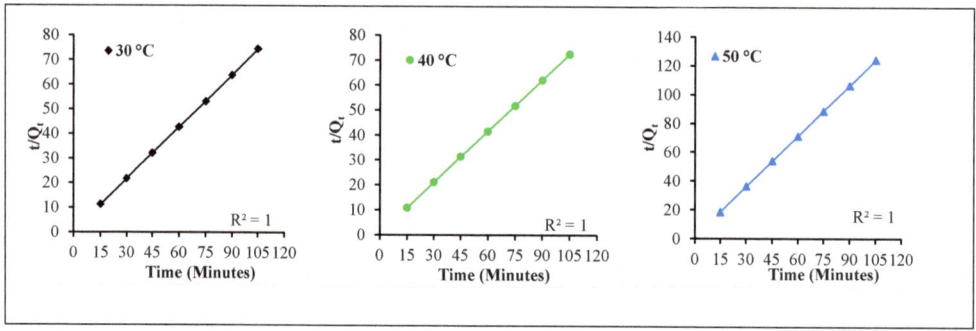

Figure 13. Ho and McKay's plot for the adsorption of Metanil Yellow over Hen Feathers at the indicated temperatures.

2.5. Mechanism of MY Adsorption over Hen Feathers

With the results mentioned above, it can be determined that the azo dye MY adsorbs over Hen Feathers via chemisorption. First, a uniform monolayer is formed, which can extend to form multilayers. The FTIR spectrum of MY-treated Hen Feather in Figure 5 confirms the presence of N=N, N–H and S=O bonds. In acidic media, the azo bond would be expected to be protonated to give the –HN$^+$=N– bond. On the other hand, FT-IR studies of the Hen Feather indicate the presence of amide linkages containing C=O and N–H bonds, and these are known to hydrogen bond to form keratin sheets in feathers. The adsorption isotherm studies and evaluated thermodynamic parameters clearly indicate that the adsorption of MY over Hen Feathers undergoes a spontaneous chemisorption process with strong interactions. Therefore, it can be determined that chemical bond formation (chemisorption) will take place between the N–H, azo groups and the sulfonyl species of the MY molecule and the C=O and N-R groups of the Hen Feathers. The presence of these bonds on the MY molecules and keratin structures would be expected to give rise to strong bond formation.

3. Experimental

3.1. Material and Methods

MY (Figure 14) is an azo dye containing the –N=N– group. The IUPAC name of MY ($C_8H_{15}N_3NaO_3S$) is sodium 3–[4anilinophenyl)diazinyl]benzene sulfonate. It is a yellow water-soluble dye with a molecular weight of 376.39 and a melting point of >250 °C. AR-grade MY was procured from M/s Merck. All working solutions of MY were prepared in double-distilled water after diluting its 1 M stock solution. The pH of the working solutions was adjusted using HCl and NaOH.

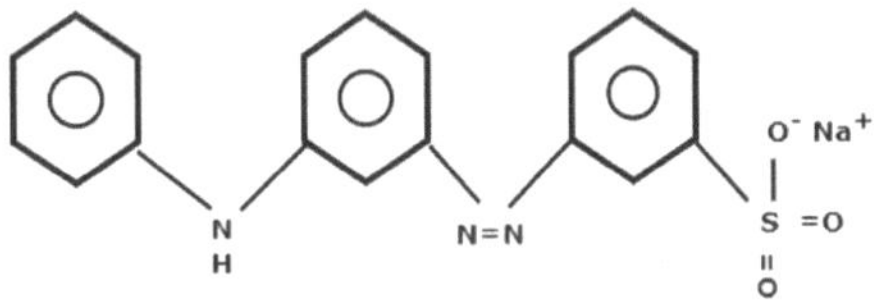

Figure 14. Chemical structure of Metanil Yellow.

The biosorbent Hen Feathers were obtained from local poultry farmers. The feathers were washed and activated before use. The characterization of Hen Feathers was carried out using a range of techniques. SEM photographs were obtained using a JEOL JSM-IT200 instrument (JEOL UK Ltd., Welwyn Garden City, UK) operating at 10 kV at a working distance of 10 mm in both secondary electron and backscattered electron modes. XRD patterns of Hen Feathers were collected on a PANalytical Empyrean instrument (Malvern Panalytical, Malvern, UK) using Cu K_{a1} radiation (1.5406 Å) in reflection mode over a 2θ range of 10–90°. XPS was carried out on a Scienta XPS spectrometer (Scienta Omicron, Uppsala, Sweden) with a monochromatic source. Using a Shimadzu IRAffinity 1S spectrometer (Kyoto, Japan), FTIR spectra were obtained over the range of 400–4000 cm^{-1}.

To carry out all adsorption studies, a water bath shaker (RSB-12) of M/s Remi (Mumbai, India) a microprocessor-based pH system (model no. 1013) of M/s ESICO (Parwanoo, India) and a double-beam spectrophotometer (M/s ESICO India) were used.

3.2. Development of Biosorbent

Hen Feathers were obtained from local poultry. These were dirty and stained in blood. Therefore, these were first cleaned with water and detergent several times. Using double-distilled water, the washed material was further rinsed. In order to remove adhering organic impurities, the feathers were kept in H_2O_2 solution for about 24 h. The material was once again submerged in double-distilled water overnight. The Hen Feathers thus obtained were dried in a hot air oven at 80 °C. Using a pair of sharp scissors, the barbs and barbules of the Hen Feathers were first separated from the shaft and cut down to very small pieces typically 1 mm in length. The material thus obtained was stored in a desiccator.

A three-step batch adsorption study was performed, which included preliminary investigations, adsorption isotherm studies and kinetic studies. Firstly, to assess the optimum values of the parameters pH, biosorbent dosage, adsorbate concentration and contact time to remove MY from its aqueous solutions, preliminary investigations were carried out. Then, adsorption isotherm studies were carried out in a wide range of dye concentrations with appropriate amounts of Hen Feather at three different temperatures (30, 40 and 50 °C) and recording uptake of the dye. To evaluate kinetic parameters, the adsorption was monitored at different time intervals.

In each batch experiment, 20 mL of the known concentration and pH of MY was taken in a well-stoppered 100 mL flask and mixed thoroughly with the chosen amount of biosorbent (Hen Feather) at a constant temperature (30, 40 and 50 °C) and shaking speed (150 rpm) for a specific time interval. The solution was then filtered, and its absorbance was recorded at a fixed wavelength (λ_{max} = 425 nm) using the ultraviolet–visible spectrophotometer to evaluate the percentage removal of the dye.

4. Conclusions

The present paper focuses on the efficacy of Hen Feathers, a waste material, which is easily available in very large quantities and can be used as an adsorbent in aqueous media without compromising the cleanliness of the water. Hen Feathers are a type of biosorbent that can be successfully and directly used without any structural alteration and exhibit effective removal of dyes. The data provided in this paper demonstrate how effective Hen Feathers are at absorbing the dye MY. Furthermore, the interpretation of these data by reference to a range of appropriate adsorption models provides detailed information relevant to evaluating the practicality, cost-effectiveness and environmental friendliness of Hen Feathers for the adsorption of MY. The best adsorption of the dye can be achieved at pH 2.0. As a result, it can be safely stated that Hen Feathers are an effective and cheap waste material for the eradication of MY from its aqueous solutions.

Author Contributions: Conceptualization, J.M., A.M. and B.G.; methodology, B.G. and S.A.A.S.; validation, A.M., J.M. and R.T.B.; formal analysis, B.G.; investigation, B.G. and J.M.; writing—original draft preparation, B.G. and R.T.B.; writing—review and editing, J.M. and A.M.; supervision, A.M., J.M. and R.T.B.; project administration, A.M. and R.T.B. funding acquisition, A.M. All authors have read and agreed to the published version of the manuscript.

Funding: Ministry of Human Resource Development (Presently Ministry of Education) of the Government of India via the SPARC initiative (project: SPARC/2018-2019/P307/SL).

Institutional Review Board Statement: Not applicable.

Informed Consent Statement: Not applicable.

Data Availability Statement: Data are contained within the article.

Acknowledgments: The authors are grateful to the Ministry of Human Resource Development (Presently Ministry of Education) of the Government of India for financial support via the SPARC initiative. One of the authors (Bharti Gaur) is thankful to MANIT, Bhopal, for providing fellowship support. XPS experiments were performed at the XPS Facility, University of St Andrews. Electron microscopy was carried out at the Electron Microscopy Facility, University of St Andrews, and we acknowledge recent funding for the Facility from the EPSRC and the EPSRC Strategic Resources Grant [EP/L017008/1, EP/R023751/1 and EP/T019298/1].

Conflicts of Interest: The authors declare no conflict of interest.

References

1. Schweitzer, L.; Noblet, J. Water contamination and pollution. In *Green Chemistry: An Inclusive Approach*; Torok, B., Dransfield, T., Eds.; Elsevier Inc.: Amsterdam, The Netherlands, 2018; pp. 261–290. [CrossRef]
2. Droste, R.L. *Theory and Practice of Water and Wastewater Treatment*; John Wiley and Sons Inc.: Hoboken, NJ, USA, 1997.
3. Zollinger, H. *Synthesis, Properties and Applications of Organic Dyes and Pigments, Color Chemistry*, 2nd ed.; VCH: New York, NY, USA, 1991.
4. Ramakrishna, K.R.; Viraraghavan, T. Dye removal using low cost adsorbent. *Water Sci. Technol.* **1997**, *36*, 189–196. [CrossRef]
5. Franklin, L.B. *Wastewater Engineering: Treatment, Disposal and Reuse*; McGraw Hill Inc.: New York, NY, USA, 1991.
6. Chung, K.T. Azo dyes and human health: A review. *J. Environ. Sci. Health C Environ. Carcinog. Ecotoxicol. Rev.* **2016**, *34*, 233–261. [CrossRef] [PubMed]
7. Dhakal, S.; Chao, K.; Schmidt, W.; Qin, J.; Kim, M.; Chan, D. Evaluation of turmeric powder adulterated with Metanil Yellow using FT-Raman and FT-IR Spectroscopy. *Foods* **2016**, *5*, 36. [CrossRef] [PubMed]
8. Mittal, J. Permissible synthetic food dyes in India. Resonance. *J. Sci. Edu.* **2020**, *25*, 567–577. [CrossRef]
9. Hazra, S.; Dome, R.N.; Ghosh, S.; Ghosh, D. Protective effect of methanolic leaves extract of coriandrum sativum against metanil yellow induced lipid peroxidation in goat liver: An in vitro study. *Intern. J. Pharmacol. Pharmaceut. Sci.* **2016**, *3*, 34–41.
10. Ramchandani, S.; Das, M.; Joshi, A.; Khanna, S.K. Effect of oral and parenteral administration of metanil yellow on some hepatic and intestinal biochemical parameters. *J. Appl. Toxicol.* **1997**, *17*, 85–91. [CrossRef]
11. Nagaraja, T.N.; Desiraju, T. Effects of chronic consumption of Metanil Yellow by developing and adult rats on brain regional levels of noradrenaline, dopamine and serotonin, on acetylcholine esterase activity and on operant conditioning. *Food Chem. Toxicol.* **1993**, *31*, 41–44. [CrossRef] [PubMed]
12. Nath, P.P.; Sarkar, K.; Mondal, M.; Paul, G. Metanil Yellow impairs the estrous cycle physiology and ovarian folliculogenesis in female rats. *Environ. Toxicol.* **2016**, *31*, 2057–2067. [CrossRef] [PubMed]
13. Islam, M.S.; Jhily, N.J.; Parvin, N.; Shampad, M.M.H.; Hossain, J.; Sarkar, S.C.; Rahman, M.M.; Islam, M.A. Dreadful practices of adulteration in food items and their worrisome consequences for public health: A review. *J. Food Saf. Hyg.* **2022**, *8*, 223–236. [CrossRef]
14. Brush, A.H. On the origin of feathers. *J. Evol. Biol.* **1996**, *9*, 131–142. [CrossRef]

15. Leeson, S.; Walsh, T. Feathering in commercial poultry II. Factors influencing feather growth and feather loss. *World's Poul. Sci. J.* **2004**, *60*, 52–63. [CrossRef]
16. Reddy, N.; Yang, Y. Structure and properties of chicken feather barbs as natural protein fibers. *J. Environ. Polym. Degrad.* **2007**, *15*, 81–87. [CrossRef]
17. Ma, B.; Qiao, X.; Hou, X.; Yang, Y. Pure keratin membrane and fibers from chicken feather. *Intern. J. Biol. Macromol.* **2016**, *89*, 614–621. [CrossRef]
18. Idris, A.; Vijayaraghavan, R.; Rana, U.A.; Fredericks, D.; Patti, A.F.; MacFarlane, D.R. Dissolution of feather keratin in ionic liquids. *Green Chem.* **2013**, *15*, 525–534. [CrossRef]
19. Khosa, M.A.; Ullah, A. In-situ modification, regeneration, and application of keratin biopolymer for arsenic removal. *J. Hazard. Mater.* **2014**, *278*, 360–371. [CrossRef] [PubMed]
20. Li, Q.; Xue, Y.; Yan, G.S. Water-assisted enol-to-keto tautomerism of a simple peptide model: A computational investigation. *J. Mol. Struct. THEOCHEM* **2008**, *868*, 55–64. [CrossRef]
21. Tesfaye, T.; Sithole, B.; Ramjugernath, D.; Chuniall, V. Valorisation of chicken feathers: Characterisation of chemical properties. *Waste Manag.* **2017**, *68*, 626–635. [CrossRef]
22. Mittal, J.; Maiyam, A.; Sakina, F.; Baker, R.T.; Sharma, A.K.; Mittal, A. Efficient Batch and Fixed-Bed Sequestration of a basic dye using a novel variant of ordered mesoporous carbon as adsorbent. *Arabian J Chem.* **2021**, *14*, 103186. [CrossRef]
23. Mittal, J.; Maiyam, A.; Sakina, F.; Baker, R.T.; Sharma, A.K.; Mittal, A. Batch and bulk adsorptive removal of anionic dye using metal/halide-free ordered mesoporous carbon as adsorbent. *J. Clean. Prod.* **2021**, *321*, 129060. [CrossRef]
24. Adamson, A.W.; Gast, A.P. *Physical Chemistry of Surfaces*, 6th ed.; Wiley Interscience: Hoboken, NJ, USA, 1997.
25. Masel, R. *Principles of Adsorption and Reaction on Solid Surfaces*; Wiley Interscience: Hoboken, NJ, USA, 1996.
26. Hutson, N.D.; Yang, R.T. Theoretical basis for the Dubinin-Radushkevitch (D-R) adsorption isotherm equation. *Adsorption* **1997**, *3*, 189–195. [CrossRef]
27. Ho, Y.S.; McKay, G. Pseudo–second order model for sorption processes. *Process Biochem.* **1999**, *34*, 451–465. [CrossRef]
28. Unuabonah, E.I.; Adebowale, K.O.; Olu-Owolabi, B.I. Kinetic and thermodynamic studies of the adsorption of lead (II) ions onto phosphate-modified kaolinite clay. *J. Hazard. Mater.* **2007**, *144*, 386–395. [CrossRef] [PubMed]

Disclaimer/Publisher's Note: The statements, opinions and data contained in all publications are solely those of the individual author(s) and contributor(s) and not of MDPI and/or the editor(s). MDPI and/or the editor(s) disclaim responsibility for any injury to people or property resulting from any ideas, methods, instructions or products referred to in the content.

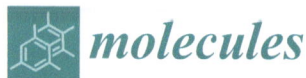

Article

Fabrication of Loose Nanofiltration Membrane by Crosslinking TEMPO-Oxidized Cellulose Nanofibers for Effective Dye/Salt Separation

Shasha Liu [1], Mei Sun [1], Can Wu [1], Kaixuan Zhu [1], Ying Hu [1], Meng Shan [1], Meng Wang [1], Kai Wu [1], Jingyi Wu [1], Zongli Xie [2,*] and Hai Tang [1,*]

[1] School of Chemical and Environmental Engineering, Anhui Polytechnic University, Wuhu 241000, China; liushasha@ahpu.edu.cn (S.L.); 2230621105@stu.ahpu.edu.cn (M.S.); wucancz@163.com (C.W.); kaixuan0080@163.com (K.Z.); huying@ahpu.edu.cn (Y.H.); 2220630110@stu.ahpu.edu.cn (M.S.); wm18855372043@163.com (M.W.); 13955064236@163.com (K.W.); wujingyi0602@163.com (J.W.)
[2] CSIRO Manufacturing, Private Bag 10, Clayton South, VIC 3169, Australia
* Correspondence: zongli.xie@csiro.au (Z.X.); tanghai@ahpu.edu.cn (H.T.)

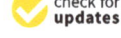

Citation: Liu, S.; Sun, M.; Wu, C.; Zhu, K.; Hu, Y.; Shan, M.; Wang, M.; Wu, K.; Wu, J.; Xie, Z.; et al. Fabrication of Loose Nanofiltration Membrane by Crosslinking TEMPO-Oxidized Cellulose Nanofibers for Effective Dye/Salt Separation. *Molecules* **2024**, *29*, 2246. https://doi.org/10.3390/molecules29102246

Academic Editor: Qingguo Shao

Received: 16 April 2024
Revised: 6 May 2024
Accepted: 8 May 2024
Published: 10 May 2024

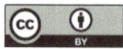

Copyright: © 2024 by the authors. Licensee MDPI, Basel, Switzerland. This article is an open access article distributed under the terms and conditions of the Creative Commons Attribution (CC BY) license (https://creativecommons.org/licenses/by/4.0/).

Abstract: Dye/salt separation has gained increasing attention in recent years, prompting the quest to find cost-effective and environmentally friendly raw materials for synthesizing high performance nanofiltration (NF) membrane for effective dye/salt separation. Herein, a high-performance loose-structured NF membrane was fabricated via a simple vacuum filtration method using a green nanomaterial, 2,2,6,6-tetramethylpiperidine-1-oxide radical (TEMPO)-oxidized cellulose nanofiber (TOCNF), by sequentially filtering larger-sized and finer-sized TOCNFs on a microporous substrate, followed by crosslinking with trimesoyl chloride. The resulting TCM membrane possessed a separating layer composed entirely of pure TOCNF, eliminating the need for other polymer or nanomaterial additives. TCM membranes exhibit high performance and effective dye/salt selectivity. Scanning Electron Microscope (SEM) analysis shows that the TCM membrane with the Fine-TOCNF layer has a tight layered structure. Further characterizations via Fourier transform infrared spectroscopy (FTIR) and X-ray diffraction (XRD) confirmed the presence of functional groups and chemical bonds of the crosslinked membrane. Notably, the optimized TCM-5 membrane exhibits a rejection rate of over 99% for various dyes (Congo red and orange yellow) and 14.2% for NaCl, showcasing a potential candidate for efficient dye wastewater treatment.

Keywords: TEMPO-oxidized cellulose nanofibers; nanofiltration membrane; dye/salt separation

1. Introduction

The rapid development of the global textile industry has heightened the urgency for treating dye wastewater and addressing environmental pollution [1]. Traditional methods for treating dye wastewater often face challenges such as low efficiency, high cost, and the generation of large amounts of by-products [2,3]. In the textile industry, the synthesis or application of dyes typically leads to the generation of high-salinity-dye wastewater [4]. The dye synthesis process yields a large amount of inorganic salt (i.e., ~5.0% NaCl) as a by-product, diminishing the dye's purity and reducing the brightness of the printed image in textile applications [5–7]. Discharging a large amount of salt along with dyes is the main issue in textile wastewater [8–10]. Therefore, effective treatment of textile wastewater is of great significance to mitigate the release of the highly polluted dye wastewater. Various approaches, including biotechnology and adsorption, have been applied to treat dye wastewater. However, most of these solutions face problems such as toxic nanomaterials leaching, limited flexibility, high cost, and complicated operating processes. Therefore, the identification of green materials and simple procedures is crucial to solving this problem.

Cellulose is a polysaccharide with a crystalline structure that is usually derived from abundant and renewable plants. As a member of the cellulose nanomaterial family, 2,2,6,6-tetramethylpiperidine-1-oxide radical (TEMPO)-oxidized cellulose nanofiber (TOCNF) is synthesized in a mild aqueous environment, followed by moderate mechanical treatment. Compared with other cellulose nanomaterials fabrication approaches, such as high-pressure homogenization and acid hydrolysis, the TEMPO-mediated oxidation method is more environmentally friendly. TOCNF has many advantages, such as a high surface-to-volume ratio, excellent mechanical stability, multi-functional surface groups, cost-effectiveness, and environmentally friendly characteristics [11]. TOCNF has made significant breakthroughs in the fields of adsorption and separation [12–15]. Through processing and functional modification of TOCNF, it can be applied to the preparation of nanofiltration (NF) or reverse osmosis (RO) membranes for dye wastewater treatment [16]. Due to its hydrogen-bonded parallel chains, TOCNF is a strong natural nanomaterial with a one-dimensional (1D) structure [17,18]. It can be combined with other two-dimensional (2D) nanomaterials to fabricate NF membranes [19,20]. Yang et al. [19] reported a mixed-dimensional NF membrane fabricated by assembling TOCNFs and covalent organic framework (COF) nanosheets. The prepared TOCNF/COF NF membrane exhibited outstanding hydrolytic stability and improved mechanical properties. Mohammed et al. [20] developed an NF membrane by incorporating graphene oxide (GO) nanosheets into the CNF matrix via the vacuum filtration method, followed by crosslinking by glutaraldehyde. The obtained GO/CNF mixed-dimensional NF membrane showed a pure solvent flux of 13.9 L m^{-2} h^{-1} bar^{-1} for water and over 90% rejections for two dyes.

Additionally, TOCNFs can serve as additives or substrates for thin composite NF/RO membrane [21–23]. Wang et al. [23] prepared a composite RO membrane with modified TOCNFs incorporated in a polyamide barrier layer based on an electrospun nanofibrous substrate. The inclusion of TOCNF improved both the flux and the rejection of the composite RO membrane and was attributed to the formation of external water channels caused by TOCNFs. In our previous work, TOCNFs were used as additives that were incorporated into the polyamide selective layer of the RO membrane to enhance the water flux and hydrophilicity of the membrane [22]. However, few researchers have focused on using pure TOCNF to fabricate a dense separating layer of an NF membrane.

Herein, we develop an environmentally friendly NF membrane with a hierarchical nanostructured TOCNF separating layer via a simple vacuum filtration method. Different diameters of TOCNFs were vacuum filtrated on polyvinylidene fluoride (PVDF) substrate membrane to form a dense NF membrane with a narrow pore size, which can effectively reject dyes. Specifically, Thick-TOCNFs (without probe ultrasonication) were vacuum-filtrated on the substrate membrane, followed by the addition of Fine-TOCNFs (with probe ultrasonication) to form a compact barrier layer of NF membrane. The Fine-TOCNFs served to further reduce the pore size of the composite membrane, consequently enhancing dye rejection rate. Furthermore, TMCs were used as a crosslinking agent to enhance the stability of the TOCNF layer. The morphology and physicochemical properties of the fabricated TOCNF NF membrane with different Fine-TOCNF concentrations were characterized, and their dye/salt separation performance was also evaluated compared with that of the neat Thick-TOCNF membrane. For better comparison, Fine-TOCNF membranes crosslinked with different concentrations of TMC were also synthesized. To the best of our knowledge, this work is the first study to use pure TOCNFs to fabricate the separating layer of NF membrane.

2. Result and Discussion

2.1. Morphology of TOCNFs and TCM Membranes

The morphologies of the Fine-TOCNFs and Thick-TOCNFs were observed by Transmission Electron Microscopy (TEM) (Figure 1). The length and diameter distributions of Fine-TOCNFs and Thick-TOCNFs are shown in Figure 1. The results show that the Thick-TOCNFs exhibit a long rod structure, while the Fine-TOCNFs show a shorter and finer rod structure. The length of Thick-TOCNFs is in the range of 300–1100 nm, and the average length is about 802 nm. The diameter of Thick-TOCNFs is 20.8 nm. After the probe ultrasonic treatment, the Fine-TOCNFs became shorter and thinner, the average length of Fine-TOCNFs reduced to 476 nm, and average width of Fine-TOCNFs decreased to 14.8 nm. The results show that compared to Thick-TOCNFs, Fine-TOCNFs became shorter and thinner, mainly due to the powerful probe ultrasonication, and thus the cellulose dispersed more evenly. In this study, Thick-TOCNFs without probe ultrasound were longer and were used to fill the big holes in the PVDF substrate membrane (pore size 220 nm). Then, Thin-TOCNFs were filtrated and crosslinked on the prefabricated membrane to form a denser layer, due to their finer diameter.

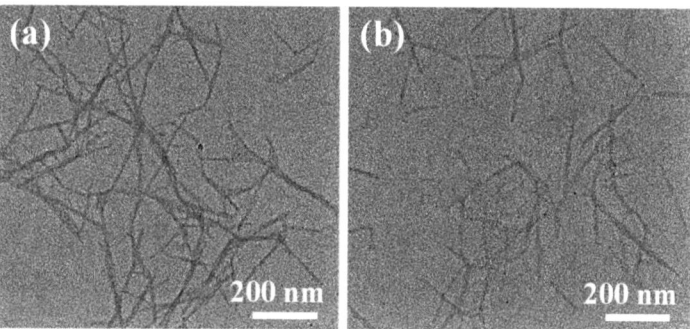

Figure 1. TEM images of (**a**) Thick-TOCNFs and (**b**) Fine-TOCNFs.

2.2. Characterization of Membranes

Figure 2 shows the Scanning Electron Microscope (SEM) surface morphology images of the PVDF substrate membrane, TCM-0 membrane (5 mL Thick-TOCNFs + 0 mL Fine-TOCNFs), TCM-5 membrane (5 mL Thick-TOCNFs + 5 mL Fine-TOCNFs), and TCM-10 membrane (5 mL Thick-TOCNFs + 10 mL Fine-TOCNFs). The average pore size of PVDF membrane is ~220 μm. Some huge pores (500~600 μm) are observed in Figure 2a, while the pore size of TCM-0 membrane (Figure 2b) became much smaller (the average pore size is ~30 nm). TCM-0 membrane was prepared by vacuum filtrating 5 mL on PVDF membrane. The Thick-TOCNFs were uniformly distributed on the surface of the PVDF membrane, with obviously reduced surface pore size. However, this pore size was still not small enough to reject the dye molecules. Therefore, Thick-TOCNFs have a great effect on narrowing the substrate pore size. Based on this Thick-TOCNFs-modified substrate, an additional 5 mL or 10 mL of Fine-TOCNFs was filtrated and followed by TMC crosslinking, by which the TCM-5 and TCM-10 membrane were obtained. Both TCM-5 and TCM-10 membranes exhibited a uniform and compact surface structure, which can provide a possibility to reject dyes. No obvious big pores could be observed in the TCM-5 and TCM-10 membranes under 50 k magnification. The pore sizes of TCM-5 and TCM-10 were about several nanometers.

Figure 3 shows a cross-sectional SEM image of the TCM membranes. Compared with the substrate membrane, TCM-0 membrane has an extra top layer (2.53 μm). As the content of Fine-TOCNFs increases, the thickness of the extra top layer of the composite membrane also increases. The top layer thicknesses of TCM-5 and TCM-10 are about 4.75 nm and 6.66 nm, respectively. This result indicates that more and more cellulose fibers assemble in the top layer with the increase in the Fine-TOCNFs concentration. Moreover, the image reveals that the top layers of TCM-5 and TCM-10 membranes are more compact, presenting a tight layered stacking structure. This is mainly due to the Fine-TOCNFs filling the pores of the Thick-TOCNFs layer, creating a denser separation layer. The compact top layer is beneficial for the high rejection rate of the membranes. The separation performance of TCM-0, TCM-5, and TCM-10 membranes shows that TCM-10 membrane possesses the highest rejection rate of Congo red (CR) dye.

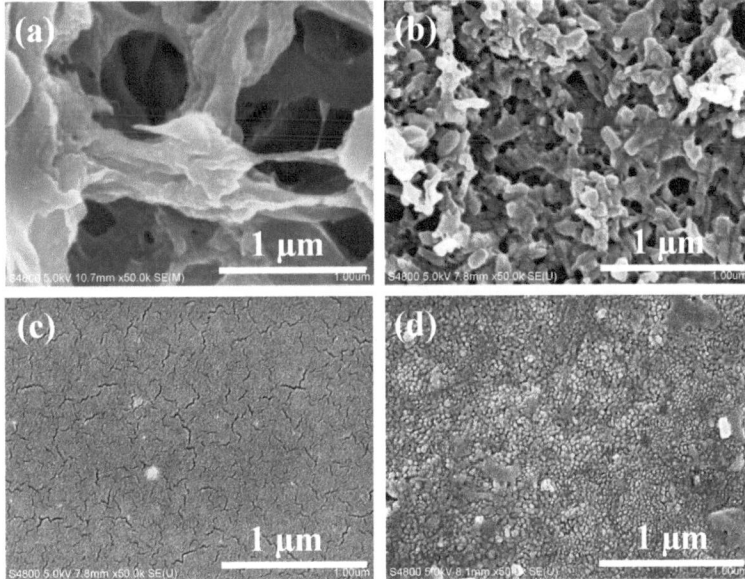

Figure 2. SEM images of membrane surface: (**a**) PVDF membrane, (**b**) TCM-0 membrane, (**c**) TCM-5 membrane, and (**d**) TCM-10 membrane.

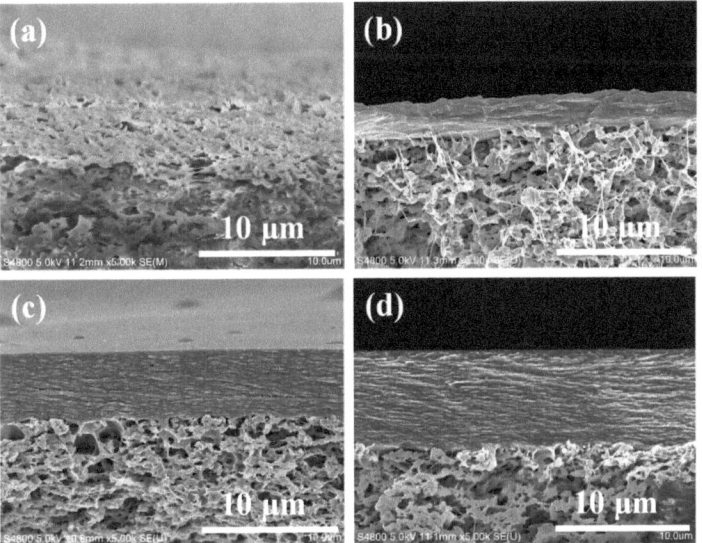

Figure 3. SEM images of membrane cross-sections: (**a**) PVDF membrane, (**b**) TCM-0 membrane, (**c**) TCM-5 membrane, and (**d**) TCM-10 membrane.

Figure 4a shows the Fourier transform infrared spectroscopy (FTIR) spectra of membrane samples, including the control (TOCNFs content equivalent to TCM-5 but without TMC crosslinking process), TCM-0 membrane, TCM-5 membrane, and TCM-10 membrane sample. The characteristic vibrational bands of TOCNFs are typically observed near 3322 cm^{-1} and 1024 cm^{-1}, corresponding to the hydroxyl and cyclic alcohol groups in CNFs, respectively [22]. Additionally, the vibrational band at 1605 cm^{-1} is the C=C ring stretching vibration. Compared to the Uncrosslinked membrane sample, all TOCNF membranes crosslinked with TMC (TCM-0, TCM-5, and TCM-10 membranes) exhibit an additional vibrational band at 1712 cm^{-1}, indicating the presence of the ester bond generated via the acylation reaction between the acyl chloride groups of the TMC and -OH groups of TOCNF [24]. This vibrational band confirms the successful crosslinking between TMC and TOCNFs on the membrane's surface. Furthermore, in comparison to the Uncrosslinked membrane without TMC crosslinking, the crosslinked membranes (TCM-0, TCM-5, and TCM-10 membranes) show lower transmittance vibrational bands near 3322 cm^{-1} and 1023 cm^{-1}, with the intensity of these two vibrational bands decreasing as the concentration of Fine-TOCNFs increases. This result suggests that the increase in -OH group concentration due to TOCNFs may increase the membrane hydrophilicity, while crosslinking agent TMC could weaken the membrane hydrophilicity.

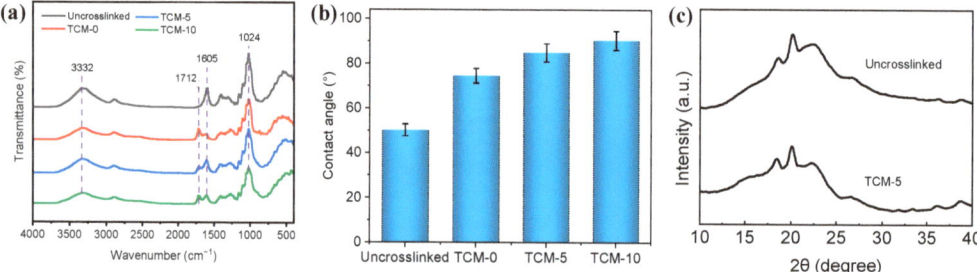

Figure 4. (**a**) FTIR, and (**b**) CA of Uncrosslinked, TCM-0, TCM-5, and TCM-10 membrane; (**c**) XRD of Uncrosslinked membrane and TCM-5 membrane.

Figure 4b shows the water contact angle of Uncrosslinked, TCM-0, TCM-5, and TCM-10 membrane samples. It can be seen that increasing the Fine-TOCNF content gradually weakens the hydrophilicity, which may be related to the increased hydrophobicity of TOCNF after TMC crosslinking. With the increase in TOCNF content, the crosslinked TOCNFs also increased, causing a slight increase in the contact angle, which was consistent with the infrared spectroscopy results.

The X-ray diffraction (XRD) patterns of TOCNF membrane before and after TMC crosslinking are shown in Figure 4c. The result shows similar peaks at 2θ = 18° and 20° for both the TOCNF membrane, with and without TMC crosslinking. However, the TOCNF membrane after TMC crosslinking shows a weaker peak at 2θ = 22.5°, corresponding to the (002) crystal plane of cellulose I [25]. This small difference may show that TMC crosslinking weakened the crystalline structure of TOCNF membrane.

2.3. The Performance of TCM Membranes

The effect of crosslinking agent (TMC) concentration on the pure water flux and Na$_2$SO$_4$ rejection performance of the composite membranes was investigated (Figure 5a). All of the membrane samples were prepared with the same method as the TCM-5 membrane sample, except for the crosslinking agent (TMC) concentration. Compared with the Uncrosslinked membrane, the membrane crosslinked with 0.1% TMC showed a decrease in pure water flux of the nanofiltration membrane from 24.87 L/m^2·h·bar to 13.89 L/m^2·h·bar, and the Na$_2$SO$_4$ rejection rate increased from 36.9% to 67.6%. This indicates an improvement in the membrane's rejection performance after TMC crosslinking, but a decrease in the water flux. This is mainly due to the consumption of hydrophilic carboxyl groups on the surface of the TMC crosslinked membrane, resulting in decreased hydrophilicity and reducing the rate of water molecule transport through the membrane, thereby decreasing the flux. With a further increase in TMC concentration, the flux slightly decreased, but the Na$_2$SO$_4$ rejection effect first increased and then decreased. This is mainly because the increase in TMC concentration helps to improve the crosslinking degree of TOCNFs and provides a denser surface, thus enhancing the membrane's rejection performance. However, a high crosslinking degree reduces the water flux, while the pore size sieving effect cannot further improve the Na_2SO_4 rejection rate. When the TOCNFs were not crosslinked with TMC, the structure formed by the hydrogen bonding between the TOCNFs was relatively loose and not strong. Therefore, when the TMC concentration was 0.3%, the nanofiltration membrane had an optimal rejection performance, with a Na_2SO_4 rejection rate of 75.5% and a pure water flux of 11.61 L/m²·h·bar.

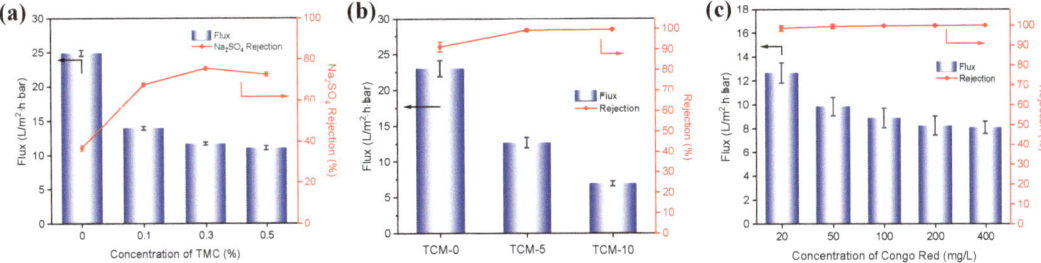

Figure 5. (a) The pure water flux and rejection of Na_2SO_4 solution (1000 ppm) of TCM membrane crosslinked with different TMC concentration. (b) The pure water flux and rejection of CR dye by TCM membranes with different Fine-TOCNF contents (TCM-0, TCM-5, TCM-10 membrane). (c) The flux and rejection of CR dye by the TCM-5 membrane at different concentrations.

The effect of the Fine-TOCNF content on the separation performance of TCM membranes can be seen in Figure 5b, where the flux decreases as the TOCNF content increases. As the SEM images (Figure 3) and contact anger test (Figure 4b) results show, with the increase in Fine-TOCNF content, the thickness of the top layer increases, and the hydrophilicity of the membranes decreases. Both the thicker selective layer and decreased hydrophilicity of the membrane may lead to more resistance for water molecules attempting to pass through the membrane. On the other hand, the rejection rate of CR increased rapidly after adding Fine-TOCNFs, and the CR rejection rate of TCM-5 membrane increased from 91.2% to 99.2% compared to TCM-0, and further increased to 99.7% for the TCM-10 membrane. This indicates that the dense pore structure produced by probe-ultrasound-treated TOCNF (Fine-TOCNF) has an excellent rejection effect on small-molecule dyes. The results show that by increasing the CNF content loaded on the membrane surface, the rejection rate of the membrane can be improved to a certain extent, but the flux decreases to a certain extent. TCM-5 membrane still has a rejection rate of 99.2% for CR while retaining a certain permeability performance (12.67 L/m²·h·bar).

The impact of different concentrations of CR on the performance of nanofiltration membranes was tested by adjusting the dye concentration from 20 to 400 ppm (Figure 5c). The flux of the TCM-5 membrane slightly decreased with the increase in the dye concentration, from 12.66 L/m²·h·bar to around 8.09 L/m²·h·bar. This is because as the dye concentration increases, the dye molecules are more likely to attach to the pores and permeation channels on the membrane surface, forming a dense layer of dye molecules which increases the transmembrane resistance of water molecules and leads to a decrease in water flux. In addition, as the dye concentration increases, the membrane's rejection rate of dye also increases slightly from 98.4% to 99.9%. This is mainly due to the formation of a "filter cake" layer on the membrane surface, which creates a spatial resistance effect that blocks the passage of dye molecules, resulting in a decrease in water flux but an increase in the membrane's rejection rate of dye.

2.4. Separation Performance of TCM Membrane for Different Salts and Dyes

The salt separation performance of the TCM-5 membrane was evaluated based on the rejection of Na_2SO_4 and NaCl salt solutions at a pressure of 0.4 MPa, and the results of the permeation flux and rejection ratios are shown in Figure 6a. The TCM-5 membrane shows a good rejection performance for divalent salt, with rejection of 71.0% for Na_2SO_4, and poor rejection for monovalent salt, with rejection of 14.2% for NaCl. The result is consistent with literature reports on negatively charged nanofiltration membrane performance [26]. According to the Donnan effect theory, the negatively charged nanofiltration membrane has a stronger repulsion force for divalent anions (SO_4^{2-}) than monovalent anions (Cl^-), resulting in a higher rejection rate of Na_2SO_4 by the membrane. This result shows that TCM-5 membrane has good $NaCl/Na_2SO_4$ selectivity. Similarly, the low rejection rate of Rhodamine B (RhB) dyes with positive charges on the negatively charged membrane surface indicates that the separation mechanism of the composite membrane is a combination of pore size screening and electrostatic effects.

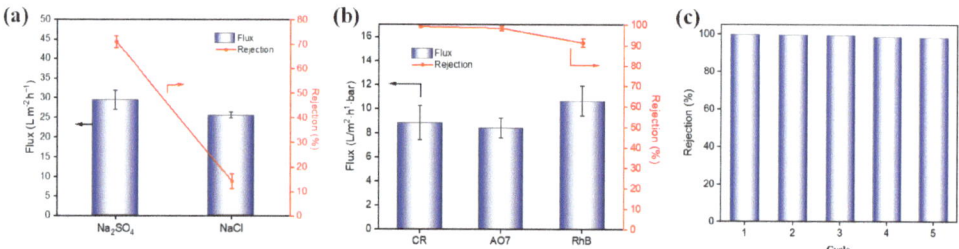

Figure 6. Separation performance of TCM-5 membrane for (**a**) Na_2SO_4 and NaCl, and (**b**) different dyes, including CR, AO7, and RhB. (**c**) Reusability test results of TCM-5 membrane against CR (200 ppm).

The dye selectivity performance of the TCM-5 membrane was evaluated by filtration of three types of dye solutions (CR, orange yellow (AO7), and RhB), and the results are shown in Figure 6b. The concentration of the dye was 200 mg/L, and the flux and dye of the membrane were tested at room temperature under 0.4 MPa using cross-flow equipment. Both CR and AO7 are cationic dyes, while RhB dye is an anodic dye. The rejection rate of TMC-5 membrane reached over 99% for both CR and AO7, while the rejection rate for RhB was only 91%. Generally, the removal rate of the membrane for these three dyes is mainly determined by their charge performance and molecular weight. Similar to the salt selectivity result shown in Figure 6a, the negatively charged NF membrane has a stronger repulsion force for cationic dyes than anodic dyes. Therefore, The TCM-5 membrane shows excellent rejection rates for CR and AO7. In terms of cationic dyes, the membrane will show higher rejection rates for dyes with larger molecular weight. Hence, the rejection rate of CR (Mw = 670 g/mol) is greater than that of AO7 (Mw = 350 g/mol). However, for RhB (Mw = 479 g/mol), the rejection rate is lower than that of AO7 with a larger molecular weight. This is mainly because the nanofiltration membrane surface is negatively charged, resulting in greater electrostatic repulsion of AO7 dye than RhB, and the combined effect of pore size and electrostatic effects leads to a lower rejection rate for RhB dye. The experimental results show that the prepared TCM-5 membrane has an excellent rejection effect for cationic dyes.

The reusability of the membrane was tested using cyclic filtration in cross-flow equipment (Figure 6c). Between each cycle, ethanol and distilled water were sequentially filtrated to wash the membrane. This washing method can remove the dyes from the membrane, due to the weaker electrostatic interactions between the dye and membrane [27]. After five cycles, the membrane still maintained a high rejection rate of 98.1%. The high rejection rate of TCM-5 membrane towards CR dye was mainly determined by pore size sieving and electrostatic interaction.

3. Experimental Section

3.1. Materials

1,3,5-benzenetriacyl chloride (TMC), 2,2,6,6-tetramethylpiperidine-1-oxide radical (TEMPO), sodium hypochlorite (NaClO), sodium bromide (NaBr), Congo red (CR), rhodamine B (RhB), orange yellow (AO7), Na_2SO_4, $MgSO_4$, NaCl, and $MgCl_2$ were purchased from Shanghai Aladdin Biochemical Co. Ltd. (Shanghai, China). Polyvinylidene fluoride (PVDF) membranes were purchased from Nantong Longjin Film Technology Co., Ltd. (Nantong, China). Kraft pulp (Kinleith Hi White) was provided by Oji Fibre Solutions Company (Jinan, China). All the chemicals were used as received without further purification. Deionized (DI) water was used to prepare all aqueous solutions.

3.2. Preparation of TOCNF

A TOCNFs suspension was synthesized using a similar method to one that was recently reported in the literature [22]. To be specific, 1g pulp was used as raw material, shredded and dissolved in 100 mL of DI water, and added to 100 mg of NaBr, 16 mg of TEMPO, and 11.16 g of NaClO (the original concentration was 12.5%). The pH of the mixed solution was adjusted to 10 and maintained for 8 h. Then, centrifugation was performed three times at 9000 rpm to remove any remaining impurities from the mixture to obtain a gel-like solid. Then, 500 mL of DI water was added to dissolve the solid, and the mixture was stirred in a homogenizer for 3 min to obtain a transparent aqueous solution. The obtained solution was named Thick-TOCNFs. Finally, some of the obtained Thick-TOCNF solution was further broken by an ultrasonic probe, using a Qsonica sonicator with a pulse of 30% and output power of 500 W-20 kHz to yield a transparent solution. The obtained transparent TOCNF solution was named Fine-TOCNF. The concentration of both the Thick-TOCNF and Fine-TOCNF was 0.2 wt%.

3.3. Preparation of TCM

A vacuum-assistant method was adopted to prepare the TOCNF membranes. The specific steps were as follows: Firstly, 5 mL Thick-TOCNF solution was filtrated onto a PVDF membrane (pore size 200 nm). Then, an additional 0, 5, or 10 mL Fine-TOCNF solution was filtered onto the membrane, respectively. After the TOCNF solutions were vacuumed, 5 mL TMC solution (0.3% in n-hexane) was poured on the membrane to crosslink the TOCNFs. Finally, the obtained TOCNF membranes were kept in an oven at 80 °C for 30 min for better crosslinking. Based on the different Fine-TOCNF dosage, the obtained membranes were named TCM-0, TCM-5, and TCM-10, respectively. As a comparison, a control membrane (Uncrosslinked membrane) was prepared in the same condition as TCM-5 but without the TMC crosslinking step. All the prepared membranes were rinsed and stored in DI water.

3.4. Characterization of Membranes

The morphologies of Thick-TOCNFs and Fine-TOCNFs were observed by TEM (FEI Tecnai F20, Hillsboro, OR, USA). Diluted Thick-TOCNFs and Fine-TOCNFs drops were dropped on copper grids. The surface and cross-section morphologies of the PVDF membrane, TCM-0, TCM-5, and TCM-10 membrane were observed by SEM. All the samples were coated with gold, and the cross-section membrane samples were fractured in liquid nitrogen to maintain the membranes' original morphology. The thickness of the membrane's top layer was measured by Nano Measurer 1.2.5 software, and the thickness value was the average value of at least ten measurements. The chemical compositions of Uncrosslinked membrane, TCM-0, TCM-5, and TCM-10 membranes were obtained through FTIR (Thermo Scientific Nicolet iS 10, Waltham, MA, USA) in the wavelength range of 400–4000 cm^{-1}. The hydrophilicity of PVDF membrane, TCM-0, TCM-5, and TCM-10 membranes was measured at room temperature using a contact-angle measuring instrument (OSA 60, Königshofen, Germany). The contact angle was tested based on a video camera image of the droplet using the drop shape analysis software (SurfaceMeter Element) supplied.

The contact angles of water drops were measured in quintuplicate to obtain the average contact angle. The crystal structure of cellulose in Uncrosslinked membrane and TCM-5 membranes were measured by a XRD (Rigaku Miniflex 600, Yamanashi, Japan). XRD patterns were determined at 40 kV and 25 mA.

3.5. Permeability Performance of TCM Membrane

The filtration performance of composite membranes was evaluated using a cross-flow filtration system. Membrane flux and rejection rate tests were conducted on an effective membrane surface area of 25.12 cm^2 at 0.4 MPa. Dye or salt solutions were used as feed solution, and the weight of the permeate solution was continuously recorded using a precision electronic balance connected to a computer. All results given are averages with standard deviations for at least three samples of each type of membrane. The pure water flow rate was calculated using Equation (1). The dye or salt rejection rate was calculated using Equation (2).

$$F = \frac{V}{A \times \Delta t}, \quad (1)$$

where F is the permeate flux (L/m^{2}h), V is the permeate volume (L), A is the membrane area (m^2), and Δt is the filtration time (h).

$$R = \left(1 - \frac{C_p}{C_f}\right) \times 100\%, \quad (2)$$

where R is the rejection, and C_p and C_f are the dye or salt concentrations of permeate and feed solution, respectively.

The dye rejection test was carried out on TCM-5 membrane using cross-flow equipment at under 0.4 MPa, and three different dyes (CR, AO7, and RhB) were used for the dye rejection test using dye solution (200 ppm). The concentration of dyes was determined by a UV spectrophotometer. For the salt rejection test, 1000 ppm Na$_2$SO$_4$ or NaCl solution was used as feed solution, and the salt concentration of the permeate and feed solution was measured by an electrical conductivity device.

4. Conclusions

In this work, TCM nanofiltration membranes were fabricated by depositing Fine-TOCNF into Thick-TOCNF structure, followed by crosslinking with TMC. The dense selective layer of the TCM nanofiltration membrane consisted entirely of pure cellulose nanofibers. The fabrication conditions were optimized, and the results show that 0.3% TMC as the crosslinking agent was the optimal concentration, and Fine-TOCNF 5 mL filtrated on the Thick-TOCNF membrane was the optimal fabrication condition. The SEM result shows that TCM-5 and TCM-10 membranes have a tighter pore structure compared with the TCM-0 membrane (without Fine-TOCNF) layer. The hydrophilicity of the TCM membranes decreased as the Fine-TOCNF content increased. The TCM-5 membrane shows a good rejection rate for divalent salt (Na$_2$SO$_4$) with a rejection rate of 71.0% and a low rejection of monovalent ion (NaCl) at only 14.2%. Meanwhile, the TCM-5 membrane shows excellent removal performance (over 90%) for all three of the tested dyes, especially for CR and AO7 (both of which showed removal of over 99.0%). These findings highlight the TCM-5 membrane's exceptional dyes/NaCl selectivity and NaCl/Na$_2$SO$_4$ selectivity. Moreover, TOCNF membranes, which are derived from sustainable resources, offer low cost and high separation efficiency, making them promising candidates to be used in the field of dye/salt wastewater treatment.

Author Contributions: Conceptualization, Z.X. and H.T.; methodology, S.L. and M.S. (Mei Sun); validation, S.L. and K.Z.; formal analysis, C.W. and M.S. (Meng Shan); investigation, Y.H. and M.W.; data curation, K.W. and J.W.; writing—original draft preparation, S.L.; writing—review and editing, Z.X. and H.T.; visualization, K.Z.; funding acquisition, S.L., Y.H. and H.T. All authors have read and agreed to the published version of the manuscript.

Funding. This work was financially supported by Natural Science Foundation of Anhui Province (2108085ME188), the Anhui Polytechnic University Startup Foundation for Introduced Talents, China (2021YQQ048), the Anhui Polytechnic University Startup Foundation for Introduced Talents, China (2022YQQ083), the Key Program of Anhui Polytechnic University, China (Xjky2022115), and the Innovation and Entrepreneurship Training Program for College Students (S202210363249).

Institutional Review Board Statement: Not applicable.

Informed Consent Statement: Not applicable.

Data Availability Statement: Data are contained within the article.

Conflicts of Interest: The authors declare no conflicts of interest.

References

1. Li, J.; Yu, Z.; Zhang, J.; Liu, C.; Zhang, Q.; Shi, H.; Wu, D. Rapid, Massive, and Green Synthesis of Polyoxometalate-Based Metal–Organic Frameworks to Fabricate POMOF/PAN Nanofiber Membranes for Selective Filtration of Cationic Dyes. *Molecules* **2024**, *29*, 1493. [CrossRef]
2. Zhao, J.; Wang, Q.; Yang, J.; Li, Y.; Liu, Z.; Zhang, L.; Zhao, Y.; Zhang, S.; Chen, L. Comb-shaped amphiphilic triblock copolymers blend PVDF membranes overcome the permeability-selectivity trade-off for protein separation. *Sep. Purif. Technol.* **2020**, *239*, 116596. [CrossRef]
3. Yang, L.; Zhang, X.; Rahmatinejad, J.; Raisi, B.; Ye, Z. Triethanolamine-based zwitterionic polyester thin-film composite nanofiltration membranes with excellent fouling-resistance for efficient dye and antibiotic separation. *J. Membr. Sci.* **2023**, *670*, 121355. [CrossRef]
4. Hu, M.; Yang, S.; Liu, X.; Tao, R.; Cui, Z.; Matindi, C.; Shi, W.; Chu, R.; Ma, X.; Fang, K.; et al. Selective separation of dye and salt by PES/SPSf tight ultrafiltration membrane: Roles of size sieving and charge effect. *Sep. Purif. Technol.* **2021**, *266*, 118587. [CrossRef]
5. Cao, X.-L.; Yan, Y.-N.; Zhou, F.-Y.; Sun, S.-P. Tailoring nanofiltration membranes for effective removing dye intermediates in complex dye-wastewater. *J. Membr. Sci.* **2020**, *595*, 117476. [CrossRef]
6. Saleem, H.; Zaidi, S.J. Nanoparticles in reverse osmosis membranes for desalination: A state of the art review. *Desalination* **2020**, *475*, 114171. [CrossRef]
7. Yang, Z.; Zhou, Y.; Feng, Z.; Rui, X.; Zhang, T.; Zhang, Z. A Review on Reverse Osmosis and Nanofiltration Membranes for Water Purification. *Polymers* **2019**, *11*, 1252. [CrossRef] [PubMed]
8. Fortunato, L.; Elcik, H.; Blankert, B.; Ghaffour, N.; Vrouwenvelder, J. Textile dye wastewater treatment by direct contact membrane distillation: Membrane performance and detailed fouling analysis. *J. Membr. Sci.* **2021**, *636*, 119552. [CrossRef]
9. Nia, M.H.; Tavakolian, M.; Kiasat, A.R.; van de Ven, T.G.M. Hybrid Aerogel Nanocomposite of Dendritic Colloidal Silica and Hairy Nanocellulose: An Effective Dye Adsorbent. *Langmuir* **2020**, *36*, 11963–11974. [CrossRef]
10. Routoula, E.; Patwardhan, S.V. Degradation of Anthraquinone Dyes from Effluents: A Review Focusing on Enzymatic Dye Degradation with Industrial Potential. *Environ. Sci. Technol.* **2020**, *54*, 647–664. [CrossRef]
11. Liu, S.; Low, Z.X.; Xie, Z.; Wang, H.J.A.M.T. TEMPO-Oxidized Cellulose Nanofibers: A Renewable Nanomaterial for Environmental and Energy Applications. *Adv. Mater. Technol.* **2021**, *6*, 2001180. [CrossRef]
12. Das, R.; Lindström, T.; Sharma, P.R.; Chi, K.; Hsiao, B.S.J.C.R. Nanocellulose for sustainable water purification. *Chem. Rev.* **2022**, *122*, 8936–9031. [CrossRef]
13. Mautner, A. Nanocellulose water treatment membranes and filters: A review. *Polym. Int.* **2020**, *69*, 741–751. [CrossRef]
14. Wang, S.; Zhang, Q.; Wang, Z.; Pu, J. Facile fabrication of an effective nanocellulose-based aerogel and removal of methylene blue from aqueous system. *J. Water Process. Eng.* **2020**, *37*, 101511. [CrossRef]
15. Liu, Y.; Bai, L.; Zhu, X.; Xu, D.; Li, G.; Liang, H.; Wiesner, M.R. The role of carboxylated cellulose nanocrystals placement in the performance of thin-film composite (TFC) membrane. *J. Membr. Sci.* **2021**, *617*, 118581. [CrossRef]
16. Norfarhana, A.; Ilyas, R.; Ngadi, N.J.C.P. A review of nanocellulose adsorptive membrane as multifunctional wastewater treatment. *Carbohyd. Polym.* **2022**, *291*, 119563. [CrossRef]
17. Abouzeid, R.E.; Salama, A.; El-Fakharany, E.M.; Guarino, V. Mineralized polyvinyl alcohol/sodium alginate hydrogels incorporating cellulose nanofibrils for bone and wound healing. *Molecules* **2022**, *27*, 697. [CrossRef]
18. Zhao, J.; Yuan, X.; Wu, X.; Liu, L.; Guo, H.; Xu, K.; Zhang, L.; Du, G.J.M. Preparation of nanocellulose-based aerogel and its research progress in wastewater treatment. *Molecules* **2023**, *28*, 3541. [CrossRef]

19. Yang, H.; Yang, L.; Wang, H.; Xu, Z.; Zhao, Y.; Luo, Y.; Nasir, N.; Song, Y.; Wu, H.; Pan, F.; et al. Covalent organic framework membranes through a mixed-dimensional assembly for molecular separations. *Nat. Commun.* **2019**, *10*, 2101. [CrossRef]
20. Mohammed, S.; Hegab, H.M.; Ou, R. Nanofiltration performance of glutaraldehyde crosslinked graphene oxide-cellulose nanofiber membrane. *Chem. Eng. Res. Des.* **2022**, *183*, 1–12. [CrossRef]
21. Wang, X.; Ma, H.; Chu, B.; Hsiao, B.S. Thin-film nanofibrous composite reverse osmosis membranes for desalination. *Desalination* **2017**, *420*, 91–98. [CrossRef]
22. Liu, S.; Low, Z.-X.; Hegab, H.M.; Xie, Z.; Ou, R.; Yang, G.; Simon, G.P.; Zhang, X.; Zhang, L.; Wang, H. Enhancement of desalination performance of thin-film nanocomposite membrane by cellulose nanofibers. *J. Membr. Sci.* **2019**, *592*, 117363. [CrossRef]
23. Wang, Q.; Hu, L.; Ma, H.; Venkateswaran, S.; Hsiao, B.S. High-flux nanofibrous composite reverse osmosis membrane containing interfacial water channels for desalination. *ACS Appl. Mater. Interfaces* **2023**, *15*, 26199–26214. [CrossRef]
24. Baroña, G.N.B.; Lim, J.; Choi, M.; Jung, B. Interfacial polymerization of polyamide-aluminosilicate SWNT nanocomposite membranes for reverse osmosis. *Desalination* **2013**, *325*, 138–147. [CrossRef]
25. Zheng, Q.; Cai, Z.; Ma, Z.; Gong, S. Cellulose Nanofibril/Reduced Graphene Oxide/Carbon Nanotube Hybrid Aerogels for Highly Flexible and All-Solid-State Supercapacitors. *ACS Appl. Mater. Interfaces* **2015**, *7*, 3263–3271. [CrossRef]
26. Bai, L.; Liu, Y.; Ding, A.; Ren, N.; Li, G.; Liang, H. Fabrication and characterization of thin-film composite (TFC) nanofiltration membranes incorporated with cellulose nanocrystals (CNCs) for enhanced desalination performance and dye removal. *Chem. Eng. J.* **2019**, *358*, 1519–1528. [CrossRef]
27. Pak, S.; Ahn, J.; Kim, H. High performance and sustainable CNF membrane via facile in-situ envelopment of hydrochar for water treatment. *Carbohyd. Polym.* **2022**, *296*, 119948. [CrossRef]

Disclaimer/Publisher's Note: The statements, opinions and data contained in all publications are solely those of the individual author(s) and contributor(s) and not of MDPI and/or the editor(s). MDPI and/or the editor(s) disclaim responsibility for any injury to people or property resulting from any ideas, methods, instructions or products referred to in the content.

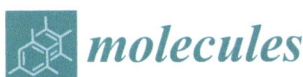

Article

High-Performance Dual-Ion Battery Based on Silicon–Graphene Composite Anode and Expanded Graphite Cathode

Guoshun Liu [†], Xuhui Liu [†], Xingdong Ma, Xiaoqi Tang, Xiaobin Zhang, Jianxia Dong, Yunfei Ma, Xiaobei Zang, Ning Cao and Qingguo Shao *

School of Materials Science and Engineering, China University of Petroleum (East China), Qingdao 266580, China; z22140037@s.upc.edu.cn (G.L.)
* Correspondence: qgshao@upc.edu.cn
† These authors contributed equally to this work.

Abstract: Dual-ion batteries (DIBs) are a new kind of energy storage device that store energy involving the intercalation of both anions and cations on the cathode and anode simultaneously. They feature high output voltage, low cost, and good safety. Graphite was usually used as the cathode electrode because it could accommodate the intercalation of anions (i.e., PF_6^-, BF_4^-, ClO_4^-) at high cut-off voltages (up to 5.2 V vs. Li^+/Li). The alloying-type anode of Si can react with cations and boost an extreme theoretic storage capacity of 4200 mAh g^{-1}. Therefore, it is an efficient method to improve the energy density of DIBs by combining graphite cathodes with high-capacity silicon anodes. However, the huge volume expansion and poor electrical conductivity of Si hinders its practical application. Up to now, there have been only a few reports about exploring Si as an anode in DIBs. Herein, we prepared a strongly coupled silicon and graphene composite (Si@G) anode through in-situ electrostatic self-assembly and a post-annealing reduction process and investigated it as an anode in full DIBs together with home-made expanded graphite (EG) as a fast kinetic cathode. Half-cell tests showed that the as-prepared Si@G anode could retain a maximum specific capacity of 1182.4 mAh g^{-1} after 100 cycles, whereas the bare Si anode only maintained 435.8 mAh g^{-1}. Moreover, the full Si@G//EG DIBs achieved a high energy density of 367.84 Wh kg^{-1} at a power density of 855.43 W kg^{-1}. The impressed electrochemical performances could be ascribed to the controlled volume expansion and improved conductivity as well as matched kinetics between the anode and cathode. Thus, this work offers a promising exploration for high energy DIBs.

Keywords: dual-ion battery; anode materials; Si nanospheres; energy density

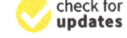

Citation: Liu, G.; Liu, X.; Ma, X.; Tang, X.; Zhang, X.; Dong, J.; Ma, Y.; Zang, X.; Cao, N.; Shao, Q. High-Performance Dual-Ion Battery Based on Silicon–Graphene Composite Anode and Expanded Graphite Cathode. *Molecules* 2023, 28, 4280. https://doi.org/10.3390/molecules28114280

Academic Editor: Lihua Gan

Received: 22 April 2023
Revised: 16 May 2023
Accepted: 22 May 2023
Published: 23 May 2023

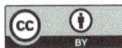

Copyright: © 2023 by the authors. Licensee MDPI, Basel, Switzerland. This article is an open access article distributed under the terms and conditions of the Creative Commons Attribution (CC BY) license (https://creativecommons.org/licenses/by/4.0/).

1. Introduction

Despite the high energy and power density of lithium ion batteries, the limited and uneven distribution of lithium and rare metal resources have led to the search of new energy storage technologies with low cost, high safety, and reliability [1–3]. DIBs are energy storage devices that store energy involving the intercalation of both anions and cations on the cathode and anode simultaneously. They feature high output voltage, low cost, and good safety [4]. Graphite was commonly used as a cathode electrode because it could accommodate intercalation of anions (i.e., PF_6^-, BF_4^-, ClO_4^-) at a high cut-off voltage (up to 5.2 V vs. Li^+/Li) [5,6]. However, the tested capacity of graphite cathodes usually ranged between 80–130 mAh g^{-1}, and it is difficult to be further increased. As for the anode side, any materials that can reversibly store cations can be used as anodes for DIBs [7]. In this case, the traditional graphite anode could be exchanged to other electrode materials with larger capacities. Recently, it was found that the replacement of the low capacity of graphite anodes with other large capacity anodes could indeed increase the capacity of the full DIBs. For instance, Wei et al. [8] assembled DIBs employing the high lithium storage capacity of

MoSe$_2$/Nitrogen-Doped Carbon (1224 mA h g^{-1}) as an anode and graphite as a cathode, and the DIBs delivered a reversible discharge capacity of 86 mA h g^{-1} at 2C after 150 cycles. Tang et al. [9] studied Al foil (theoretical lithium storage capacity is 2235 mAh g^{-1}) as an anode, and, when coupled with graphite cathode, the DIBs showed a reversible capacity of ≈100 mAh g^{-1} and a capacity retention of 88% after 200 charge–discharge cycles. Wang et al. [10] designed a high capacity Ge/CNFs anode (2614 mA h g^{-1}), and the assembled Ge/CNFs-Graphite DIBs showed a high discharge capacity of 281 mA h g^{-1} at a discharge current of 0.25 A g^{-1}, which greatly surpassed those of most of the reported DIBs. Therefore, in order to take full advantage of the DIBs, further optimization of the anode materials is also important.

According to the cation storage mechanisms, the anode materials can be divided into three types: the intercalation type, conversion type, and alloying type. However, the intercalation-type anode (such as graphite, soft carbon, hard carbon, Na$_2$Ti$_3$O$_7$, etc.) usually exhibits low capacity, and the conversion-type anode (such as MoS$_2$, MoSe$_2$, Co$_3$O$_4$, etc.) suffers from low reaction kinetics and shows unimpressed rate performance. The alloying-type anode (such as Al, P, Si, Sn, Ge, etc.) reacts with cations to boost an extreme specific capacity [11–13]. The silicon anode materials possess a high theoretic Lithium storage capacity of 4200 mAh g^{-1} [14–16]. Therefore, it is an efficient method to improve the energy density of DIBs by combining graphite cathode with high-capacity silicon anode. However, the huge volume expansion (>300%) of silicon throughout alloying and de-alloying must be controlled [17–20]. Moreover, the poor electrical conductivity of silicon is also an important factor that hinders its development [21–23]. Up to now, there are only a few reports about exploring Si as an anode in DIBs. Shao et al. [24] prepared a Si/C anode by adding a little amount of Si (7.6 wt%) into graphite and used it in full DIBs with enhanced energy densities. Wang et al. [25] investigated pre-lithiated Si as an anode with the intention of tailoring the voltage to match the cathode. Tang et al. [26] cleverly designed a flexible interface between Si and a conducting soft polymer substrate to modulate the alloying stress of the silicon anode in DIBs, achieving excellent flexible electrochemical properties. Despite the above efforts, to fully take advantage of the large capacity of an Si anode, it is still a challenge to further design a new Si-based anode material with a controlled volume expansion effect and improved conductivity, as well as matched kinetics with the cathode side.

Herein, we prepared a strongly coupled silicon and graphene composite (Si@G) anode through in-situ electrostatic self-assembly and a post-annealing reduction process and investigated it as an anode in full DIBs. Home-made expanded graphite (EG) with a larger inter-layer distance was employed as a cathode with fast intercalation kinetic to accommodate anions (Figure 1). Half-cell tests showed that the as-prepared Si@G anode could retain a maximum specific capacity of 1182.4 mAh g^{-1} after 100 cycles, whereas the bare Si anode only maintained a low capacity of 435.8 mAh g^{-1}. Moreover, the full Si@G//EG DIBs achieved a high energy density of 367.84 Wh kg^{-1} at a power density of 855.43 W kg^{-1}. The impressed electrochemical performances could be ascribed to the following aspects: (i) the composite structure greatly suppressed the stress/strain induced by volume change and alleviated the pulverization during charging and discharging; (ii) the graphene layer adhered on the surface of Si nanospheres could weaken volume expansion and prevent the inter-agglomeration of Si with high surface energy; (iii) the electron migration during the charge/discharge process was promoted by highly conductive graphene; (iv) the improved rate ability of the Si@G anode matched well with the fast kinetics of the EG cathode.

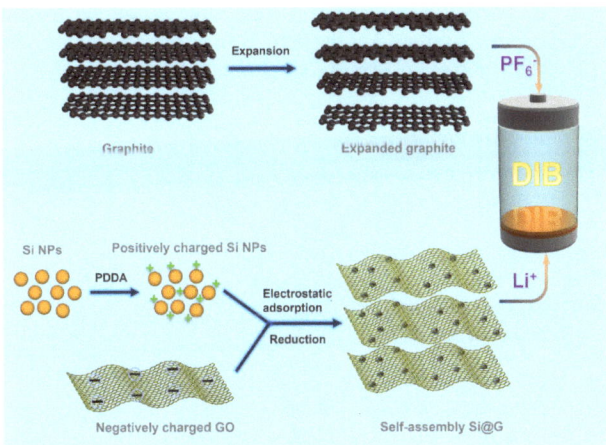

Figure 1. Diagram of the preparation process.

2. Results and Discussion

2.1. Structure and Morphology Analysis

Figure 2a is the XRD comparison of Si@G-1, Si@G-5 and Si@G-10. Evident diffraction peaks are observed at 28.46, 47.26, 56.20, 69.12, and 76.28°, corresponding to the (111), (220), (311), (400), and (331) crystallographic planes of silicon, respectively. The characteristic diffraction peaks of Si@G-5 and Si@G-10 correspond almost exactly to the standard cards, and almost no diffraction peaks of graphene appear, which is attributed to the comparatively low content of graphene in the composite. The weak peak of Si@G-1 at 25.58° corresponds to the (002) characteristic crystallographic plane of the graphene, implying that GO has been successfully reduced, and the product is free of byproducts such as SiC [27,28]. The spectrogram of the unreduced GO is shown in Figure 2b. After self-assembly, the graphene bonded well to silicon during the high-temperature reduction process, which mainly showed the characteristic peaks of Si. Figure 2c shows the Raman plot of composites. Si@G-1, Si@G-5, and Si@G-10 nanocomposites all have characteristic peaks at about 511 and 942.7 cm^{-1}, corresponding to the characteristic peaks of nano-silicon. For Si@G-1, relatively weak graphene characteristic peaks at 1360 and 1580 cm^{-1} were observed. At the same time, no other byproducts appeared. The whole nanocomposite exhibited high crystallinity.

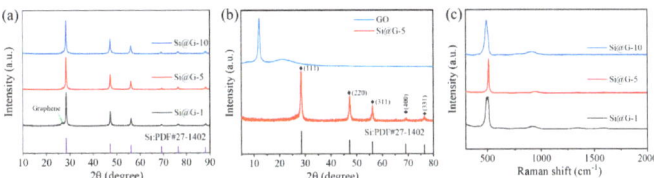

Figure 2. (**a**) XRD comparison of Si@G-1, Si@G-5, and Si@G-10, (**b**) XRD of Si@G-5 and GO, (**c**) Raman plot comparison of Si@G-1, Si@G-5, and Si@G-10.

Figure 3a shows the nitrogen adsorption and desorption curves of Si@G-1, Si@G-5, and Si@G-10, and it is evident that the curves all show typical type IV isotherms. The climbing of the H$_3$ hysteresis loop at a relative pressure (P/Po) of 0.8 to 1.0 is evidence of the presence of mesoporous structures, which may originate from the voids between the adjacent graphene. Apparently, the specific surface area of Si@G-1 is higher than that of Si@G-5 and Si@G-10 due to the relatively more disordered arrangement of graphene. The specific surface areas of Si@G-5 and Si@G-10 are comparable, and the less graphene content cannot change the silicon arrangement. In addition, the pore diameter distribution curves (Figure 3b) show that the pore diameter is mainly around 5 nm, which is favorable for the migration of Li$^+$ to Si@G inside the composites [29].

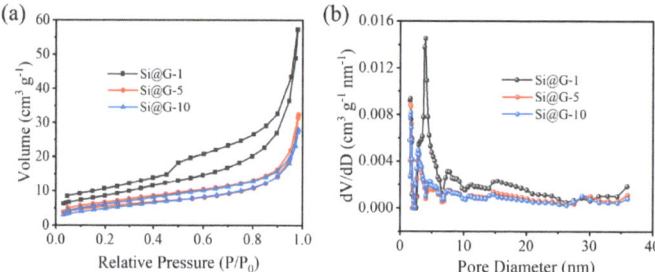

Figure 3. (**a**) Comparison of BET nitrogen adsorption and desorption curves for Si@G-1, Si@G-5, and Si@G-10 samples, (**b**) pore diameter distribution.

To characterize the morphology of the Si@G composites, SEM was performed. Figure 4a–c show the morphology of Si@G-1 sample. As can be observed, silicon nanoparticles (range of 50–100 nm) were anchored on graphene nanosheets, and the size of the graphene sheets was between 1 and 10 um. The silicon nanoparticles were completely encapsulated by the graphene nanosheets, and the agglomeration of silicon and the folding and stacking of graphene sheets created many voids that facilitated electrolyte penetration and Li$^+$ transport [30,31]. At the same time, the silicon-loaded nanosheets were interconnected to provide additional electronic pathways. Figure 4d–f show the SEM images of the Si@G-5 composites, where more silicon nanoparticles mask the presence of graphene, but the graphene sheets can still be observed by higher magnification, as shown in Figure 4f. For the Si@G-10 sample, the extremely high content of silicon makes graphene not observable in the SEM images.

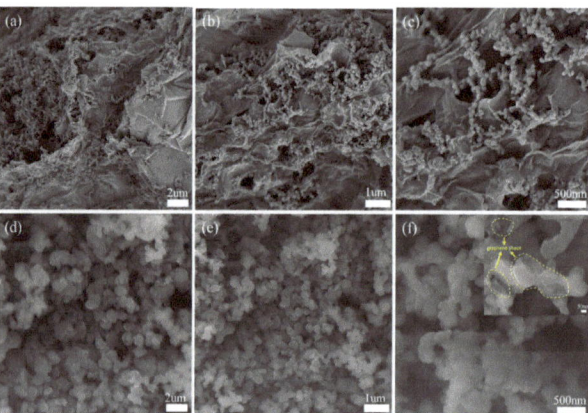

Figure 4. SEM comparison at different magnifications: (**a**–**c**) Si@G-1, (**d**–**f**) Si@G-5.

TEM was applied to further examine the structure of the Si@G-5 material. TEM images (Figure 5a,b) clearly demonstrate the presence of graphene sheets and silicon nanoparticles, with a few layers of large diameter graphene completely wrapping the silicon nanoparticles. It is evident that silicon nanoparticles are firmly anchored on graphene sheets due to the electrostatic binding effect. Figure 5c shows the HRTEM image of the silicon–graphene composite. The spacing of (111) is 0.31 nm, and a sheet of graphene tightly attached to the Si shells and amorphous carbon deposited on the surface of the composite can also be observed from the HRTEM image. From the dark-field diffraction image (Figure 5d), it is possible to derive each crystallographic plane of the Si nanoparticles, which confirms that the crystallinity of the Si nanoparticles is mostly preserved.

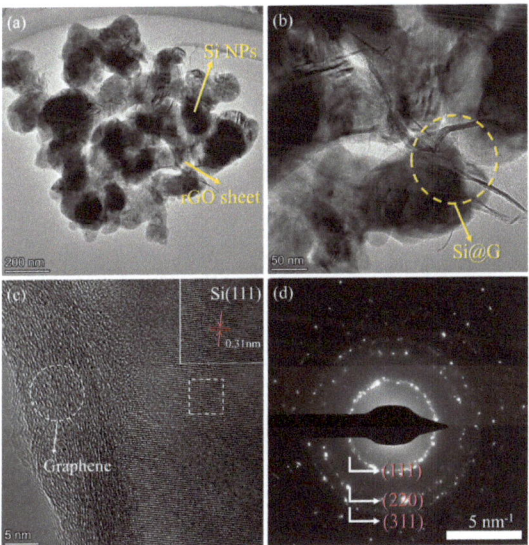

Figure 5. (**a**,**b**) TEM images of Si@G-5 material at different magnifications, (**c**) HRTEM of silicon–graphene composites, (**d**) Dark-field diffraction images of Si@G-5.

2.2. Electrochemical Studies

Structure and morphology analysis indicated that the Si@G-5 composite exhibited high crystallinity, proper specific surface area, and better integration. Thus, it was chosen to be tested as an electrode for the lithium half-cell, lithium-ion full cell, and dual-ion full battery. The half-cell was firstly assembled to evaluate the lithium storage capacity of the Si@G composite electrode using Si@G as the working electrode and lithium metal as the reference electrode. The CV curves of Si@G-5 are displayed in Figure 6a. Two cathodic peaks appeared in the first cycle. The broad peak at 0.69 V was attributed to the formation of the solid electrolyte interphase (SEI) and the contribution of graphene sheets [32,33]. Another cathodic peak out near 0.23 V was attributed to the transformation of the silicon structure from crystalline to amorphous [34]. In contrast, the two anodic peaks at 0.39 and 0.52 V corresponded to the de-lithiation process of amorphous Li_xSi to Si.

Figure 6b shows the first three GCD curves of Si@G-5 anode at 0.1 A g^{-1}. Due to the formation of SEI films, the ICE is 69.94%. In the second and third cycles, the curves overlap almost completely, and the specific discharge capacity is about 4100 mAh g^{-1}. This is consistent with the CV results, indicating that the Si@G-5 has excellent reversibility. Figure 6c shows the curve of the 100 cycles of nano-silicon and Si@G-5 with the same current density. Apparently, the Si@G-5 material had a specific capacity of 1182.40 mAh g^{-1} after 100 cycles, with a capacity retention of 59.12%, much higher than the pure silicon sample of 435.8 mAh g^{-1} and 20.94%. Figure 6d shows the GCD curves under different cycle numbers. Except for the low CE of the first cycle, the subsequent CEs are higher than 95%, indicating that Si@G-5 has excellent stability and electrochemical reversibility. This is due to the strong binding force produced by electrostatic action, which makes the volume expansion of Si@G-5 in the cycle process is significantly inhibited [35].

The rate performance of pure silicon and Si@G-5 were tested, as shown in Figure 6e. At 0.1, 0.2, 0.5, 1.0, and 2.0 A g^{-1}, the discharge capacities were 3348.8/3520.3, 2567.1/2874.4, 1999.5/2369.4, 1672.1/1973.4, and 1390/1600 mAh g^{-1}, respectively. Evidently, Si@G-5 performed better than pure silicon samples at each current density. When the current density was restored to 0.1 A g^{-1} again, the Si@G-5 specific capacity was restored to 2801.6 mAh g^{-1}, the capacity retention was 83.66%, and the pure silicon sample was only 60.09%. Figure 6f shows the charge–discharge curves of Si@G-5 under different current densities. As the current density increased, the specific capacity decreased. However, the voltage difference between charging and discharging platforms was still small, which indicated that Si@G-5 had small polarization, high reversibility, and electrode stability. These excellent properties could be attributed to the introduction of graphene to enhance the charge transfer ability, and the graphene sheets could effectively inhibit the internal stress caused by the silicon volume expansion.

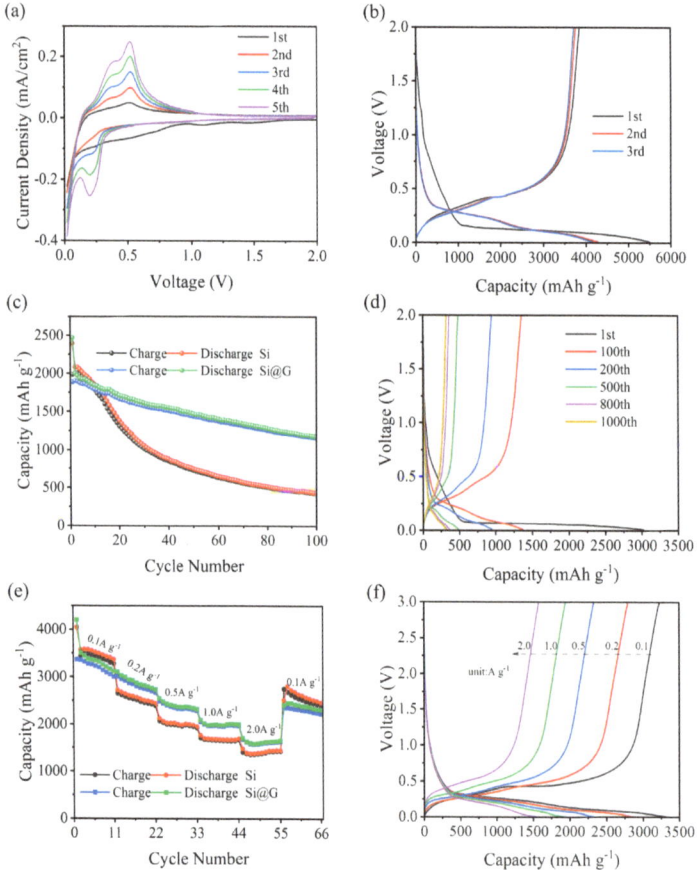

Figure 6. (a) CV curves of the first five cycles of the Si@G-5 electrode at 0.5 mV s^{-1}, (b) Charge-discharge curves of the first three cycles of the Si@G-5 electrode at 0.1 A g^{-1}, (c) GCD comparisons between pure silicon and Si@G-5 at 0.2 A g^{-1}, (d) GCD curves of Si@G-5 at 1 A g^{-1} for different cycles, (e) Comparison of rate performance between pure silicon and Si@G-5, (f) Charge–discharge curves of Si@G-5 at different current densities.

In addition to the excellent rate performance, the Si@G-5 electrode also demonstrated excellent long-term cycling stability. As shown in Figure 7, after 1000 cycles at 1.0 A g^{-1}, the reversible specific capacity remained at 325.1 mAh g^{-1}, while the pure silicon sample failed after 1000 cycles due to volume expansion [36].

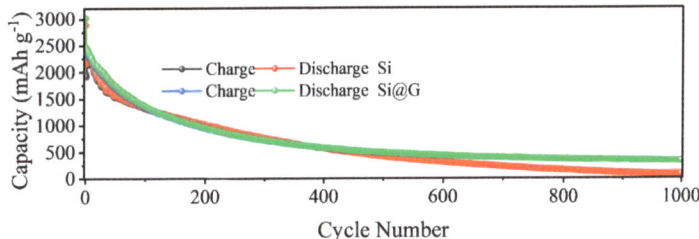

Figure 7. Comparison of long-term cycle performance of pure Si and Si@G-5 at 1.0 A g^{-1}.

To verify the performance of the Si@G-5 in the DIB, the full cell of a lithium-based DIB was assembled, with Si@G-5 as the anode and (expanded graphite) EG as the cathode (Figure 8a). EG was selected because it possessed an enhanced interlaying distance, which could accommodate more PF$_6^-$ intercalation. The detailed structure and electrochemical PF$_6^-$ storage performances of the EG are shown in Figures S1–S3. Figure 8b shows the CV curves of the EG//Si@G-5 DIB, which almost entirely overlap, indicating the excellent electrochemical reversibility. Three evident oxidation peaks appeared around 4.29, 4.60, and 4.83 V, which were the initial electrochemical processes occurring jointly at the cathode and anode, corresponding to different intercalation processes of PF$_6^-$ [37]. The first three cycles of the GCD curve of the EG//Si@G-5 DIB at 1 C are shown in Figure 8c, and the first charging specific capacity was up to 388.23 mAh g^{-1}. However, the initial coulomb efficiency (ICE) was 24.31%, due to the formation of SEI films and side reactions [38]. Thereafter, the curves converge in terms of specific capacity and CE. The rate performance of the full cell is shown in Figure 8d. After 10 cycles at 2, 4, 6, 8, 10, 20, and 2 C in sequence, the discharge specific capacity recovered to 64.66 mAh g^{-1}, with a capacity retention of 74.39%, and all CEs were around 95%. Figure 8e shows the GCD curves at different current densities. The cells have evident and similar charging and discharging plateaus, which correspond to the results of the CV curves. The capacity was 48.35 mAh g^{-1} after 100 cycles at 2 C, with a capacity retention of 57.18% (Figure 8f), and the capacity fade was also relatively slow. These were attributed to the synergistic effect of the cathode and anode, emphasizing the improved structure of the silicon-based electrode in the DIBs.

In addition, we also assembled a LiFePO$_4$//Si@G-5 LIB full cell to compare the electrochemical performance of the LIB and DIB. The GCD curves and cycling curves of LiFePO$_4$//Si@G-5 LIB are shown in Figures S4 and S5, respectively. The results show that its electrochemical performance was much less than EG//Si@G-5 DIB.

To further study the kinetic properties of the EG//Si@G-5 DIB, EIS was performed. Figure 9a shows the EIS plots of the EG//Si@G-5 DIB in the uncycled state, after 50 cycles, and after 200 cycles. The charge transfer resistance (R$_{ct}$) was 34.03 Ω when uncycled (Figure 9b). After cycling, there was a different degree of increase in R$_{ct}$ (Figure 9c). This may have been due to the creation of SEI films in the first cycle and was also responsible for the irreversible capacity and cell performance degradation in the first cycle [39]. In the low-frequency region, the curve flattened out, owing to the decreasing rate of diffusion. However, a high ion migration rate could be maintained after 200 cycles. The fitted curves were calculated as σ_0 = 170.51, σ_{50} = 669.40, and σ_{200} = 1328.49, resulting in Li$^+$ diffusion coefficients of 1.37 × 10^{-21}, 8.90 × 10^{-23}, and 2.26 × 10^{-23} cm^2 s^{-1} for the three, respectively (please refer to Equation (S1) for the detailed calculation procedure).

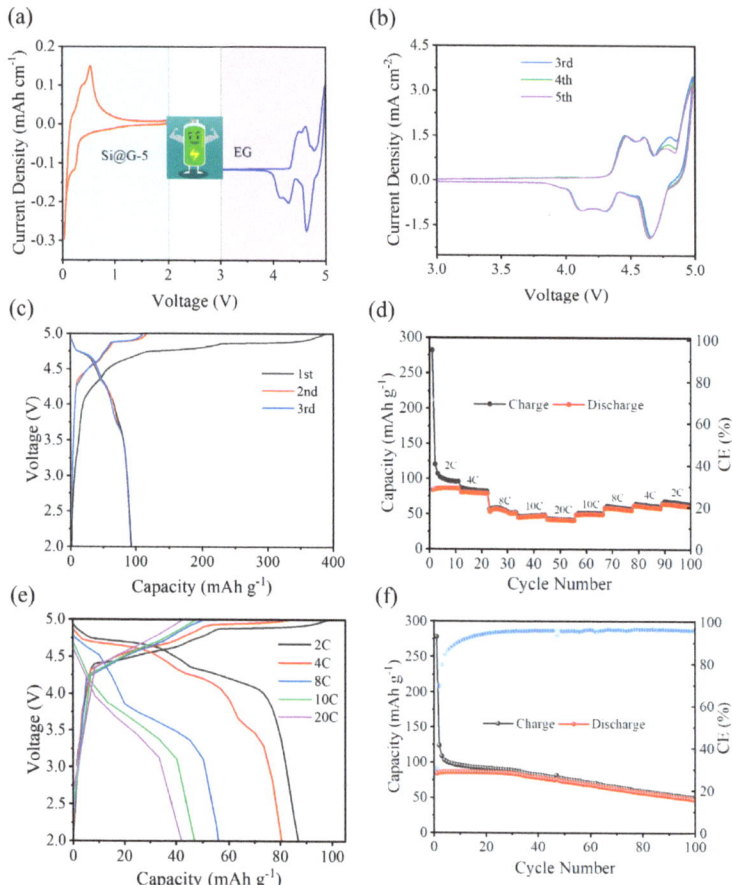

Figure 8. Electrochemical performance of EG//Si@G-5 DIB: (**a**) selection of voltage range, (**b**) CV curves at 0.5 mV s^{-1}, (**c**) the first three GCD curves at 1 C, (**d**) rate performance, (**e**) GCD curves at different current densities, (**f**) 100 cycles performance at 2 C.

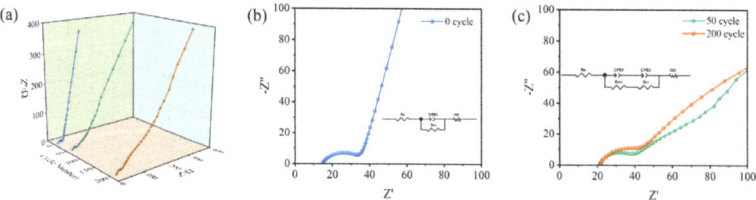

Figure 9. EG//Si@G-5 DIB kinetic analysis: (**a**) EIS comparison at different cycle times, (**b**) EIS without cycle, (**c**) EIS comparison after 50 and 200 cycles (The inset is the equivalent circuit diagram).

To evaluate the value of the EG//Si@G-5 DIB for practical applications, we calculated the energy density and power density at different current densities (Tables S1 and S2 and Equation (S2)). The EG//Si@G-5 DIB achieved an energy density of 367.84 Wh kg^{-1} at 2 C, while the LiFePO$_4$//Si@G-5 LIB showed only a low energy density of 93.58 Wh kg^{-1}. Moreover, the EG//Si@G-5 DIB could maintain a high energy density of 138.37 Wh kg^{-1}

even at 20 C. These results demonstrated that the EG//Si@G-5 DIB held great potential for a high-performance energy storage device.

3. Materials and Methods

3.1. Chemicals and Reagents

For the synthesis of Si@G and EG materials, the following reagents were used: silicon powder (Si, cell grade), purchased from Shenzhen Huaqing Material Technology Co. (Shenzhen, China); natural graphite (C, purity ≥ 99%), purchased from Shenzhen Kejing Technology Co. (Shenzhen, China); Poly dimethyl diallyl ammonium chloride ($(C_8H_{16}ClN)_n$, AR), sodium nitrate ($NaNO_3$, AR), concentrated sulfuric acid (H_2SO_4, AR), potassium permanganate ($KMnO_4$, AR), hydrogen peroxide (H_2O_2, AR), and anhydrous ethanol (C_2H_6O, AR), all the above chemical reagents were purchased from Sinopharm Chemical Reagent Co. (Shanghai, China). All chemical reagents used in this work were not further purified.

3.2. Material Preparation

3.2.1. Preparation of Si@G Anode Material

First, 100 mg Si powder was weighed and fully stirred in 50 mL deionized water for 30 min, and then 2 mL 20 wt% PDDA solution (Poly dimethyl diallyl ammonium chloride) was added. The solution was stirred and ultrasonically dispersed for 1 h. Then, the above solution was centrifuged at 10,000 rpm for 5 min, and the excess PDDA was removed three times to obtain a positively charged Si precipitate. In total, 100 mg of graphite oxide (GO) was weighed, 100 mL of deionized water was added, mixed, stirred, and sonicated for 1 h to obtain the GO solution (1.0 mg mL^{-1}).

The prepared aqueous Si-PDDA solution was slowly added to the GO solution and stirred for 12 h. The solution was filtered to obtain Si@GO filter cake, which was then dried under vacuum at 80 °C for 12 h. The dried filter cake was ground into powder and then calcined at 900 °C under 10% H_2/Ar atmosphere for 2 h. Finally, the Si@G-1 sample (for comparison, the addition of 500 mg and 1000 mg of silicon powder were noted as Si@G-5 and Si@G-10) was obtained. As illustrated in Figure 1, the fabrication process is clearly shown.

3.2.2. Preparation of EG Cathode Material

In total, 1 g of natural graphite and 0.5 g of $NaNO_3$ were weighed and slowly added to 23 mL of concentrated H_2SO_4, while the temperature was controlled to below 5 °C. After stirring in a water bath for 30 min, the temperature was increased to 35 °C, and then 0.5 g of $KMnO_4$ of different masses was added and kept stirred for 2 h. After that, 46 mL of deionized water was added, heated to 98 °C, and stirred continuously for 30 min. In total, 130 mL of deionized water and 10 mL of H_2O_2 were added.

The above solution was added to anhydrous ethanol and deionized water and continuously filtered at least four times to make the pH neutral. The filter cake was transferred to a vacuum oven and dried at 80 °C for 12 h. Subsequently, it was heated to 600 °C in N_2 atmosphere and held for 5 h. Finally, EG was obtained.

3.3. Material Characterization

The crystal structure and composition were determined by X-ray diffraction (XRD, Ultima IV, using Cu Kα) at a scan rate of 10° min^{-1}. The morphology was characterized by scanning electron microscopy (SEM, Hitachi SU8000, Hitachi, Tokyo, Japan). The microstructure was characterized by transmission electron microscopy (TEM, JEOL-2100F Plus, JEOL, Osaka, Japan). Raman spectroscopy was performed on a Raman spectrometer system (JY HR-800 Lab Ram), with a laser wavelength of 532 nm. The specific surface area, pore volume, and pore size distribution of the materials were tested by a specific surface area and porosity analyzer (BET, Micromeritics ASAP 2460, Norcross, GA, USA), with nitrogen adsorption and desorption tests at 77.3 K.

3.4. Electrochemical Characterization

The Si@G or EG, binder carboxymethyl cellulose (CMC), and conductive agent Super P were weighed in the ratio of 7:2:1, mixed and ground, and then anhydrous ethanol and deionized water was added in a 1:1 solution as a solvent and stirred for 12 h. After that, the resulting slurry was daubed on the aluminum foil, dried under vacuum at 80 °C for 12 h, and cut into 14 mm diameter round pole pieces after drying.

The CR2032 button cell was made in an argon-filled glove box. Half-cell was assembled to evaluate the lithium storage capacity of Si@G composite. Si@G was used as working electrodes. Lithium metal was used as both counter and reference electrode. Celgard-2400 was used as the separator. In total, 1 M $LiPF_6$ and 10 wt% fluoroethylene carbonate (FEC) in a 1:1:1 (volume ratio) mixture of ethylene carbonate (EC), diethyl carbonate (DEC), and dimethyl carbonate (DMC) was used as the electrolyte. In full-DIB assembly, EG was used as the cathode, Si@G was used as anode, and the electrolyte was changed to 4 M $LiPF_6$ and 2.0% VC in the ethyl methyl carbonate (EMC). The higher lithium salt concentration induced the solvent molecules to complex with $LiPF_6$. At high voltage, the complexed solvent molecules had stronger antioxidant properties, and the electrolyte was more stable. In addition, the VC in the electrolyte as an additive could preferentially form a SEI film with excellent performance on the graphite electrode, which could effectively inhibit the continuous decomposition of solvent molecules on the electrode surface. Cyclic voltammetry (CV) was performed on ModuLab XM ECS-type electrochemical workstation at scan rates of 0.5 mV s^{-1} between 3.00–5.00 V. Charge/discharge tests (GCD) at different current densities at 3.00–5.00 V were performed with the NEWARE 8.0 battery test system. Electrochemical impedance spectroscopy (EIS) was performed on a ModuLab XM ECS-type electrochemical workstation, with a frequency of 0.01 Hz–100 kHz and an amplitude of 5 mV.

4. Conclusions

In summary, we prepared a silicon and graphene composite (Si@G) anode through in-situ electrostatic self-assembly and a post-annealing reduction process and investigated it as an anode in full DIBs, together with home-made expanded graphite (EG) as a fast kinetic cathode. The composite structure could suppress the stress/strain induced by volume change and alleviated the pulverization during charging and discharging. In addition, the graphene layer adhered on the surface of Si nanospheres could weaken volume expansion, prevent the inter-agglomeration of Si, and improve the conductivity. Benefiting from that, the as-prepared Si@G anode could retain a maximum specific capacity of 1182.4 mAh g^{-1} after 100 cycles, while the bare Si anode only maintained at 435.8 mAh g^{-1}. Moreover, the full Si@G//EG DIBs achieved a high energy density of 367.84 Wh kg^{-1} at a power density of 855.43 W kg^{-1}. Thus, this work shed some light on the practical applications of high energy DIBs.

Supplementary Materials: The following supporting information can be downloaded at: https://www.mdpi.com/article/10.3390/molecules28114280/s1, Figure S1: XRD and Raman plot of graphite and EG; Figure S2: GCD curves and rate diagrams for graphite and EG; Figure S3: GCD curves at different current densities; Figure S4: GCD curves of $LiFePO_4$//Si@G-5 LIB at different current densities; Figure S5: Cycle curve of $LiFePO_4$//Si@G-5 LIB; Table S1: Energy density and power density of EG//Si@G-5 DIB at different current densities; Table S2: Energy density and power density of $LiFePO_4$//Si@G-5 LIB at different current densities.

Author Contributions: Conceptualization, Q.S., G.L. and X.L.; methodology, G.L. and X.L.; software, X.M.; validation, X.T.; formal analysis, X.Z. (Xiaobin Zhang); investigation, J.D. and Y.M.; writing—original draft preparation, Q.S.; writing—review and editing, X.L.; supervision, N.C. and Q.S.; project administration, Q.S.; funding acquisition, X.Z. (Xiaobei Zang). All authors have read and agreed to the published version of the manuscript.

Funding: This work was supported by the Natural Science Foundation of Shandong Province with grant (ZR2020QE048) and the National Natural Science Foundation of China with grant (21905304).

Institutional Review Board Statement: The study did not require ethical approval.

Informed Consent Statement: Not applicable.

Data Availability Statement: Data will be made available on request.

Conflicts of Interest: The authors declare that they have no conflict of interest.

Sample Availability: Samples are available from the authors upon request.

References

1. Hadjipaschalis, I.; Poullikkas, A.; Efthimiou, V. Overview of current and future energy storage technologies for electric power applications. *Renew. Sustain. Energy Rev.* **2009**, *13*, 1513–1522. [CrossRef]
2. Naik, M.V. Recent advancements and key challenges with energy storage technologies for electric vehicles. *Int. J. Electr. Hybrid Veh.* **2021**, *13*, 256–288. [CrossRef]
3. Niu, J.; Zhang, S.; Niu, Y.; Song, H.; Chen, X.; Zhou, J. Silicon-Based Anode Materials for Lithium-Ion Batteries. *Prog. Chem.* **2015**, *27*, 1275–1290.
4. Ji, B.; Zhang, F.; Song, X.; Tang, Y. A Novel Potassium-Ion-Based Dual-Ion Battery. *Adv. Mater.* **2017**, *29*, 1700519. [CrossRef]
5. Wang, S.; Jiao, S.; Tian, D.; Chen, H.-S.; Jiao, H.; Tu, J.; Liu, Y.; Fang, D.-N. A Novel Ultrafast Rechargeable Multi-Ions Battery. *Adv. Mater.* **2017**, *29*, 1606349. [CrossRef]
6. Sui, Y.; Liu, C.; Masse, R.C.; Neale, Z.G.; Atif, M.; AlSalhi, M.; Cao, G. Dual-ion batteries: The emerging alternative rechargeable batteries. *Energy Storage Mater.* **2020**, *25*, 1–32. [CrossRef]
7. Wang, M.; Tang, Y. A Review on the Features and Progress of Dual-Ion Batteries. *Adv. Energy Mater.* **2018**, *8*, 1703320. [CrossRef]
8. Zheng, C.; Wu, J.; Li, Y.; Liu, X.; Zeng, L.; Wei, M. High-Performance Lithium-Ion-Based Dual-Ion Batteries Enabled by Few-Layer $MoSe_2$/Nitrogen-Doped Carbon. *ACS Sustain. Chem. Eng.* **2020**, *8*, 5514–5523. [CrossRef]
9. Zhang, X.; Tang, Y.; Zhang, F.; Lee, C.-S. A Novel Aluminum–Graphite Dual-Ion Battery. *Adv. Energy Mater.* **2016**, *6*, 1502588. [CrossRef]
10. Zhou, J.; Zhou, Y.; Zhang, X.; Cheng, L.; Qian, M.; Wei, W.; Wang, H. Germanium-based high-performance dual-ion batteries. *Nanoscale* **2020**, *12*, 79–84. [CrossRef]
11. Luo, P.; Zheng, C.; He, J.; Tu, X.; Sun, W.; Pan, H.; Zhou, Y.; Rui, X.; Zhang, B.; Huang, K. Structural Engineering in Graphite-Based Metal-Ion Batteries. *Adv. Funct. Mater.* **2021**, *32*, 2107277. [CrossRef]
12. Zhang, L.; Wang, H.; Zhang, X.; Tang, Y. A Review of Emerging Dual-Ion Batteries: Fundamentals and Recent Advances. *Adv. Funct. Mater.* **2021**, *31*, 2010958. [CrossRef]
13. Ou, X.; Gong, D.; Han, C.; Liu, Z.; Tang, Y. Advances and Prospects of Dual-Ion Batteries. *Adv. Energy Mater.* **2021**, *11*, 2102498. [CrossRef]
14. Han, Y.; Qi, P.; Feng, X.; Li, S.; Fu, X.; Li, H.; Chen, Y.; Zhou, J.; Li, X.; Wang, B. In Situ Growth of MOFs on the Surface of Si Nanoparticles for Highly Efficient Lithium Storage: Si@MOF Nanocomposites as Anode Materials for Lithium-Ion Batteries. *ACS Appl. Mater. Interfaces* **2015**, *7*, 2178–2182. [CrossRef] [PubMed]
15. Zheng, P.; Sun, J.; Liu, H.; Wang, R.; Liu, C.; Zhao, Y.; Li, J.; Zheng, Y.; Rui, X. Microstructure Engineered Silicon Alloy Anodes for Lithium-Ion Batteries: Advances and Challenges. *Batter. Supercaps* **2023**, *6*, e202200481. [CrossRef]
16. Raić, M.; Mikac, L.; Marić, I.; Štefanić, G.; Škrabić, M.; Gotić, M.; Ivanda, M. Nanostructured Silicon as Potential Anode Material for Li-Ion Batteries. *Molecules* **2020**, *25*, 891. [CrossRef]
17. Shi, C.; Chen, J.; Guo, T.; Luo, G.; Shi, H.; Shi, Z.; Qin, G.; Zhang, L.; He, X. Controllable Preparation to Boost High Performance of Nanotubular SiO_2@C as Anode Materials for Lithium-Ion Batteries. *Batteries* **2023**, *9*, 107. [CrossRef]
18. Fang, H.; Liu, Q.; Feng, X.; Yan, J.; Wang, L.; He, L.; Zhang, L.; Wang, G. Carbon-Coated Si Nanoparticles Anchored on Three-Dimensional Carbon Nanotube Matrix for High-Energy Stable Lithium-Ion Batteries. *Batteries* **2023**, *9*, 118. [CrossRef]
19. Duan, H.; Xu, H.; Wu, Q.; Zhu, L.; Zhang, Y.; Yin, B.; He, H. Silicon/Graphite/Amorphous Carbon as Anode Materials for Lithium Secondary Batteries. *Molecules* **2023**, *28*, 464. [CrossRef]
20. Shi, F.; Song, Z.; Ross, P.N.; Somorjai, G.A.; Ritchie, R.O.; Komvopoulos, K. Failure mechanisms of single-crystal silicon electrodes in lithium-ion batteries. *Nat. Commun.* **2016**, *7*, 11886. [CrossRef]
21. Jung, H.; Park, M.; Yoon, Y.-G.; Kim, G.-B.; Joo, S.-K. Amorphous silicon anode for lithium-ion rechargeable batteries. *J. Power Sources* **2003**, *115*, 346–351. [CrossRef]
22. Du, F.-H.; Wang, K.-X.; Chen, J.-S. Strategies to succeed in improving the lithium-ion storage properties of silicon nanomaterials. *J. Mater. Chem. A* **2016**, *4*, 32–50. [CrossRef]
23. Chae, S.; Ko, M.; Kim, K.; Ahn, K.; Cho, J. Confronting Issues of the Practical Implementation of Si Anode in High-Energy Lithium-Ion Batteries. *Joule* **2017**, *1*, 47–60. [CrossRef]
24. He, S.; Wang, S.; Chen, H.; Hou, X.; Shao, Z. A new dual-ion hybrid energy storage system with energy density comparable to that of ternary lithium ion batteries. *J. Mater. Chem. A* **2020**, *8*, 2571–2580. [CrossRef]
25. Li, C.; Ju, Y.; Yoshitake, H.; Yoshio, M.; Wang, H. Preparation of Si-graphite dual-ion batteries by tailoring the voltage window of pretreated Si-anodes. *Mater. Today Energy* **2018**, *8*, 174–181. [CrossRef]
26. Jiang, C.; Xiang, L.; Miao, S.; Shi, L.; Xie, D.; Yan, J.; Zheng, Z.; Zhang, X.; Tang, Y. Flexible interface design for stress regulation of a silicon anode toward highly stable dual-ion batteries. *Adv. Mater.* **2020**, *32*, 1908470. [CrossRef]

27. Feng, K.; Ahn, W.; Lui, G.; Park, H.W.; Kashkooli, A.G.; Jiang, G.; Wang, X.; Xiao, X.; Chen, Z. Implementing an in-situ carbon network in Si/reduced graphene oxide for high performance lithium-ion battery anodes. *Nano Energy* **2016**, *19*, 187–197. [CrossRef]
28. Fatima, A.; Majid, A.; Haider, S.; Akhtar, M.S.; Alkhedher, M. First principles study of layered silicon carbide as anode in lithium ion battery. *Int. J. Quantum Chem.* **2022**, *122*, e26895. [CrossRef]
29. Wang, C.; Zhang, C.; Xue, Q.; Li, C.; Miao, J.; Ren, P.; Yang, L.; Yang, Z. Atomic mechanism of the distribution and diffusion of lithium in a cracked Si anode. *Scr. Mater.* **2021**, *197*, 113807. [CrossRef]
30. Han, C.; Si, H.; Sang, S.; Liu, K.; Liu, H.; Wu, Q. Achieving fully reversible conversion in Si anode for lithium-ion batteries by design of pomegranate-like Si@C structure. *Electrochem. Acta* **2021**, *389*, 138736. [CrossRef]
31. Zhang, X.; Wang, D.; Qiu, X.; Ma, Y.; Kong, D.; Müllen, K.; Li, X.; Zhi, L. Stable high-capacity and high-rate silicon-based lithium battery anodes upon two-dimensional covalent encapsulation. *Nat. Commun.* **2020**, *11*, 3826. [CrossRef] [PubMed]
32. Kim, W.-S.; Choi, J.; Hong, S.-H. Meso-porous silicon-coated carbon nanotube as an anode for lithium-ion battery. *Nano Res.* **2016**, *9*, 2174–2181. [CrossRef]
33. Zheng, Z.; Wu, H.-H.; Chen, H.; Cheng, Y.; Zhang, Q.; Xie, Q.; Wang, L.; Zhang, K.; Wang, M.-S.; Peng, D.-L.; et al. Fabrication and understanding of Cu_3Si-Si@ carbon@ graphene nanocomposites as high-performance anodes for lithium-ion batteries. *Nanoscale* **2018**, *10*, 22203–22214. [CrossRef] [PubMed]
34. Ke, C.-Z.; Liu, F.; Zheng, Z.-M.; Zhang, H.-H.; Cai, M.-T.; Li, M.; Yan, Q.-Z.; Chen, H.-X.; Zhang, Q.-B. Boosting lithium storage performance of Si nanoparticles via thin carbon and nitrogen/phosphorus co-doped two-dimensional carbon sheet dual encapsulation. *Rare Met.* **2021**, *40*, 1347–1356. [CrossRef]
35. Xu, Y.; Yin, G.; Ma, Y.; Zuo, P.; Cheng, X. Nanosized core/shell silicon@carbon anode material for lithium ion batteries with polyvinylidene fluoride as carbon source. *J. Mater. Chem.* **2010**, *20*, 3216–3220. [CrossRef]
36. Wan, X.; Tang, Z.; Chen, J.; Xue, Y.; Zhang, J.; Guo, X.; Liu, Y.; Kong, Q.; Yuan, A.; Fan, H. Molten Salt-assisted Magnesiothermic Reduction Synthesis of Spherical Si Hollow Structure as Promising Anode Materials of Lithium Ion Batteries. *Chem. Lett.* **2019**, *48*, 1547–1550. [CrossRef]
37. Matsuo, Y.; Sekito, K.; Ashida, Y.; Inamoto, J.; Tamura, N. Factors Affecting the Electrochemical Behaviors of Graphene-like Graphite as a Positive Electrode of a Dual-Ion Battery. *ChemSusChem* **2023**, *16*, e202201127. [CrossRef]
38. Li, X.; Sun, X.; Hu, X.; Fan, F.; Cai, S.; Zheng, C.; Stucky, G.D. Review on comprehending and enhancing the initial Coulombic efficiency of anode materials in lithium-ion/sodium-ion batteries. *Nano Energy* **2020**, *77*, 105143. [CrossRef]
39. Lei, H.; Wang, H.; Cheng, B.; Zhang, F.; Liu, X.; Wang, G.; Wang, B. Anion-Vacancy Modified WSSe Nanosheets on 3D Cross-Networked Porous Carbon Skeleton for Non-Aqueous Sodium-Based Dual-Ion Storage. *Small* **2023**, *19*, e2206340. [CrossRef]

Disclaimer/Publisher's Note: The statements, opinions and data contained in all publications are solely those of the individual author(s) and contributor(s) and not of MDPI and/or the editor(s). MDPI and/or the editor(s) disclaim responsibility for any injury to people or property resulting from any ideas, methods, instructions or products referred to in the content.

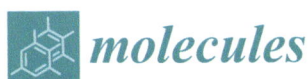

Article

Supramolecular Gels Based on C_3-Symmetric Amides: Application in Anion-Sensing and Removal of Dyes from Water

Geethanjali Kuppadakkath, Sreejith Sudhakaran Jayabhavan and Krishna K. Damodaran *

Department of Chemistry, Science Institute, University of Iceland, Dunhagi 3, 107 Reykjavík, Iceland
* Correspondence: krishna@hi.is; Tel.: +354-525-4846; Fax: +354-552-8911

Abstract: We modified C_3-symmetric benzene-1,3,5-*tris*-amide (BTA) by introducing flexible linkers in order to generate an N-centered BTA (N-BTA) molecule. The N-BTA compound formed gels in alcohols and aqueous mixtures of high-polar solvents. Rheological studies showed that the DMSO/water (1:1, v/v) gels were mechanically stronger compared to other gels, and a similar trend was observed for thermal stability. Powder X-ray analysis of the xerogel obtained from various aqueous gels revealed that the packing modes of the gelators in these systems were similar. The stimuli-responsive properties of the N-BTA towards sodium/potassium salts indicated that the gel network collapsed in the presence of more nucleophilic anions such as cyanide, fluoride, and chloride salts at the MGC, but the gel network was intact when in contact with nitrate, sulphate, acetate, bromide, and iodide salts, indicating the anion-responsive properties of N-BTA gels. Anion-induced gel formation was observed for less nucleophilic anions below the MGC of N-BTA. The ability of N-BTA gels to act as an adsorbent for hazardous anionic and cationic dyes in water was evaluated. The results indicated that the ethanolic gels of N-BTA successfully absorbed methylene blue and methyl orange dyes from water. This work demonstrates the potential of the N-BTA gelator to act as a stimuli-responsive material and a promising candidate for water purification.

Keywords: LMWGs; C_3-symmetric amides; stimuli-responsive; water remediation; dye adsorption

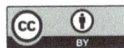

Citation: Kuppadakkath, G.; Jayabhavan, S.S.; Damodaran, K.K. Supramolecular Gels Based on C_3-Symmetric Amides: Application in Anion-Sensing and Removal of Dyes from Water. *Molecules* 2024, 29, 2149. https://doi.org/10.3390/molecules29092149

Academic Editor: Qingguo Shao

Received: 31 March 2024
Revised: 26 April 2024
Accepted: 3 May 2024
Published: 5 May 2024

Copyright: © 2024 by the authors. Licensee MDPI, Basel, Switzerland. This article is an open access article distributed under the terms and conditions of the Creative Commons Attribution (CC BY) license (https://creativecommons.org/licenses/by/4.0/).

1. Introduction

The quantity of contaminants of emerging concern (CECs) [1,2], which are chemicals and toxic materials in wastewater, has dramatically increased since the pre-industrial era. The synthetic dyes found in wastewater are mostly generated from industries such as textiles, cosmetics, paper, pharmaceuticals, and paint, and these can be considered as CECs due to their toxicity to ecological or human health [3]. The non-biodegradable nature of synthetic dyes leads to ecological problems due to their accumulation on land and in aquatic environments [4]. This problem resulted in the development of various techniques to remove dyes from wastewater [5], such as adsorption, photodegradation, oxidative or biochemical degradation, chemical precipitation, ion exchange, and electrocoagulation. Adsorption techniques can be considered among the best techniques for removing dyes from wastewater [6] because most adsorbents can be recycled due to their non-reactive nature to toxic substances. In this process, dyes interact with the adsorbent via chemical or non-bonding interactions, separating them from the mixture [7]. Several adsorbents [8] based on activated carbon, zeolites, mineral clay, chitosan, and waste biomass have been employed for the wastewater dye removal process. The drawbacks of pollutant uptake and selectivity, the cost involved in activating the adsorbent for recycling, and the enormous amount of toxic sludge generated prompted researchers to explore alternative methods for dye adsorption. Supramolecular gels based on low-molecular-weight gelators (LMWGs) [9–13] are excellent candidates for use in adsorption studies due to their porous networks and stimuli-responsive properties [14–19]. LMWGs display superior adsorption capacities for dyes [20–23], but the majority of LMWGs reported for the removal of dyes are metallogels or pH-dependent [14,24–28].

LMWGs have gained considerable attention during the last two decades as soft materials due to their intriguing potential applications, such as in stimuli-responsive materials, media for synthesis and crystallization, drug delivery, tissue engineering, and environmental clean-up, including oil spills and the removal of toxic chemicals [9–13]. LMWGs are fibrous networks arising from the self-assembly of gelator molecules in the presence of a solvent medium, which is stabilized by non-covalent interactions, and the solvent molecules are trapped within these networks. These networks are stabilized by various non-covalent interactions such as hydrogen bonding, van der Waals interactions, π–π stacking, and halogen bonding. The nature of these interactions is responsible for the stimuli-responsive behavior of LMWGs, where the gelation process can be turned ON/OFF in the presence of an external stimulus (temperature, pH, sound, salts/ions, or additives) [15–19]. LMWGs resemble protein structures in terms of solvent content and their porous nature grants better dye adsorption properties than traditional adsorbents [29]. However, predicting the formation of a supramolecular gel is a challenging task because the self-assembly process depends on the dynamic nature of the non-bonding interactions, the nature of the functional groups, and the balance between the hydrophilic and hydrophobic interactions [9–13]. The formation of a one-dimensional (1-D) fibrous architecture capable of entangling into a 3-D network in the presence of a solvent is considered one of the important criteria for gel network formation. Introducing hydrogen bonding groups, such as amide, urea, thiourea, amino acids, and hydrazone moieties, into LMWGs [30–35] can induce 1-D self-assembly via various non-bonding interactions, which results in a myriad of LMWGs with intriguing properties.

Several reports on LMWGs with tunable properties are based on amide moieties [36]. Amide-based compounds display complementary N−H···O=C interactions, arising from the donor (N-H) and acceptor (C=O) of the amide moieties, to form a 1-D fibril structure, and these 1-D chains self-assemble to 3-D porous architecture, within which the solvent molecules are entrapped [36,37]. These cooperative and unidirectional hydrogen bonding interactions arising from the amide units play a crucial role in the self-assembly process of LMWGs, and these moieties can interact with anions, leading to stimuli-responsive materials [15–19]. Supramolecular gels based on C_3-symmetric amides display versatile gelation abilities due to their hydrogen-bonded helical columnar structures, which are stabilized by hydrogen bonding and π–π stacking. An example of this is benzene-1,3,5-*tris*-amide (BTA) [15–19]. However, C_3-symmetric amides have rarely been used to remove dyes, presumably due to the absence of suitable porous architectures and a lack of selectivity for substrates [38,39]. Separation and selectivity can be improved by introducing/modifying functional groups to the supramolecular gels in order to produce LMWGs with better adsorption capacities. The post-modification of the functional groups via covalent capture can be used to tune their stability and robustness, leading to better adsorption performances [40,41]. Qiu et al. showed a folic acid-gelatin hybrid gel obtained by introducing gelatin into folic acid improved the specific surface and porosity of the hybrid gel, making it a better adsorbent for dye adsorption [41]. In this work, we have modified the C_3-symmetric N-centered BTA with flexible linkers to explore its stimuli-responsive properties and ability to act as an adsorbent of both cationic and anionic dyes in water.

2. Results and Discussion

2.1. Synthesis of C_3-Symmetric N-Centered BTA (N-BTA)

Supramolecular gels based on C_3-symmetric BTA can be classified as either C=O centered or N-centered BTA molecules based on their connection to the aromatic platform, and these compounds display similar 1-D columnar structures stabilized by the hydrogen bonding interactions between the amide functionalities [42]. Haldar et al. analyzed the role of the spatial orientation of the amide bonds in the self-assembly process of C=O centered and N-centered C_3-symmetric tripeptides gels and studied the dye adsorption ability of the gels [38]. The C=O-centered C_3-symmetric BTA compounds (benzene-1,3,5-tricarboxylic amide) display versatile gelation abilities in a wide range of solvents, [43–45] but the LMWGs based on the corresponding C_3-symmetric N-centered BTA are rare, presumably due to the unavailability of the amine precursor or difficulties in synthesizing benzene-1,3,5-triamine. We designed a C_3-symmetric N-centered BTA (N-BTA) by introducing a methylene group between the aromatic core and the amine. We reported that adding/modifying the functional groups produces LMWGs with tuneable properties [34,46–48]. The C_3-symmetric N-BTA was synthesized by reacting benzene-1,3,5-triyltrimethanamine with 4-(ethoxycarbonyl)benzoic acid chloride (Scheme 1). The ester group was selected because the self-assembly mode of the amide group was preserved by introducing the ester derivatives, flanking the hydrogen bonding between amide and carboxylate functionalities.

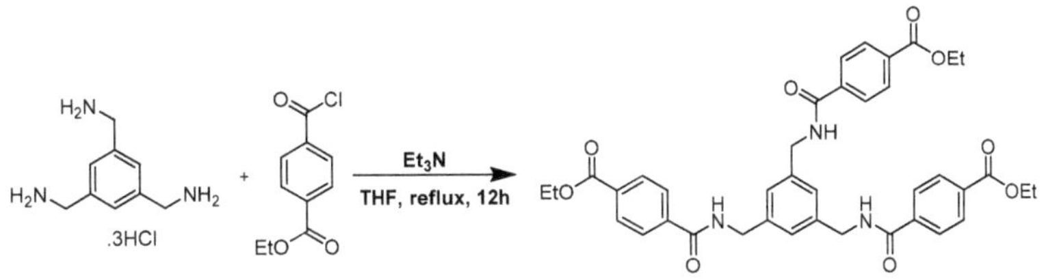

Scheme 1. Synthesis of N-centered C_3-symmetric *tris*-amide (N-BTA).

2.2. Gelation Studies

Solvent screening was undertaken to identify the ideal solvents/solvent mixtures for use in gelation by following a standardized protocol. The required amount of the compound was introduced into a standard 7.0 mL sealed vial, followed by the addition of 1.0 mL of the corresponding solvent. The resulting mixture was sonicated and heated until it formed a clear solution, then it was allowed to cool to room temperature and left undisturbed for 24.0 h. Gel formation was confirmed by a vial inversion test. The results indicated that gelation was observed for N-BTA in alcohols such as methanol, ethanol, isopropanol, and *n*-butanol, but failed to form gels in aliphatic and apolar aromatic solvents (toluene, xylenes, and mesitylene), presumably due to their poor solubility (Table S1). We also tested the gelation abilities of N-BTA in high-polar solvents, but gels were not formed in these solvents. This prompted us to perform gelation studies in aqueous mixtures of high-polar solvents by introducing water as an anti-solvent because N-BTA is insoluble in water. Gelation was observed in an aqueous mixture (1:1, v/v) of high-polar solvents, such as DMF, DMSO, DMA, and DEA.

The minimum gelator concentration (MGC), which indicates the minimum quantity of gelator necessary for forming a stable gel network in a specific solvent, was evaluated by varying the quantity of the gelator (Table 1). The MGCs were similar for the aqueous mixtures of DMF, DMA, and DEA, but higher for DMSO. The MGCs for N-BTA in alcohols were similar but lower than those in aqueous mixtures, presumably due to the insolubility of N-BTA in the antisolvent.

Table 1. Minimum Gelator Concentration (MGC) and T_{gel} (4.0 wt/v%) of the gelator.

Solvent	MGC (wt/v%)	T_{gel} (°C)
Methanol	1.9	79.9
Ethanol	1.9	82.9
Isopropanol	2.0	94.3
n-butanol	2.0	96.1
DMF/water (1:1, v/v)	2.8	92.8
DMSO/water (1:1, v/v)	3.6	99.1
DMA/water (1:1, v/v)	2.5	58.3
DEA/water (1:1, v/v)	2.7	83.9

2.3. Thermal Stability

The thermal stability of the N-BTA gels was evaluated by monitoring the transition temperature (T_{gel}) at which the gel transformed into a liquid phase (gel–sol transition). All gels were prepared at the same concentration (4.0 wt/v%) in methanol, ethanol, isopropanol, n-butanol, and aqueous mixtures (1:1, v/v) of DMF, DMSO, DMA, and DEA in order to compare their thermal stabilities (Table 1). The gel–sol transition temperature in methanol was significantly lower than that of the gels in higher alcohols, indicating that increasing the chain length of the alcohols increased the stability of the gel network, leading to a significantly stronger network. The experiments performed with the aqueous mixtures (1:1, v/v) of DMF, DMA DEA, and DMSO indicated that the thermal stabilities of gels in DMSO/water (1:1, v/v) were slightly higher than the DMF/water (1:1, v/v) gels, but significantly higher compared to the other gels. The lower thermal stability of DMA/water (1:1, v/v) gel could be attributed to the better solubility of N-BTA in DMA.

2.4. Rheology

Rheology is a valuable tool for studying the rigidity, deformation, and flow properties of gels, offering valuable insights into the underlying structural features of the gel network [46,47]. The mechanical strength of the gels was analyzed by performing amplitude and frequency-sweep experiments in methanol, ethanol, and aqueous mixtures (1:1, v/v) of DMF and DMSO at 4.0 wt/v%. Initially, a strain sweep was performed to identify the linear viscoelastic region (LVR), maintaining a constant frequency of 1.0 Hz, and the elastic modulus (G') was independent of the applied strain. All the gels displayed a constant G' up to 0.1% strain (Figures S1–S4). The point at which the elastic gel transforms into a viscous fluid, marked by a sudden decline in the G', is referred to as the crossover point. Frequency-sweep experiments were conducted with a constant strain of 0.01% (within LVR) over a frequency range of 0.1–10.0 Hz, and the results displayed constant elastic (G') and viscous (G'') moduli under varying frequencies. The comparison of mechanical strengths revealed that the gel in DMSO/water (1:1, v/v) exhibited higher storage modulus values compared to all other gels, suggesting a relatively stronger gel network (Figure 1).

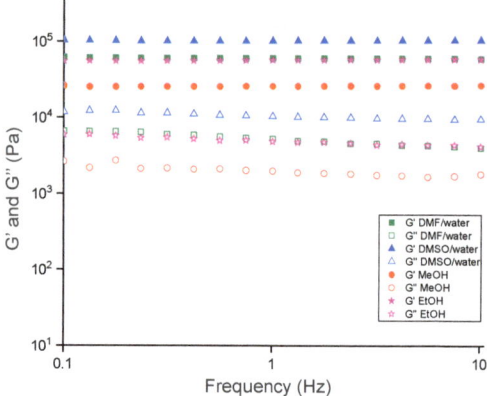

Figure 1. Frequency sweep experiments of gels in various solvents/solvent mixtures at 4.0 wt/v% at 20.0 °C with a constant strain of 0.01%.

2.5. Gel Morphology

The morphologies of the gel fibers can be visualized using modern microscopic techniques. Scanning electron microscopy (SEM) is one of the most useful techniques for elucidating gel fiber morphologies [48], which helps to evaluate the nanostructures of the LMWGs. The surface morphology of the fibrous network was analyzed by performing SEM on the dried gel samples, which were structurally similar to the actual gel network.

However, artifacts of the drying process sometimes affect the structure; therefore, these measurements are not a perfect representation of the gel network [49]. The morphology of the gel network obtained by drying the gels of N-BTA from methanol (2.0 wt/v%) displayed zoetic features (Figure 2a), but flake-like morphologies with fiber dimensions ranging from 0.1 to 1.0 μm (Figure 2b) were observed for ethanol xerogels.

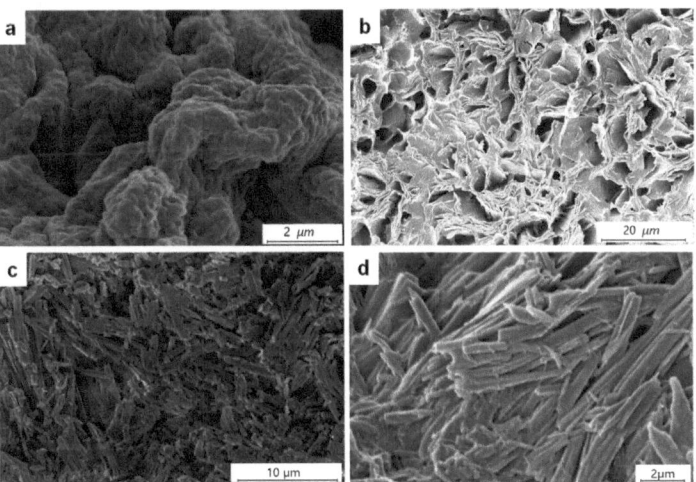

Figure 2. SEM images of N-BTA xerogels (2.0 wt/v%) from (**a**) methanol and (**b**) ethanol, and xerogels from (**c**) DMF/water and (**d**) DMSO/water (1:1, v/v) at 4.0 wt/v%, respectively.

Similar morphologies were observed for isopropanol and n-butanol xerogels at 2.0 wt/v% (Figure S5). The xerogels obtained from the aqueous mixtures (1.1, v/v) of DMF and DMSO at 4.0 wt/v% displayed needle-shaped morphologies (Figure 2c,d) with thicknesses ranging from 0.2 to 1.5 μm.

2.6. Powder X-ray Powder Diffraction (PXRD)

Powder X-ray diffraction (PXRD) is an important tool for confirming the phase purity of a material. PXRD can be used to analyze the molecular packing and the self-assembly process of LMWGs [35,48,50–52]. Our group showed that comparing the PXRD pattern of the xerogels with the simulated pattern of the gelator structure could yield valuable insights into the fundamental interactions within the gel network architecture [35,50–52]. This was a promising approach, but sometimes the drying process led to morphological changes or the phase transition of the fibrous networks [49]. We used PXRD to evaluate the self-assembly modes of N-BTA in various solvents by comparing the PXRD patterns of the xerogels for the corresponding solvents. The comparison of the PXRD patterns of the xerogels (4.0 wt/v%) taken from the aqueous solutions of DMF, DMSO, DEA, and DMA revealed that the patterns were superimposable (Figure 3).

However, the PXRD patterns obtained from the xerogels from the alcohols displayed broad peaks, presumably due to poor crystallinity of the gelators in these solvents, but most of the peaks matched with the PXRD patterns obtained for the aqueous mixtures (Figure S6) and the bulk material. These results indicate that a similar gel network for N-BTA xerogels was observed, irrespective of the solvents used.

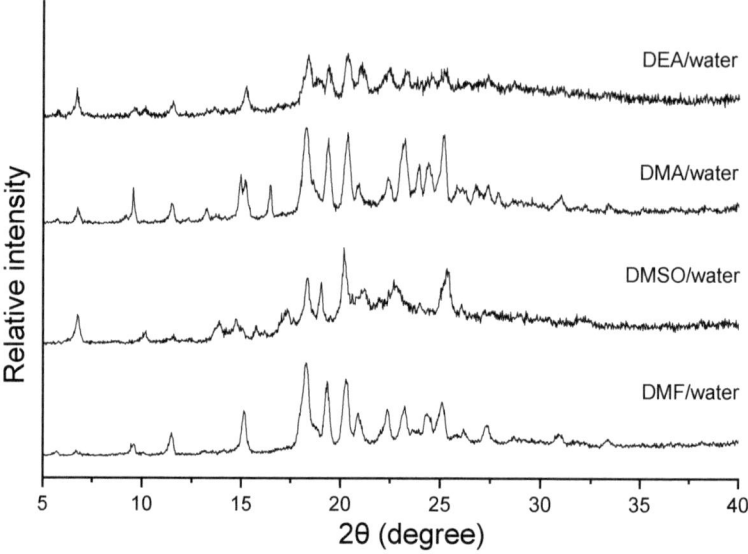

Figure 3. PXRD patterns of the dried gels (4.0 wt/v%) from the aqueous solutions of DMF, DMSO, DEA, and DMA (1:1, v/v).

2.7. Stimuli-Responsive Properties

Supramolecular gels are an excellent class of stimuli-responsive materials, as their gelation process can be modulated by various external stimuli like pH, light, sound, and redox reactions, as well as by the introduction of external factors such as salts or ions [15–19]. The interactions between cation/anions and gelator molecules can be either constructive or destructive, depending on the electrostatic interaction and acidic/basic characteristics of the cations/anions [15,53]. A positive interaction has the potential to start or enhance the process of gelation, whereas a negative interaction might result in the dissolution or collapse of the gel network [15–19]. LMWGs based on amide moieties are promising candidates for anions sensing [15–19,54], and we have reported the anion-sensing capabilities of amide-based gelators [55,56]. The presence of amide moieties in the gelators prompted us to evaluate the anion-sensing abilities of the N-BTA gelator. The stimuli-responsive properties of the gels were analyzed by treating the gels with various anions of sodium and potassium salts. The gels were prepared at MGC (3.6 wt/v%) using sodium/potassium (1.0 equiv.) halides, nitrate, sulphate, acetate, and cyanide ions in a DMSO/water mixture (1:1, v/v), and the gel state properties were compared to those of the native gelator. The fluoride, chloride and cyanide salts disrupted the gel network, but the gel network remained intact in the presence of nitrate, sulphate, acetate, bromide, and iodide salts (Figures 4 and S7). The ability of anions to induce gelation was tested by performing gelation below MGC (3.0 wt/v%) and gel formation in the presence of nitrate, sulphate, acetate, bromide, and iodide salts (1.0 equiv.) confirmed the occurrence of anion-induced gelation (Figure S8).

These results indicate that smaller and more nucleophilic anions, such as cyanide, fluoride, and chloride ions, disrupt hydrogen bonding networks (destructive interaction), but larger and less nucleophilic anions such as bromide, iodide, nitrate, sulphate and acetate enhance (constructive interaction) the formation of gel networks. The stimuli-responsive nature (ON/OFF gelation) of the N-BTA gelator towards anions indicates that the size of the anion is crucial for ensuring the effective interaction of the gelator with the anion [57–59]. Thus, N-BTA compound can be considered to be size-selective anion-responsive supramolecular gels, which can detect cyanide, fluoride and chloride ions in aqueous solution by monitoring the gel-to-sol transition. The mechanical and thermal strength of these gels was evaluated in order to observe the effect of anions on the stability of gel networks (Figure 5 and Table S2), and the results indicated that the presence of anions enhanced the thermal and mechanical stability of the LMWGs.

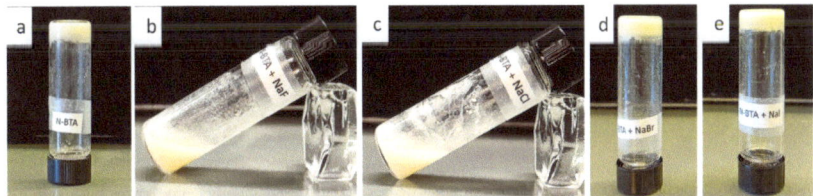

Figure 4. Stimuli-responsive properties of the (**a**) N-BTA gels in DMSO/water mixture (1:1, v/v) with sodium halides (1.0 equiv.), such as (**b**) fluoride, (**c**) chloride, (**d**) bromide, and (**e**) iodide salts.

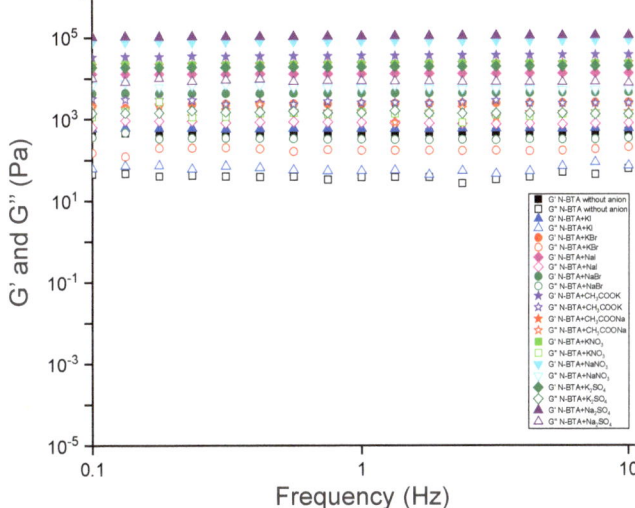

Figure 5. Frequency sweep experiments of N-BTA gels (3.6 wt/v%) in the presence of various sodium/potassium salts of bromide, iodide, nitrate, acetate, and sulphate.

2.8. Dye Adsorption Studies

For the dye adsorption studies, we chose methylene blue (MB), a widely recognized cationic dye that is extensively utilized in the textile, clothing, paper, pharmaceutical, cosmetics, and leather industries [60]. Furthermore, its limited biodegradability and its mutagenic and carcinogenic properties make the water purification process challenging. Water contamination by MB is a threat to both human health and plant life. In humans, exposure to the dye can result in a range of afflictions, including vomiting, jaundice, cyanosis, and increased heart rates. Similarly, the presence of MB causes growth inhibition and the reduction of pigments in plants [60]. We also chose methyl orange (MO), an anionic azo dye found in effluents from the textile, printing, culinary, pharmaceutical, and paper industries, as well as research labs [61]. The presence of MO and its degradation products is highly carcinogenic and toxic to land and aquatic environments [62].

The concentration of the dyes in water was optimized by performing the UV-vis experiments and the maximum absorbance of methylene blue (7.5×10^{-6} M) was 665 nm (Figure 6a). The gels prepared from ethanol (2.0 wt/v%) were loaded carefully into a solution of the MB (10.0 mL) in a 25.0 mL beaker, and the absorbance was recorded over 8 days at pH 4.2 and 21.0 °C (Figure 6a). We observed a decrease in absorbance with

MB in the solution after a span of 2 days. The blue-colored MB solution turned colorless after 5 days (Figure 6b), and the absorbance peaks almost disappeared after 7 days. The adsorbed amount of MB was calculated using UV-vis absorption and we observed that the concentration of MB gradually decreased over 8 days, with an adsorption rate of 97.9% (Figure S9).

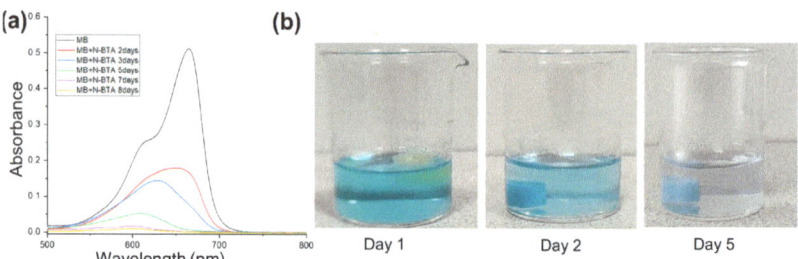

Figure 6. (a) UV-vis experiments of MB (7.5×10^{-6} M) in deionized water and (b) upon adding the N-BTA gel prepared in ethanol (2.0 wt/v%) to MB (7.5×10^{-6} M).

The UV-vis experiments performed at an optimized concentration of MO (5.0×10^{-5} M) in water at pH 3.5 and 21.0 °C revealed the maximum absorbance was 465 nm (Figure 7a). The procedure for the dye adsorption process was similar to that for MB adsorption. The experiments showed a decrease in absorbance after 2 days with a color change from yellow to orange over time and a shift in absorbance maxima towards higher wavelengths. The color change and the shift in absorbance might have been due to the change in pH from 5.0 (MO solution) to 3.5 after adding N-BTA gels to the MO solution [63]. After 5 days, the absorbance was further reduced (Figure 7a,b), and around 60.0% of the dye was removed within 8 days (Figure S10). The dye adsorption of N-BTA was confirmed by a series of experiments with N-BTA and the dyes under various conditions. Initially, dry N-BTA (5.0 mg) was dispersed in an aqueous solution of MB and MO, and no color change was observed for MB. However, the yellow color was transformed into orange in the case of MO, which was similar to what occurred in the gel state experiments (Figure S11). We repeated the MO dye adsorption experiments with N-BTA gels in different solvents such as isopropanol, n-butanol, and DMSO/water, and similar color changes/shifts in absorbance maxima were observed (Figure S12). We were unable to perform the re-adsorption studies with N-BTA gels because the recovered gels from both dyes were not reusable.

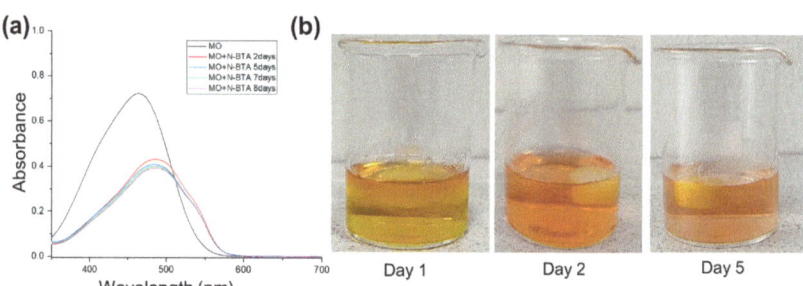

Figure 7. UV-vis: (a) UV-vis experiments of MO (5.0×10^{-5} M) in deionized water and (b) upon adding the N-BTA gel prepared in ethanol (2.0 wt/v%) to MO (5.0×10^{-5} M).

The adsorption capacity (Q_t) and adsorption efficiency (R_e) of N-BTA when used on the dye were calculated (Table 2) from the concentration of dyes before and after adsorption using the following equations [23]:

$$Q_t = \frac{V(C_0 - C_t)}{m} \text{ (mg/g)}$$

$$R_e = \frac{(C_0 - C_t)}{C_0} \times 100\%$$

where C_0 is the initial dye concentration in solution (mg/L), C_t is the residual dye concentration in solution at time t (mg/L), V is the solution volume (L), and m is the mass of the dry adsorbent (g).

Table 2. Comparison of adsorption capacity (Q_t) and adsorption efficiency (R_e) of N-BTA when used on MB and MO.

Day	Adsorption Capacity (mg/g)		Adsorption Efficiency (%)	
	MB	MO	MB	MO
2	0.78	4.92	64.94	60.11
5	1.07	5.09	89.58	62.19
7	1.15	5.14	96.64	62.81
8	1.17	5.21	97.87	63.61

The adsorption efficiency with respect to the concentration of the gelator was studied by varying the quantity of N-BTA from 20.0 to 60.0 mg. The N-BTA gels were immersed in 10.0 mL of dye solutions, the absorbance was recorded over a span of 2, 5, and 7 days, and we calculated the adsorption efficiency (Figures 8 and S13–S18). The results showed that adsorption efficiency increased with the concentration of N-BTA and reached a plateau (Figure 8b). The adsorption ratio of MB remained at approximately 94.5% when the concentration of N-BTA was 6.0 mg/mL. The adsorption ratio of MO was approximately 76.5% when the concentration of N-BTA was 6.0 mg/mL (Figure S18). These experiments reveal the ability of the N-BTA gel to adsorb MB and MO dyes from water.

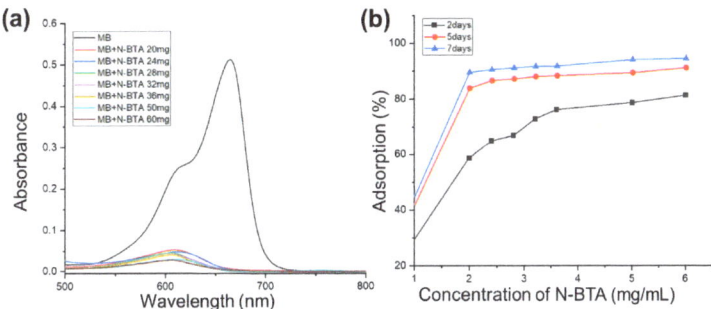

Figure 8. (a) UV-vis experiments of MB (7.5×10^{-5} M) in deionized water with varying concentrations of N-BTA after 7 days and (b) adsorption ratio of MB with varying concentrations of N-BTA after 2, 5, and 7 days.

Our adsorption studies indicate that N-BTA gel is more efficient in terms of removing cationic methylene blue dye than the anionic methyl orange. These results demonstrate that the C_3-symmetric BTA (N-BTA) LMWGs can interact with both cationic and anionic dyes in water, which reveals the versatile properties of N-BTA gel as a selective anion sensor and dye adsorber. As mentioned in the introduction, synthesizing N-BTA molecules is challenging, and we have shown that simple alteration of the functional group will lead to C_3-symmetric compounds with intriguing properties.

3. Materials and Methods

The starting materials and solvents were purchased commercially from Sigma-Aldrich (MEDOR ehf, Reykjavik, Iceland), Fluorochem UK, and TCI-Europe (Boereveldseweg, Belgium) and were utilized as supplied. Deionized water was used for the gelation tests. We characterized the molecules using ^{1}H and ^{13}C NMR spectra (Figures S19–S22), which were recorded in a Bruker Avance 400 spectrometer (Rheinstetten, Germany), and the SEM images (Carl Zeiss, Oberkochen, Germany) were recorded on a Leo Supra 25 microscope. The rheological experiments were performed on an Anton Paar modular compact rheometer MCR 302 (Graz, Austria). Powder X-ray diffraction (PXRD) experiments were performed with bulk compounds and xerogel using a PANalytical instrument (Almelo, The Netherlands).

3.1. Synthesis of Ligands

We synthesized the 1,3,5-tris(azidomethyl)benzene by modifying the reported procedure for obtaining a similar reaction [64].

3.1.1. Synthesis of Benzene-1,3,5-Triyltrimethanamine

The corresponding azide (2.7 g, 11.1 mmol) was dissolved in a mixture of 60.0 mL of THF and 7.5 mL of water. This solution was treated with triphenylphosphine (14.6 g, 55.5 mmol) and then stirred at room temperature for 15 h. The completion of the reaction was monitored using a TLC, and the mixture was concentrated to ~10.0 mL. The mixture was treated with 2.0 M HCl (20.0 mL), resulting in a hydrochloride salt of the amine, which was washed with DCM (3 × 30 mL) to remove the other organic impurities. The aqueous layer was evaporated in a fume hood to obtain a white powder, which was washed with DCM to yield the amine hydrochloride. Yield: 2.89 g, 95.0%. ^{1}H NMR (400 MHz, DMSO-d_6) δ (ppm): 8.65 (s, 9H), 7.66 (s, 3H), and 4.01 (s, 6H). ^{13}C {^{1}H} NMR (100 MHz, DMSO-d_6) δ (ppm): 134.61, 129.68, and 42.06. MS (ESI): calcd for $C_9H_{15}N_3Na$ [M + Na]$^+$, 188.1158; found, 188.1146.

3.1.2. Synthesis of Triethyl 4,4′,4″-(((benzene-1,3,5-triyltris(methylene))tris(azanediyl))tris(carbonyl))tribenzoate (N-BTA)

The benzene-1,3,5-triyltrimethanamine hydrochloride (0.89 g, 3.2 mmol) sample was dissolved in 70.0 mL of THF by adding triethylamine (3.1 mL, 22.6 mmol) under a nitrogen atmosphere and the product was kept in an ice bath. The acid chloride of 4-(ethoxycarbonyl)benzoic acid (2.7 g, 11.1 mmol) was then added dropwise after being dissolved in 50.0 mL of THF and stirred at room temperature for an hour. The mixture was refluxed overnight, cooled, and evaporated to dryness. The crude mixture was kept in the fume hood for a day and then stirred with 5.0% sodium bicarbonate for 12.0 h. The mixture was filtered, washed with copious amounts of water, and dried to obtain the corresponding amide as a white powder. The product was then recrystallized in ethanol. Yield: 1.6 g, 71.5%. ^{1}H NMR (400 MHz, DMSO-d_6) δ (ppm): 9.22 (t, J = 6.1 Hz, 3H), 7.93 (q, J = 8.7 Hz, 12H), 7.17 (s, 3H), 4.47 (d, J = 6.0 Hz, 6H), 4.34 (q, J = 7.1 Hz, 6H), 1.34 (t, J = 7.1 Hz, 9H). ^{13}C {^{1}H} NMR (100 MHz, DMSO-d_6) δ (ppm): 170.63, 170.37, 144.90, 143.59, 137.21, 134.23, 132.75, 129.55, 66.25, 47.75, 19.32. MS (ESI): calcd for $C_{39}H_{39}N_3O_9Na$ [M + Na]$^+$, 716.2579; found, 716.2564.

3.2. Gelation Studies

We added 10.0 mg of N-BTA and 1.0 mL of the solvent to a standard 7.0 mL vial (ID = 15.0 mm), and the vial was sealed. The mixture was sonicated and heated gradually to produce a transparent solution, and the mixture was kept undisturbed for 24.0 h. A gelation confirmation test was performed using an inversion test. Gelation experiments were also performed in a 1:1, v/v mixed aqueous system, where 10.0 mg of the N-BTA was dissolved in 0.5 mL of the suitable solvent in a standard 7.0 mL vial. Subsequently, 0.5 mL of deionized water was added to the solution. The vial was sealed, and the solution was subjected to sonication and heated slowly to achieve a clear solution. The solution was kept undisturbed, and gel formation was confirmed using a vial inversion test. The experiments were replicated, using higher doses of the compound (up to 50.0 mg) to check gel formation at higher concentrations.

3.2.1. Minimum Gelator Concentration (MGC)

The MGC experiment was conducted using appropriate solvents, where different quantities of the compounds were weighed in a standard 7.0 mL vial. Then, 1.0 mL of solvent or solvent mixture was added. The vial was sealed, sonicated, and heated gradually to achieve complete dissolution. Subsequently, the solution was maintained at room temperature to facilitate gel formation. The minimum quantity of the compound necessary for the formation of a stable gel within a 24.0 h period was determined as the MGC.

3.2.2. T_{gel} Experiments

The necessary quantity of gelator and 1.0 mL of solvent were added to a 7.0 mL standard vial. The solution was subjected to sonication and heated slowly until it dissolved, and the product was then allowed to gel without any disturbance. Following 24.0 h, a ball-drop method was employed to observe the gel-to-sol transition temperature (T_{gel}). A spherical-shaped glass ball was positioned on the gel surface and the vials were sealed before being submerged in an oil bath. The oil bath equipped with a magnetic stirrer was gradually heated at a rate of 10.0 °C per minute, and a thermometer was utilized to monitor the temperature of the oil bath. As the ambient temperature was reached, the glass ball gradually became submerged within the gels, and the temperature at which the ball made contact with the lower surface of the vial was recorded as T_{gel}. The experiments were repeated three times, and the average was taken to be the T_{gel}.

3.3. Rheology

Rheological measurements were conducted using an Anton Paar Modular Compact Rheometer MCR 302 and the experiments were repeated three times for each sample. Mechanical strength was measured using a 2.5 cm stainless-steel parallel-plate geometry setup. In all instances, oscillatory measurements were performed under a constant temperature of 20.0 °C. A Peltier temperature control hood was used as a solvent trap, which maintained a temperature of 20.0 °C for frequency and amplitude sweeps. A suitable quantity of the respective gelator was dissolved in 1.0 mL of solvent to make the gels. After 24 h, the studies were conducted by transferring the gel onto the plate. A consistent frequency of 1.0 Hz was preserved during the amplitude sweep, while the logarithmic ramp strain (Y) ranged between 0.01 and 100%. The frequency sweep was conducted inside the linear viscoelasticity domain (0.01% strain) between 0.1 and 10.0 Hz.

3.4. Scanning Electron Microscopy (SEM)

A Leo Supra 25 microscope was used to perform the SEM imaging to analyze the surface morphologies of the xerogels. Gels of the compound were prepared in methanol, ethanol, isopropanol, and n-butanol at 2.0 wt/v%, and in aqueous mixtures (1:1, v/v) of DMF and DMSO at 4.0 wt/v%. The gels were filtered after 24 h and dried under a fume hood to obtain xerogels. A small amount of xerogel was put on a pin mount with the carbon tab on top. It was subsequently coated with gold for 5–6 min (12.0 nm thickness) to keep the surface from charging and was then loaded. mages were taken at a working distance of 3.0–4.0 mm and an operating voltage of 3.0 kV. The SEM picture was taken with an in-lens detector.

3.5. Powder X-ray Diffraction

We obtained samples of microcrystalline material of N-BTA in ethanol (20.0 mg in 2.0 mL). The crystalline material was filtered, dried in air, and ground down to a fine powder. The xerogels of the compound were prepared from corresponding gels made from methanol, ethanol, isopropanol, and n-butanol, and from aqueous mixtures of DMSO, DMF, DMA, and DEA at 4.0 wt/v%. Gels were further filtered and dried in a fume hood to obtain xerogels. All the tests were conducted using a PANalytical instrument with a Cu anode (Almelo, The Netherlands), with a step size of 0.025 and a range of 2θ, running from 4.0 to 50.0.

3.6. Stimuli-Responsive Properties

We dissolved 36.0 mg of N-BTA (MGC) in 0.5 mL of DMSO and dissolved sodium/potassium halides, nitrate, carbonate, cyanide, sulphate, and acetate (1.0 equiv.) in 0.5 mL water. The solutions were mixed, heated until they dissolved, and left undisturbed for gel formation. We performed thermal analysis of the obtained gels using T_{gel} studies, and the mechanical properties were recorded using rheological measurements (frequency sweep) following the procedures described in Sections 3.2.2 and 3.3, respectively, and the experiments were repeated two times for each anion.

3.7. UV–Visible Spectroscopy

UV-vis absorptions were recorded on the Agilent Cary UV-vis Multicell Peltier spectrometer. The MB and MO dye solutions were prepared in water (10.0 mL) at a concentration of 7.5×10^{-6} M and 5.0×10^{-5} M via dilution from a higher known concentration. In the dye adsorption experiment, data was collected with a bandwidth of 2.0 nm. Initially, we prepared the solution of the dye in water in a 25.0 mL beaker at the required concentration, and then the absorbance was recorded. We then carefully immersed the gel in a dye solution, sealed the beaker, and recorded the absorbance of the solution after 2 to 8 days.

3.7.1. Dye Adsorption Studies with Varying Concentrations of N-BTA

Gels of the compound were prepared at various concentrations (wt/v%) of N-BTA (2.0, 2.4, 2.8, 3.2, 3.6, 5.0 and 6.0) in ethanol and immersed in 10.0 mL aqueous solutions of MB (7.5×10^{-6} M) and MO (5.0×10^{-5} M). The absorbance was recorded after 2, 5, and 7 days.

3.7.2. Dye Adsorption Studies of MO with N-BTA Gel from Other Solvents

Gels of the compound were prepared at 4.0 wt/v% in *n*-butanol, isopropanol, and DMSO/water mixture (1:1, *v/v*) and immersed in an aqueous solution (10.0 mL) of MO. The absorbance was recorded after 2 days.

4. Conclusions

We successfully synthesized C_3-symmetric N-centered BTA (N-BTA) by modifying BTA molecules with flexible linkers. Our gelation studies revealed that N-BTA formed gels in alcohols and aqueous mixtures of high-polar solvents. We characterized the gels using standard gelation techniques and analyzed their morphologies using SEM. The comparison of mechanical strength in different solvents revealed that the gel from DMSO/water (1:1, *v/v*) mixture displayed a stronger gel network, which correlated well with the thermal stability experiments. The xerogels from aqueous mixtures displayed needle-shaped morphologies, whereas the xerogels from alcohols displayed zoetic and flake-like morphologies. The comparison of the PXRD patterns of the xerogels obtained from the aqueous mixtures found that they perfectly matched, suggesting a similar mode of packing. The xerogels from the alcohols were less crystalline, displaying broad peaks, but most of the peaks matched with those of the aqueous mixtures and bulk material. The anion-sensing properties of N-BTA were evaluated in the presence of sodium and potassium salts in a DMSO/water mixture (1:1, *v/v*) at MGC and below. The gel network was disrupted by cyanide, chloride and fluoride salts, but remained intact in the presence of nitrate, sulphate, acetate, bromide and iodide salts. The experiments performed below MGC revealed that nitrate, sulphate, acetate, bromide and iodide salts induced gelation. Analysis of the mechanical and thermal strengths of these gels in comparison with the native gelator revealed that the N-BTA gels exhibited improved thermal and mechanical stability in the presence of nitrate, sulphate, acetate, bromide and iodide salts. The dye adsorption capability of N-BTA was analyzed by dispersing the ethanolic gel in an aqueous solution of MB and MO, resulting in a colorless solution of MB after 5 days. The UV-vis absorption studies revealed a reduction in absorbance for MB within 2 days, which was mostly absorbed within 8 days. Similarly, the MO solution also showed a decrease in absorbance after 8 days, but the adsorption of MO from water by the N-BTA gel was lower compared to that of the cationic MB dye. In summary, this study highlights the potential of C_3-symmetric N-BTA for application in anion-sensing and dye removal from wastewater treatment. This study demonstrates an easy synthetic route for synthesizing N-centered BTA molecules with intriguing properties by altering functional groups.

Supplementary Materials: The following supporting information can be downloaded at: https://www.mdpi.com/article/10.3390/molecules29092149/s1, Figure S1. Amplitude sweep measurement was performed for the N-BTA gel in EtOH at 4.0 wt/v%; Figure S2. Amplitude sweep measurement was performed for the N-BTA gel in MeOH at 4.0 wt/v%; Figure S3. Amplitude sweep measurement was performed for the N-BTA gel in DMSO/water at 4.0 wt/v%: Figure S4. Amplitude sweep measurement was performed for the N-BTA gel in DMF/water at 4.0 wt/v%; Figure S5. SEM images of N-BTA xerogels (2.0 wt/v%) in (a) isopropanol and (b) *n*-butanol; Figure S6. Comparison of PXRD patterns of the dried gels (4.0 wt/v%) from alcohols, DMF/water, and bulk material; Figure S7. Stimuli-responsive properties of the N-BTA gels with various anions (1.0 eq) at MGC in DMSO/water (1:1, v/v); (a) potassium halides, (b) sodium and (c) potassium salts of cyanide, sulphate, nitrate and acetate anions, respectively; Figure S8. (a) N-BTA gels below MGC in DMSO/water (1:1, v/v) and anion induced gelation with (b) sodium and (c) potassium salts such as bromide, iodide, nitrate, sulphate and acetate ions (1.0 eq.); Figure S9. The time-dependent adsorption of MB by N-BTA gel; Figure S10. The time-dependent adsorption of MO by N-BTA gel; Figure S11. Aqueous solution of (a) MB and MO before and after the addition of dry N-BTA; Figure S12. UV-vis experiments of MO (5.0×10^{-5} M) with N-BTA gel from n-butanol, isopropanol, and DMSO/water; Figure S13. UV-vis experiments of MB (7.5×10^{-6} M) with different concentrations of N-BTA after 2 days; Figure S14. UV-vis experiments of MB (7.5×10^{-6} M) with different concentrations of N-BTA after 5 days; Figure S15. UV-vis experiments of MO (5.0×10^{-5} M) with different concentrations of N-BTA after 2 days; Figure S16. UV-vis experiments of MO (5.0×10^{-5} M) with different concentrations of N-BTA after 5 days; Figure S17. UV-vis experiments of MO (5.0×10^{-5} M) with different concentrations of N-BTA after 7 days; Figure S18. Adsorption ratio of MO with varying concentrations of N-BTA after 2, 5, and 7 days; Figure S19. ^{1}H NMR spectrum of benzene-1,3,5-triyltrimethanamine; Figure S20. ^{13}C NMR spectrum of benzene-1,3,5-triyltrimethanamine, Figure S21; ^{1}H NMR spectrum of N-BTA; Figure S22. ^{13}C NMR spectrum of N-BTA; Table S1. Gelation Experiments; Table S2. T_{gel} studies with the gels in DMSO/water (1:1, v/v) in the presence potassium and sodium salts (1.0 equiv.).

Author Contributions: Conceptualization, K.K.D.; methodology, G.K. and S.S.J.; software, G.K., and S.S.J.; validation, G.K., S.S.J. and K.K.D.; formal analysis, G.K., S.S.J. and K.K.D.; investigation, G.K. and S.S.J.; resources, K.K.D.; data curation, G.K. and K.K.D.; visualization, G.K., S.S.J. and K.K.D.; supervision, K.K.D.; project administration, K.K.D.; funding acquisition, K.K.D.; writing—original draft preparation, K.K.D.; writing—review and editing, G.K., S.S.J. and K.K.D. All authors have read and agreed to the published version of the manuscript.

Funding: This research was funded by the Icelandic Research Fund (IRF-228902-051) Rannís Iceland.

Institutional Review Board Statement: Not applicable.

Informed Consent Statement: Not applicable.

Data Availability Statement: All the details are given in the Supplementary Materials.

Acknowledgments: We thank the University of Iceland Research Fund and Icelandic Research Fund (IRF-228902-051) Rannís Iceland for funding. We acknowledge Sigríður Jónsdóttir, University of Iceland, for NMR and mass spectrometry, and Friðrik Magnus, University of Iceland, for powder X-ray diffraction analysis. We thank Rannís Iceland for the infrastructure grant (191763-0031) for the rheometer and (210521-901) for the UV-VIS spectrometer.

Conflicts of Interest: The authors declare no conflicts of interest.

References

1. Prasad, M.N.V.; Elchuri, S.V. Environmental Contaminants of Emerging Concern: Occurrence and Remediation. *Chem. Didact. Ecol. Metrol.* **2023**, *28*, 57–77. [CrossRef]
2. Feng, W.; Deng, Y.; Yang, F.; Miao, Q.; Ngien, S.K. Systematic Review of Contaminants of Emerging Concern (CECs): Distribution, Risks, and Implications for Water Quality and Health. *Water* **2023**, *15*, 3922. [CrossRef]
3. Al-Tohamy, R.; Ali, S.S.; Li, F.; Okasha, K.M.; Mahmoud, Y.A.G.; Elsamahy, T.; Jiao, H.; Fu, Y.; Sun, J. A critical review on the treatment of dye-containing wastewater: Ecotoxicological and health concerns of textile dyes and possible remediation approaches for environmental safety. *Ecotoxicol. Environ. Saf.* **2022**, *231*, 113160. [CrossRef]
4. Berradi, M.; Hsissou, R.; Khudhair, M.; Assouag, M.; Cherkaoui, O.; El Bachiri, A.; El Harfi, A. Textile finishing dyes and their impact on aquatic environs. *Heliyon* **2019**, *5*, e02711. [CrossRef] [PubMed]
5. Alsukaibi, A.K.D. Various Approaches for the Detoxification of Toxic Dyes in Wastewater. *Processes* **2022**, *10*, 1968. [CrossRef]
6. Dutta, S.; Gupta, B.; Srivastava, S.K.; Gupta, A.K. Recent advances on the removal of dyes from wastewater using various adsorbents: A critical review. *Mater. Adv.* **2021**, *2*, 4497–4531. [CrossRef]
7. Mudhoo, A.; Ramasamy, D.L.; Bhatnagar, A.; Usman, M.; Sillanpää, M. An analysis of the versatility and effectiveness of composts for sequestering heavy metal ions, dyes and xenobiotics from soils and aqueous milieus. *Ecotoxicol. Environ. Saf.* **2020**, *197*, 110587. [CrossRef] [PubMed]
8. Jadhav, A.C.; Jadhav, N.C. Chapter Ten—Treatment of textile wastewater using adsorption and adsorbents. In *Sustainable Technologies for Textile Wastewater Treatments*; Muthu, S.S., Ed.; Woodhead Publishing: Sawston, UK, 2021; pp. 235–273.
9. de Loos, M.; Feringa, B.L.; van Esch, J.H. Design and Application of Self-Assembled Low Molecular Weight Hydrogels. *Eur. J. Org. Chem.* **2005**, *2005*, 3615–3631. [CrossRef]
10. Kumar, D.K.; Steed, J.W. Supramolecular gel phase crystallization: Orthogonal self-assembly under non-equilibrium conditions. *Chem. Soc. Rev.* **2014**, *43*, 2080–2088. [CrossRef]
11. Steed, J.W. Anion-tuned supramolecular gels: A natural evolution from urea supramolecular chemistry. *Chem. Soc. Rev.* **2010**, *39*, 3686–3699. [CrossRef]
12. Smith, D.K. Supramolecular gels—A panorama of low-molecular-weight gelators from ancient origins to next-generation technologies. *Soft Matter* **2024**, *20*, 10–70. [CrossRef] [PubMed]
13. Adams, D.J. Personal Perspective on Understanding Low Molecular Weight Gels. *J. Am. Chem. Soc.* **2022**, *144*, 11047–11053. [CrossRef] [PubMed]
14. Okesola, B.O.; Smith, D.K. Applying low-molecular weight supramolecular gelators in an environmental setting—Self-assembled gels as smart materials for pollutant removal. *Chem. Soc. Rev.* **2016**, *45*, 4226–4251. [CrossRef] [PubMed]
15. Li, L.; Sun, R.; Zheng, R.; Huang, Y. Anions-responsive supramolecular gels: A review. *Mater. Des.* **2021**, *205*, 109759. [CrossRef]
16. Panja, S.; Adams, D.J. Stimuli responsive dynamic transformations in supramolecular gels. *Chem. Soc. Rev.* **2021**, *50*, 5165–5200. [CrossRef] [PubMed]
17. Chu, C.-W.; Schalley, C.A. Recent Advances on Supramolecular Gels: From Stimuli-Responsive Gels to Co-Assembled and Self-Sorted Systems. *Org. Mater.* **2021**, *3*, 025–040. [CrossRef]
18. Jones, C.D.; Steed, J.W. Gels with sense: Supramolecular materials that respond to heat, light and sound. *Chem. Soc. Rev.* **2016**, *45*, 6546–6596. [CrossRef] [PubMed]
19. Yang, X.; Zhang, G.; Zhang, D. Stimuli responsive gels based on low molecular weight gelators. *J. Mater. Chem.* **2012**, *22*, 38–50. [CrossRef]
20. Patel, A.M.; Bhardwaj, V.; Ray, D.; Aswal, V.K.; Ballabh, A. A library of benzimidazole based amide and urea derivatives as supramolecular gelators—A comparative study. *J. Mol. Liq.* **2024**, *395*, 123858. [CrossRef]
21. Cheng, N.; Hu, Q.; Guo, Y.; Wang, Y.; Yu, L. Efficient and Selective Removal of Dyes Using Imidazolium-Based Supramolecular Gels. *ACS Appl. Mater. Interfaces* **2015**, *7*, 10258–10265. [CrossRef]
22. Roy, R.; Adalder, T.K.; Dastidar, P. Supramolecular Gels Derived from the Salts of Variously Substituted Phenylacetic Acid and Dicyclohexylamine: Design, Synthesis, Structures, and Dye Adsorption. *Chem. Asian J.* **2018**, *13*, 552–559. [CrossRef] [PubMed]
23. Li, L.; Chen, J.; Wang, Z.; Xie, L.; Feng, C.; He, G.; Hu, H.; Sun, R.; Zhu, H. A supramolecular gel made from an azobenzene-based phenylalanine derivative: Synthesis, self-assembly, and dye adsorption. *Colloids Surf. A Physicochem. Eng. Asp.* **2021**, *628*, 127289. [CrossRef]
24. Ray, S.; Das, A.K.; Banerjee, A. pH-Responsive, Bolaamphiphile-Based Smart Metallo-Hydrogels as Potential Dye-Adsorbing Agents, Water Purifier, and Vitamin B12 Carrier. *Chem. Mater.* **2007**, *19*, 1633–1639. [CrossRef]

25. Samai, S.; Biradha, K. Chemical and Mechano Responsive Metal–Organic Gels of Bis(benzimidazole)-Based Ligands with Cd(II) and Cu(II) Halide Salts: Self Sustainability and Gas and Dye Sorptions. *Chem. Mater.* **2012**, *24*, 1165–1173. [CrossRef]
26. Wang, H.; Xu, W.; Song, S.; Feng, L.; Song, A.; Hao, J. Hydrogels Facilitated by Monovalent Cations and Their Use as Efficient Dye Adsorbents. *J. Phys. Chem. B* **2014**, *118*, 4693–4701. [CrossRef] [PubMed]
27. Bhavya, P.V.; Soundarajan, K.; Malecki, J.G.; Mohan Das, T. Sugar-Based Phase-Selective Supramolecular Self-Assembly System for Dye Removal and Selective Detection of Cu^{2+} Ions. *ACS Omega* **2022**, *7*, 39310–39324. [CrossRef] [PubMed]
28. Okesola, B.O.; Smith, D.K. Versatile supramolecular pH-tolerant hydrogels which demonstrate pH-dependent selective adsorption of dyes from aqueous solution. *Chem. Commun.* **2013**, *49*, 11164–11166. [CrossRef] [PubMed]
29. Samsami, S.; Mohamadizaniani, M.; Sarrafzadeh, M.-H.; Rene, E.R.; Firoozbahr, M. Recent advances in the treatment of dye-containing wastewater from textile industries: Overview and perspectives. *Process Saf. Environ. Prot.* **2020**, *143*, 138–163. [CrossRef]
30. Weiss, R.G.; Terech, P. (Eds.) *Molecular Gels: Materials with Self-Assembled Fibrillar Networks*; Springer: Dordrecht, The Netherlands, 2006; p. 978.
31. Fages, F.; Voegtle, F.; Zinic, M. Systematic design of amide- and urea-type gelators with tailored properties. *Top. Curr. Chem.* **2005**, *256*, 77–131.
32. Moulin, E.; Armao, J.J.; Giuseppone, N. Triarylamine-Based Supramolecular Polymers: Structures, Dynamics, and Functions. *Acc. Chem. Res.* **2019**, *52*, 975–983. [CrossRef]
33. Wang, Y.; de Kruijff, R.M.; Lovrak, M.; Guo, X.; Eelkema, R.; van Esch, J.H. Access to Metastable Gel States Using Seeded Self-Assembly of Low-Molecular-Weight Gelators. *Angew. Chem. Int. Ed.* **2019**, *58*, 3800–3803. [CrossRef] [PubMed]
34. Ghosh, D.; Chaudhary, P.; Pradeep, A.; Singh, S.; Rangasamy, J.; Damodaran, K.K. Structural modification induced hydrogelation and antibacterial properties in supramolecular gels. *J. Mol. Liq.* **2023**, *382*, 122023. [CrossRef]
35. Ghosh, D.; Farahani, A.D.; Martin, A.D.; Thordarson, P.; Damodaran, K.K. Unraveling the Self-Assembly Modes in Multicomponent Supramolecular Gels Using Single-Crystal X-ray Diffraction. *Chem. Mater.* **2020**, *32*, 3517–3527. [CrossRef]
36. Dastidar, P. Supramolecular gelling agents: Can they be designed? *Chem. Soc. Rev.* **2008**, *37*, 2699–2715. [CrossRef] [PubMed]
37. Estroff, L.A.; Hamilton, A.D. Water gelation by small organic molecules. *Chem. Rev.* **2004**, *104*, 1201–1218. [CrossRef] [PubMed]
38. Kumar, S.; Bera, S.; Nandi, S.K.; Haldar, D. The effect of amide bond orientation and symmetry on the self-assembly and gelation of discotic tripeptides. *Soft Matter* **2021**, *17*, 113–119. [CrossRef] [PubMed]
39. Yang, Z.; Wu, G.; Gan, C.; Cai, G.; Zhang, J.; Ji, H. Effective adsorption of arsenate, dyes and eugenol from aqueous solutions by cationic supramolecular gel materials. *Colloids Surf. A Physicochem. Eng. Asp.* **2021**, *616*, 126238. [CrossRef]
40. Fang, H.; Qu, W.-J.; Yang, H.-H.; He, J.-X.; Yao, H.; Lin, Q.; Wei, T.-B.; Zhang, Y.-M. A self-assembled supramolecular gel constructed by phenazine derivative and its application in ultrasensitive detection of cyanide. *Dyes Pigm.* **2020**, *174*, 108066. [CrossRef]
41. Hao, C.; Gao, J.; Wu, Y.; Wang, X.; Zhao, R.; Mei, S.; Yang, J.; Zhai, X.; Qiu, H. Design of folic acid based supramolecular hybrid gel with improved mechanical properties in NMP/H_2O for dye adsorption. *React. Funct. Polym.* **2018**, *122*, 140–147. [CrossRef]
42. Lou, X.; Lafleur, R.P.M.; Leenders, C.M.A.; Schoenmakers, S.M.C.; Matsumoto, N.M.; Baker, M.B.; van Dongen, J.L.J.; Palmans, A.R.A.; Meijer, E.W. Dynamic diversity of synthetic supramolecular polymers in water as revealed by hydrogen/deuterium exchange. *Nat. Commun.* **2017**, *8*, 15420. [CrossRef]
43. Lynes, A.D.; Hawes, C.S.; Ward, E.N.; Haffner, B.; Möbius, M.E.; Byrne, K.; Schmitt, W.; Pal, R.; Gunnlaugsson, T. Benzene-1,3,5-tricarboxamide n-alkyl ester and carboxylic acid derivatives: Tuneable structural, morphological and thermal properties. *CrystEngComm* **2017**, *19*, 1427–1438. [CrossRef]
44. Daly, R.; Kotova, O.; Boese, M.; Gunnlaugsson, T.; Boland, J.J. Chemical Nano-Gardens: Growth of Salt Nanowires from Supramolecular Self-Assembly Gels. *ACS Nano* **2013**, *7*, 4838–4845. [CrossRef]
45. Kumar, D.K.; Jose, D.A.; Dastidar, P.; Das, A. Nonpolymeric Hydrogelators Derived from Trimesic Amides. *Chem. Mater.* **2004**, *16*, 2332–2335. [CrossRef]
46. Goodwin, J.W.; Hughes, R.W. *Rheology for Chemists: An Introduction*; Royal Society of Chemistry: London, UK, 2008.
47. Guenet, J.-M. *Organogels: Thermodynamics, Structure, Solvent Role, and Properties*; Springer: Berlin/Heidelberg, Germany, 2016.
48. Yu, L.; Yan, X.; Han, C.; Huang, F. Characterization of supramolecular gels. *Chem. Soc. Rev.* **2013**, *42*, 6697–6722. [CrossRef] [PubMed]
49. Adams, D.J. Does Drying Affect Gel Networks? *Gels* **2018**, *4*, 32. [CrossRef] [PubMed]
50. Ghosh, D.; Lebedytė, I.; Yufit, D.S.; Damodaran, K.K.; Steed, J.W. Selective gelation of N-(4-pyridyl)nicotinamide by copper(ii) salts. *CrystEngComm* **2015**, *17*, 8130–8138. [CrossRef]
51. Ghosh, D.; Mulvee, M.T.; Damodaran, K.K. Tuning Gel State Properties of Supramolecular Gels by Functional Group Modification. *Molecules* **2019**, *24*, 3472. [CrossRef]
52. Ghosh, D.; Deepa; Damodaran, K.K. Metal complexation induced supramolecular gels for the detection of cyanide in water. *Supramol. Chem.* **2020**, *32*, 276–286. [CrossRef]
53. Piepenbrock, M.-O.M.; Lloyd, G.O.; Clarke, N.; Steed, J.W. Metal- and Anion-Binding Supramolecular Gels. *Chem. Rev.* **2010**, *110*, 1960–2004. [CrossRef]
54. Ghosh, A.; Das, P.; Kaushik, R.; Damodaran, K.K.; Jose, D.A. Anion responsive and morphology tunable tripodal gelators. *RSC Adv.* **2016**, *6*, 83303–83311. [CrossRef]

55. Sudhakaran Jayabhavan, S.; Kuppadakkath, G.; Damodaran, K.K. The Role of Functional Groups in Tuning the Self-Assembly Modes and Physical Properties of Multicomponent Gels. *ChemPlusChem* **2023**, *88*, e202300302. [CrossRef]
56. Jayabhavan, S.S.; Kristinsson, B.; Ghosh, D.; Breton, C.; Damodaran, K.K. Stimuli-Responsive Properties of Supramolecular Gels Based on Pyridyl-N-oxide Amides. *Gels* **2023**, *9*, 89. [CrossRef]
57. Zhang, X.; Liu, J.; Gao, Y.; Hao, J.; Hu, J.; Ju, Y. Multi-stimuli-responsive hydrogels of gluconamide-tailored anthracene. *Soft Matter* **2019**, *15*, 4662–4668. [CrossRef] [PubMed]
58. Panja, A.; Ghosh, S.; Ghosh, K. A sulfonyl hydrazone cholesterol conjugate: Gelation, anion interaction and its application in dye adsorption. *New J. Chem.* **2019**, *43*, 10270–10277. [CrossRef]
59. Pati, C.; Ghosh, K. A 1,8-naphthalimide–pyridoxal conjugate as a supramolecular gelator for colorimetric read out of F− ions in solution, gel and solid states. *New J. Chem.* **2019**, *43*, 2718–2725. [CrossRef]
60. Yang, Y.; Zhu, Q.; Peng, X.; Sun, J.; Li, C.; Zhang, X.; Zhang, H.; Chen, J.; Zhou, X.; Zeng, H.; et al. Hydrogels for the removal of the methylene blue dye from wastewater: A review. *Environ. Chem. Lett.* **2022**, *20*, 2665–2685. [CrossRef]
61. Dutta, S.K.; Amin, M.K.; Ahmed, J.; Elias, M.; Mahiuddin, M. Removal of toxic methyl orange by a cost-free and eco-friendly adsorbent: Mechanism, phytotoxicity, thermodynamics, and kinetics. *S. Afr. J. Chem. Eng.* **2022**, *40*, 195–208. [CrossRef]
62. Iwuozor, K.O.; Ighalo, J.O.; Emenike, E.C.; Ogunfowora, L.A.; Igwegbe, C.A. Adsorption of methyl orange: A review on adsorbent performance. *Curr. Res. Green Sustain. Chem.* **2021**, *4*, 100179. [CrossRef]
63. Fortunato, A.; Mba, M. A Peptide-Based Hydrogel for Adsorption of Dyes and Pharmaceuticals in Water Remediation. *Gels* **2022**, *8*, 672. [CrossRef]
64. Mancuso, L.; Knobloch, T.; Buchholz, J.; Hartwig, J.; Möller, L.; Seidel, K.; Collisi, W.; Sasse, F.; Kirschning, A. Preparation of Thermocleavable Conjugates Based on Ansamitocin and Superparamagnetic Nanostructured Particles by a Chemobiosynthetic Approach. *Chem. Eur. J.* **2014**, *20*, 17541–17551. [CrossRef]

Disclaimer/Publisher's Note: The statements, opinions and data contained in all publications are solely those of the individual author(s) and contributor(s) and not of MDPI and/or the editor(s). MDPI and/or the editor(s) disclaim responsibility for any injury to people or property resulting from any ideas, methods, instructions or products referred to in the content.

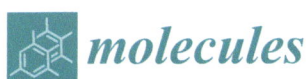

Article

Enhanced Stability of Dimethyl Ether Carbonylation through Pyrazole Tartrate on Tartaric Acid-Complexed Cobalt–Iron-Modified Hydrogen-Type Mordenite

Guangtao Fu and Xinfa Dong *

Guangdong Provincial Key Laboratory of Green Chemical Product Technology, School of Chemistry and Chemical Engineering, South China University of Technology, Guangzhou 510640, China; ce202120124494@mail.scut.edu.cn
* Correspondence: cexfdong@scut.edu.cn

Abstract: In this study, pyrazole tartrate (Pya·DL) and tartaric acid (DL) complexed with cobalt–iron bimetallic modified hydrogen-type mordenite (HMOR) were prepared using the ion exchange method. The results demonstrate that the stability of the dimethyl ether (DME) carbonylation reaction to methyl acetate (MA) was significantly improved after the introduction of Pya·DL to HMOR. The Co·Fe·DL·Pya·DL-HMOR (0.8) sample exhibited sustainable stability within 400 h DME carbonylation, exhibiting a DME conversion rate of about 70% and MA selectivity of above 99%. Through modification with the DL-complexed cobalt–iron bimetal, the dispersion of cobalt–iron was greatly enhanced, leading to the formation of new metal Lewis acidic sites (LAS) and thus a significant improvement in catalysis activity. Pya·DL effectively eliminated non-framework aluminum in HMOR, enlarged its pore size, and created channels for carbon deposition diffusion, thereby preventing carbon accumulation and pore blockage. Additionally, Pya·DL shielded the Bronsted acid sites (BAS) in the 12 MR channel, effectively suppressing the side reactions of carbon deposition and reducing the formation of hard carbon deposits. These improvements collectively contribute to the enhanced stability of the DME carbonylation reaction.

Keywords: hydrogen-type mordenite; DME carbonylation; pyrazole tartrate; cobalt–iron; Bronsted acid sites

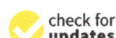

Citation: Fu, G.; Dong, X. Enhanced Stability of Dimethyl Ether Carbonylation through Pyrazole Tartrate on Tartaric Acid-Complexed Cobalt–Iron-Modified Hydrogen-Type Mordenite. *Molecules* **2024**, *29*, 1510. https://doi.org/10.3390/molecules29071510

Academic Editors: Michael A. Beckett and Qingguo Shao

Received: 23 January 2024
Revised: 6 March 2024
Accepted: 26 March 2024
Published: 28 March 2024

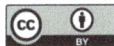

Copyright: © 2024 by the authors. Licensee MDPI, Basel, Switzerland. This article is an open access article distributed under the terms and conditions of the Creative Commons Attribution (CC BY) license (https://creativecommons.org/licenses/by/4.0/).

1. Introduction

Ethanol, highly regarded for its cleanliness and environmental friendliness, is a crucial energy source that can substitute or augment traditional fuels, thereby contributing to the mitigation of fossil fuel overconsumption [1]. The rapid growth of the fuel ethanol market has promoted the development of production methodologies embracing alternative carbonaceous sources, such as coal, biomass, or natural gas syngas. Notably, the process involved in the carbonylation of DME to produce MA, followed by hydrogenation to yield ethanol, has garnered significant attention from researchers because of its exceptional atom economy, high selectivity, and potential for widespread industrial implementation [2–4]. DME coupling with CO over acidic zeolites facilitates non-noble metal catalysis and a halide-free process to upgrade the widely available C1 intermediates into high value-added MA, which can be facilely hydrogenated to ethanol [5–9]. Thus, DME carbonylation is also considered the key step in ethanol synthesis, and it has attracted considerable attention over the past decade.

Iglesia et al. [10] found that HMOR zeolite exhibits unparalleled carbonylation activity in DME carbonylation reactions due to its unique skeletal composition. HMOR comprises a parallel 12-membered ring (12 MR) (0.70 × 0.67 nm) and 8 MR (0.57 × 0.26 nm) channels interconnected through 8 MR side pockets (0.48 × 0.34 nm) [11,12]. Notably, the carbonylation of DME mainly occurs within the 8 MR channel of HMOR, benefitting from its unique quantum domain-limiting effect. In contrast, the 12 MR channels housing Bronsted acid (BAS) serve as carbon-accumulating reactive sites prone to carbon deposition, thereby hastening the deactivation of HMOR during carbonylation [13]. To improve carbonylation activity and stability, it is necessary to manipulate the BAS distribution in HMOR precisely or to target the shielding of BAS in the 12 MR channel.

Scientists have been working to regulate the structure of HMOR in order to enhance its efficacy and stability in DME carbonylation. Li et al. [14] hydrothermally synthesized cerium-containing MOR samples. The substitution of aluminum in the zeolite framework with Ce^{3+} species increased the concentration of BAS in the 8 MR, enhancing carbonylation activity. Wang et al. [15] used the ion exchange method to modify HMOR with transition metals such as Ni, Co, Cu, Zn, and Ag, resulting in enhanced DME conversion and MA selectivity in the majority of the samples. Liu et al. [16] utilized trimethylamine cation (TMA^+) for HMOR ion exchange, maintaining catalytic activity during three rounds of experiments. However, the specific surface area decreased significantly with each exchange, with it reaching less than 1/10 of the original surface area after three exchanges, accompanied by reduced DME conversion rates. In another study, Liu et al. [17] employed plate-like alkyl imidazolium ions for selective ion exchange in HMOR. The introduction of 1,3-dimethyl imidazolium ions allowed for the selective removal of BAS in the 12 MR channel, substantially improving the stability and activity of HMOR.

At present, although the stability of HMOR has been enhanced to some extent by shielding the BAS in the 12 MR channel, the regeneration of BAS still occurs in 12 MR, which poses a challenge in maintaining the prolonged high carbonylation activity and stability of HMOR. Ma et al. [18] found that the introduction of Co^{2+} into the 8 MR pore channel could improve the adsorption of CO and DME molecules, thereby enhancing reactivity. Zhou et al. [19] showed that incorporating Fe into the initial hydrothermal gel could reduce the intensity and density of BAS in the 12 MR, mitigating coke formation. Alternatively, pyrazole is a smaller nitrogen-containing heterocyclic compound with a molecular diameter of 0.434 nm. It would be more difficult for it to pass through the 8 MR tunnel and easier for it to enter the 12 MR tunnel to shield the active sites of carbon deposits [20]. Moreover, weakly basic pyrazole reacts with hydrochloric acid to form an aqueous solution of pyrazole hydrochloride (Pya·HCl), which can achieve the same function of removing non-framework aluminum in HMOR as nitric acid [21]. Liu et al. [20] found that Pya·HCl could selectively enter 12 MR in the ion exchange process, and, in turn, the stability of the modified HMOR was improved. Tartaric acid is highly acidic, and its boiling point is as high as 399.3 °C, which is much higher than the reaction temperature of DME carbonylation. Compared with other pyrazole salts, the use of pyrazole tartrate to modify HMOR could significantly retard pyrazole desorption during the reaction, making BAS difficult to regenerate in the pore channel and effectively suppressing the side reaction of carbon deposition on 12 MR, thereby substantially improving the stability of HMOR. In this study, combined with the characteristics and synergistic effect of tartaric acid-complexed cobalt–iron and pyrazole tartrate modification, a DME carbonylation catalyst with enhanced activity and better stability was successfully prepared through the incorporation of pyrazole tartrate and tartaric acid-complexed cobalt–iron bimetal modification on HMOR using the ion exchange method. The structure and properties of HMOR before and after modification were investigated using XRD, BET, NH_3-TPD, Py-IR, FT-IR, and TG, and the fundamental reasons for the improvement in the activity and stability of modified HMOR catalysts are preliminarily explained.

2. Results and Discussion

2.1. Catalytic Performance

The unmodified hydrogen-type mordenite (HMOR) was prepared from ammonia-type mordenite (NH_4MOR) via calcination. The samples Co·Fe·DL-HMOR and Co·Fe·DL-Pya·DL-HMOR (x) (x = 0.4, 0.6, 0.8, 1.0) were synthesized using the ion exchange method (Section 3.1).

Figure 1a depicts the DME conversion curves over time in the carbonylation reaction of HMOR, Co·Fe·DL-HMOR, and Co·Fe·DL-Pya·DL-HMOR (x) (x = 0.4, 0.6, 0.8, 1.0) catalysts. As illustrated in Figure 1a, the DME conversion rate of unmodified HMOR reaches 35.5%. In contrast, the DME conversion rate significantly increases to 95% for Co·Fe·DL-HMOR, which is two-fold higher than the unmodified HMOR. However, these two catalysts were rapidly deactivated in the DME carbonylation reaction after 6 h. With further modification of the catalysts with Pya·DL via ion exchange, even though the DME conversion rate of Co·Fe·DL-Pya·DL-HMOR (x) slightly decreased compared to Co·Fe·DL-HMOR, the stability of DME carbonylation was significantly improved. As the concentration of Pya·DL gradually increased, the DME conversion rate exhibited a trend of first increasing and then decreasing. Interestingly, the DME conversion rate of the samples Co·Fe·DL-Pya·DL-HMOR (x) (x = 0.4, 0.6, 1.0) showed a slight downward trend with a prolonged reaction time. Notably, the DME conversion rate of Co·Fe·DL-Pya·DL-HMOR (0.8) consistently displayed an upward trend and exceeded that of Co·Fe·DL-Pya·DL-HMOR (0.6) at 180 h, indicating higher activity and better stability.

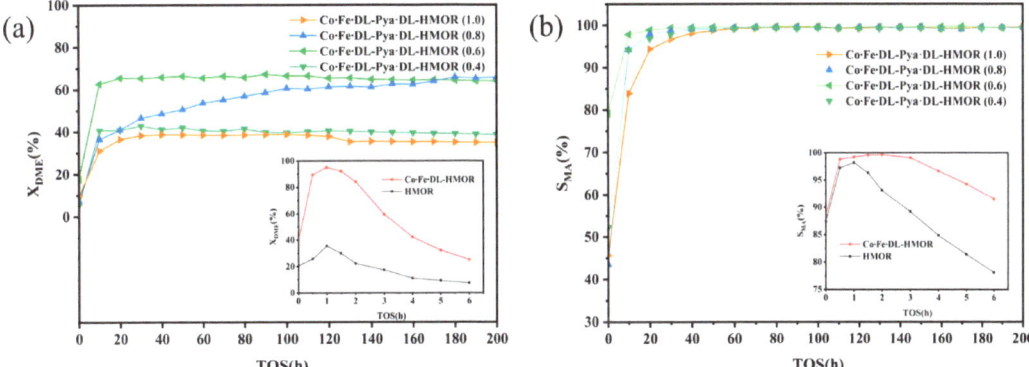

Figure 1. DME conversion rate (**a**) and MA selectivity rate (**b**) of HMOR, Co·Fe·DL-HMOR, and Co·Fe·DL-Pya·DL-HMOR (x) (x = 0.4, 0.6, 0.8, 1.0).

Figure 1b illustrates the curves of MA selectivity over time in the carbonylation reaction of HMOR, Co·Fe·DL-HMOR, and Co·Fe·DL-Pya·DL-HMOR (x) (x = 0.4, 0.6, 0.8, 1.0) catalysts. Although the MA selectivity of Co·Fe·DL-HMOR was enhanced compared to the unmodified HMOR, the MA selectivities of HMOR and Co·Fe·DL-HMOR declined rapidly after reaching their peak. Co·Fe·DL-Pya·DL-HMOR (x) displayed significantly enhanced MA selectivity after ion-exchange modification with Pya·DL, with it maintaining a stable level of more than 99%.

In order to further investigate the performance of Co·Fe·DL-Pya·DL-HMOR (0.8), a 400 h experiment was conducted. Figure 2 depicts the DME conversion and MA selectivity for the carbonylation reaction over the Co·Fe·DL-Pya·DL-HMOR (0.8) catalyst over the 400 h experimental period. The Co·Fe·DL-Pya·DL-HMOR (0.8) catalyst exhibited exceptional stability over the 400 h testing period. The DME conversion rate steadily increased, reaching about 73%, and it did not show a declining trend during the experimental period. Simultaneously, the MA selectivity remained consistently above 99%, confirming the sustained high activity and stability of the catalyst. Moreover, a comparison of the DME carbonylation performance of the HMOR modified via selective shielding and the removal of BAS within the 12 MR in recent years is provided in Table S1 as supporting information. Compared with the other modified HMOR samples, Co·Fe·DL-Pya·DL-HMOR (0.8) not only has higher DME carbonylation activity but also exhibits superior stability and a longer service life.

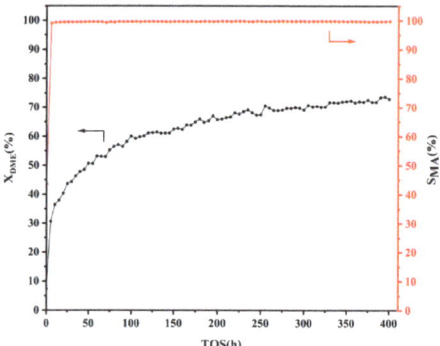

Figure 2. DME conversion and MA selectivity versus time for the Co·Fe·DL-Pya·DL-HMOR (0.8) carbonylation reaction over 400 h.

2.2. XRD Analysis

Figure 3 presents the XRD spectra of HMOR, Co·Fe·DL-HMOR, and Co·Fe·DL-Pya·DL-HMOR (x) (x = 0.4, 0.6, 0.8, 1.0). All of the modified samples exhibited a typical HMOR structure, and no crystalline phase related to cobalt and iron was observed, indicating superior dispersion of cobalt and iron ions in the zeolite structure. However, the change in the peak intensity of the modified HMOR indicates the significant influence of the DL complex cobalt–iron bimetallic modification and the Pya·DL ion exchange on the crystal structure and crystallinity. The characteristic peak intensity of Co·Fe·DL-HMOR was significantly enhanced, suggesting an improvement in crystallinity, likely attributed to the complexation effect of DL. This prevents the incorporation of Co^{2+} and Fe^{3+} ions into the zeolite framework, thereby preventing the destruction of the zeolite structure, thus further enhancing the dispersion and orderliness of cobalt and iron [22]. However, after further ion exchange modification with Pya·DL, Co·Fe·DL-Pya·DL-HMOR (x) (x = 0.4, 0.6, 0.8) exhibits a slightly reduced intensity of characteristic peaks compared to Co·Fe·DL-HMOR. The intensity of the characteristic peaks is slightly diminished, possibly attributed to the introduction of Pya·DL ions, causing a certain degree of zeolite framework collapse and pore channel blockage [17]. Notably, the intensity of characteristic peaks in Co·Fe·DL-Pya·DL-HMOR (1.0) was significantly weakened, signifying a substantial reduction in crystallinity, which may be attributed to the high concentration of Pya·DL, causing pore clogging and skeletal collapse [17]. This result is consistent with the observed decrease in DME conversion and carbonylation activity during the carbonylation activity test.

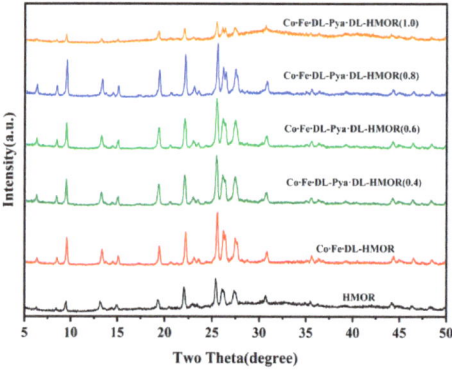

Figure 3. XRD spectrum of HMOR, Co·Fe·DL-HMOR, and Co·Fe·DL-Pya·DL-HMOR (x) (x = 0.4, 0.6, 0.8, 1.0).

In addition, XRD tests were conducted on spent Co·Fe·DL-Pya·DL-HMOR (0.8) samples, as presented in Figure S1. The spent Co·Fe·DL-Pya·DL-HMOR (0.8) sample shows similar characteristic diffraction peaks to the fresh sample, and no other related crystal phases of cobalt–iron are observed. The crystallinity of the spent sample is significantly reduced. This may be due to the formation of carbon deposits during the reaction, which causes blockage of the pore channels and a collapse of the skeleton [17].

2.3. BET Test

The specific surface area and pore size distribution of the unmodified HMOR, Co·Fe·DL-HMOR, and Co·Fe·DL-Pya·DL-HMOR (x) (x = 0.4, 0.6, 0.8, 1.0) samples were determined through N_2 adsorption–desorption experiments. As shown in Figure S2 in the Supporting Information, all samples exhibited distinctive type I isothermal adsorption curves with evident hysteresis loops, indicating typical microporous and irregular mesoporous structures [23]. It is worth noting that the pore size distributions of the various samples differed greatly, as can be seen in Figure 4. The pores of approximately 0.67 nm in size are attributed to the primary 12 MR channel, while pores of around 0.51 nm in size correspond to the 8 MR channel [24,25]. The pore structure information of both the 8 MR and the 12 MR can be obtained for unmodified HMOR and Co·Fe·DL-HMOR, which indicates effective cobalt–iron ion dispersion on the Co·Fe·DL-HMOR [18,19]. However, it was observed that the pore size of the Co·Fe·DL-Pya·DL-HMOR (x) (x = 0.4, 0.6, 0.8, 1.0) samples significantly increased with the increase in the concentration of Pya·DL. Furthermore, as the concentration of Pya·DL increased, the pore size gradually expanded. This can be attributed to the removal of non-skeletal aluminum from HMOR during acidic Pya·DL treatment, leading to an expansion in pore size and the creation of additional mesoporous structures [26]. The increase in pore size facilitates the timely diffusion of deposited carbon from the zeolite pores, preventing further coalescence and pore blockage [27]. Consequently, the Co·Fe·DL-Pya·DL-HMOR (x) (x = 0.4, 0.6, 0.8, 1.0) samples exhibit enhanced stability, aligning with the results of their carbonylation activity tests. Notably, the Co·Fe·DL-Pya·DL-HMOR (1.0) sample showed a lack of discernible micropore distribution, potentially attributed to the introduction of excessive Pya·DL ions, causing pore clogging and skeletal collapse, consistent with the carbonylation activity and XRD patterns.

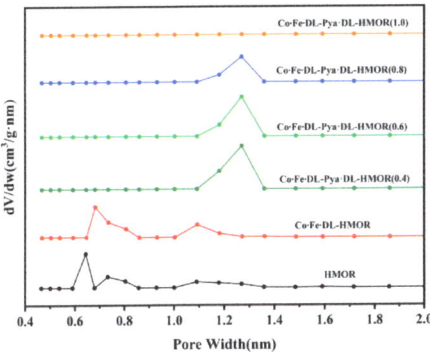

Figure 4. Pore size distribution of HMOR, Co·Fe·DL-HMOR, and Co·Fe·DL-Pya·DL-HMOR (x) (x = 0.4, 0.6, 0.8, 1.0).

Table 1 summarizes the BET-specific surface area and pore volume of the unmodified HMOR, Co·Fe·DL-HMOR, and Co·Fe·DL-Pya·DL-HMOR (x) (x = 0.4, 0.6, 0.8, 1.0) samples. The Co·Fe·DL-Pya·DL-HMOR (x) (x = 0.4, 0.6, 0.8, 1.0) samples exhibited a significant decrease in specific surface area and microporous volume. The observed changes are attributed to the substitution of H^+ ions in the 12 MR pores with larger pyrazole ions [16].

Higher Pya·DL concentrations result in increased BAS replacement in the 12 MR pores, which effectively suppress carbon accumulation reactions on the 12 MR and enhance catalyst stability. However, excessive Pya·DL introduction leads to decreased surface area and pore volume, hindering reactant and product diffusion and causing a significant decline in catalytic activity.

Table 1. Specific surface area and micropore volume of HMOR, Co·Fe·DL-HMOR, and Co·Fe·DL-Pya·DL-HMOR (x) (x = 0.4, 0.6, 0.8, 1.0).

Sample	$S_{BET}/(m^2/g)$	$V_{total}/(cm^3/g)$
HMOR	352	0.257
Co·Fe·DL-HMOR	335	0.211
Co·Fe·DL-Pya·DL-HMOR (0.4)	238	0.171
Co·Fe·DL-Pya·DL-HMOR (0.6)	142	0.118
Co·Fe·DL-Pya·DL-HMOR (0.8)	53.1	0.087
Co·Fe·DL-Pya·DL-HMOR (1.0)	6.07	0.043

2.4. NH$_3$-TPD Analysis

Figure 5 illustrates the NH$_3$-TPD plots of the unmodified HMOR, Co·Fe·DL-HMOR, and Co·Fe·DL-Pya·DL-HMOR (x) (x = 0.4, 0.6, 0.8) samples. Each sample exhibits two desorption peaks, a low-temperature peak (150–300 °C) associated with weak acid desorption and a high-temperature peak (400–700 °C) related to strong acid desorption [28]. Compared to the unmodified HMOR, the low-temperature desorption peaks for the Co·Fe·DL-HMOR and Co·Fe·DL-Pya·DL-HMOR (x) (x = 0.4, 0.6, 0.8) samples shifted to higher temperatures, indicating enhanced weak acidity resulting from DL-complexed cobalt–iron bimetallic and Pya·DL ion-exchange modification. This enhanced weak acidity further promotes carbonylation reactivity, which is consistent with the results of the carbonylation activity tests.

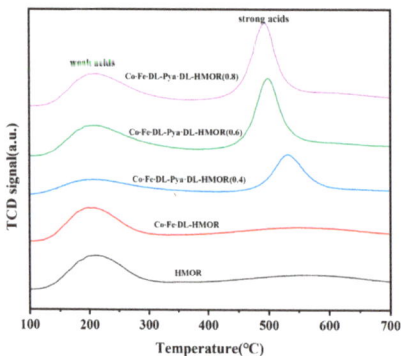

Figure 5. NH$_3$-TPD profiles of HMOR, Co·Fe·DL-HMOR, and Co·Fe·DL-Pya·DL-HMOR (x) (x = 0.4, 0.6, 0.8).

As can be seen in Figure 5, the high-temperature desorption peak for the Co·Fe·DL-HMOR sample slightly shifts to a lower temperature, suggesting that additional metal Lewis acidic sites (LAS) are generated after the modification treatment with the DL complex cobalt–iron bimetal, which enhances the acidic sites of the zeolite [29]. This increase in acidic sites contributes to the heightened conversion rate of DME, consistent with the results of the carbonylation activity test. Moreover, the high-temperature desorption peak center of the Co·Fe·DL-Pya·DL-HMOR (x) (x = 0.4, 0.6, 0.8) samples further shifts to lower temperatures with increasing Pya·DL concentration, which may be ascribed to the ion-exchange treatment with acidic Pya·DL aiding in the removal of non-skeletal aluminum from HMOR, resulting in a decrease in the strength of the strong acid [16]. The decrease in strong acid strength has the potential to inhibit side reactions, minimize carbon formation, and prolong the catalyst lifespan, consistent with the results of the carbonylation activity test.

2.5. Py-IR Analysis

Basic NH_3 molecules can combine with BAS or LAS on the outer surface of mordenite and in the pores. However, NH_3-TPD cannot determine whether the acidic sites come from the 8 MR or 12 MR of HMOR [30]. Pyridine, with a kinetic diameter of 0.585 nm, can enter the 12 MR channel of mercerized zeolite. However, it cannot enter its 8 MR channel [29,31]. Pyridine can only adsorb to the outer surface of HMOR and the acidic sites within the 12 MR pores [32]. Consequently, Py-IR analysis was utilized to provide a detailed examination and characterization of the acid content within the 12 MR pores. Figure 6 displays the Py-IR spectra of the unmodified HMOR and Co·Fe·DL-Pya·DL-HMOR (x) (x = 0.4, 0.6, 0.8) samples. Distinct peaks at 1540 cm^{-1} represent BAS, whereas peaks at 1450 cm^{-1} indicate Lewis acid sites (LAS), and the peaks at 1490 cm^{-1} arise from the combined influence of BAS and LAS [19,33]. The acid amounts in the 12 MR calculated from the peak areas at 1540 cm^{-1} and 1450 cm^{-1} reveal a significant reduction in the amount of BAS acid in the 12 MR of the Co·Fe·DL-Pya·DL-HMOR (x) samples (Table 2). Combined with the NH_3-TPD data, one can conclude that the increased number of acid sites in the modified HMOR is derived from the LAS of the 8 MR; therefore, the carbonylation activity is enhanced. As the concentration of Pya·DL increases, the amount of BAS acid in the 12 MR progressively decreases. The Py-IR spectra indicate that the non-skeletal aluminum in the 12 MR of HMOR was removed via the ion exchange treatment with Pya·DL. Thus, the BAS, which was the active center of the carbon accumulation side reaction, was replaced by Pya·DL molecules. Higher concentrations of Pya·DL lead to improved shielding of BAS in the 12 MR, resulting in a substantial improvement in carbonylation stability, which is consistent with the NH_3-TPD test results, carbonylation activity test, and stability test.

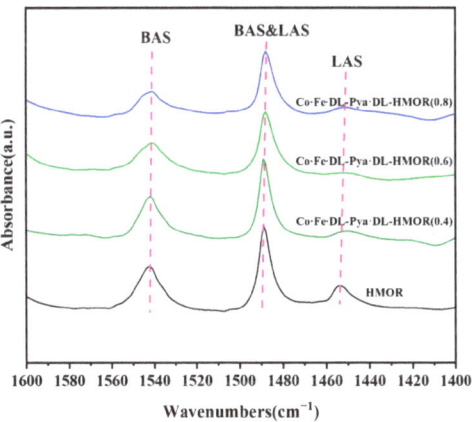

Figure 6. Py-IR spectra of HMOR and Co·Fe·DL-Pya·DL-HMOR (x) (x = 0.4, 0.6, 0.8).

Table 2. Quantities of the acidic sites for HMOR and Co·Fe·DL-Pya·DL-HMOR (x) (x = 0.4, 0.6, 0.8).

Sample	BAS in the 12 MR/(μmol/g)	LAS in the 12 MR/(μmol/g)	BAS and LAS in the 12 MR/(μmol/g)
HMOR	237	57	294
Co·Fe·DL-Pya·DL-HMOR (0.4)	172	28	200
Co·Fe·DL-Pya·DL-HMOR (0.6)	113	18	131
Co·Fe·DL-Pya·DL-HMOR (0.8)	58	16	74

2.6. FT-IR Analysis

In order to further analyze the catalytic active species of Co·Fe·DL-Pya·DL-HMOR (0.8) during carbonylation and the changes in acid sites after the reaction, FT-IR tests were carried out on the fresh and spent Co·Fe·DL-Pya·DL-HMOR (0.8) samples, as shown in Figure 7. As can be seen in Figure 7a, the peaks at 3050 cm^{-1} and 2970 cm^{-1} correspond to the asymmetric stretching vibration of -CH$_3$, which indicates that DME adsorbs on hydroxy aluminum (AlOH) to form methoxy [34]. The peak at 1680 cm^{-1} corresponds to the stretching vibration of acetyl zeolite intermediates, indicating that CO reacts with methoxy groups to form acetyl groups [2]. The peak at 1745 cm^{-1} corresponds to the stretching vibration of the reaction product MA, which indicates the productivity of MA after the reaction of acetyl groups with DME [31]. The peak at 1450 cm^{-1} corresponds to the stretching vibration of coke species, indicating that the reaction process is accompanied by carbon deposition side reactions [35]. The above results clearly indicate that methoxy and acetyl groups are the catalytic active species in the carbonylation reaction over the Co·Fe·DL-Pya·DL-HMOR (0.8) sample.

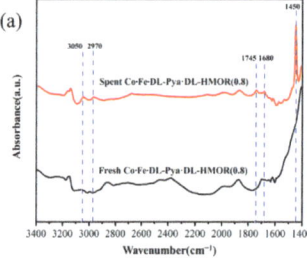
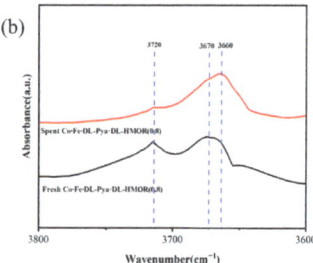

Figure 7. FT-IR spectra of the fresh and spent Co·Fe·DL-Pya·DL-HMOR (0.8) catalyst: (**a**) wavenumber in 1400~3400 cm^{-1} and (**b**) wavenumber in 3600~3800 cm^{-1}.

As can be seen from Figure 7b, the peak at wavenumber 3660~3670 cm^{-1} corresponds to the -OH stretching vibration of BAS in mordenite, and the peak at 3720 cm^{-1} corresponds to the -OH stretching vibration of the terminal silanol group. Moreover, the characteristic bands of 3660~3670 cm^{-1} can be divided into high-frequency bands corresponding to the OH group in the 12 MR and low-frequency bands corresponding to the OH group in the 8 MR [36–38]. The intensity of the characteristic peak at 3720 cm^{-1} of the spent Co·Fe·DL-Pya·DL-HMOR (0.8) sample was significantly weakened, while the characteristic peak intensity at 3660~3670 cm^{-1} was evidently enhanced and moved toward the low-frequency direction. This indicates that the BAS levels of the 8 MR increased in the spent Co·Fe·DL-Pya·DL-HMOR (0.8) sample, meaning that the carbonylation activity of the catalyst will gradually increase with the progression of the reaction, which is consistent with the results of the stability test of the Co·Fe·DL-Pya·DL-HMOR (0.8) sample.

2.7. TG Analysis

It is generally believed that the BAS acid site of 12 MR is responsible for the formation of coke. DME reacts with methoxy adsorption states in 12 MR channels to form trimethoxyonium cations (TMO+), and TMO+ is generally considered to be the precursor of hydrocarbons [39]; therefore, BAS in the 12 MR channels will lead to rapid coke formation. Moreover, DME may only enter the active sites in the 8 MR hole through the 12 MR; thus, the 12 MR channel is very important for DME diffusion into and MA diffusion out of the active sites in the 8 MR hole [40,41]. In order to probe the carbon deposition in the 12 MR of the modified HMOR, we carried out TG tests on the fresh/spent HMOR and Co·Fe·DL-Pya·DL-HMOR (0.8), as shown in Figure 8.

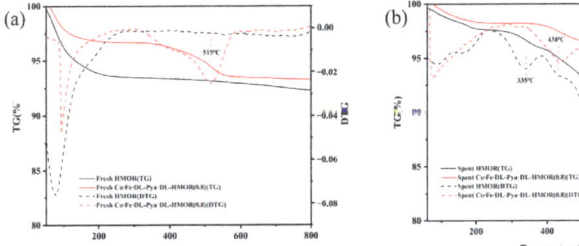

Figure 8. TG and DTG curves of (**a**) the fresh HMOR and Co·Fe·DL-Pya·DL-HMOR (0.8) samples and (**b**) the spent HMOR and Co·Fe·DL-Pya·DL-HMOR (0.8) catalysts.

Figure 8a illustrates the TG and DTG curves for the HMOR and Co·Fe·DL-Pya·DL-HMOR (0.8) samples. The weight loss observed below 250 °C corresponds to the evaporation of adsorbed water [16]. HMOR exhibits no significant weight loss peaks beyond 250 °C, indicating the removal of most internal organic templates during calcination. However, the DTG curves of the fresh Co·Fe·DL-Pya·DL-HMOR (0.8) samples do not exhibit a clear weight loss plateau at temperatures of 180–350 °C, suggesting the tight binding of pyrazole to HMOR, which is challenging to desorb after Pya·DL ion exchange modification. Moreover, a notable weight loss peak at 515 °C in the DTG curve of the unreacted Co·Fe·DL-Pya·DL-HMOR (0.8) is attributed to the combustion and carbonization of pyrazole [16].

Figure 8b illustrates the TG and DTG curves of HMOR after 10 h of reaction and the Co·Fe·DL-Pya·DL-HMOR (0.8) sample after 400 h of reaction. The weight loss rate of spent Co·Fe·DL-Pya·DL-HMOR (0.8) is lower than that of the spent HMOR. When the temperature exceeds 250 °C, the DTG curves reveal two weight loss peaks for the spent HMOR: a small peak at 335 °C from soft carbon combustion and a more prominent peak at 565 °C from hard carbon combustion [16]. This indicates that unmodified HMOR accumulates substantial hard carbon, which severely hinders the molecular diffusion process and leads to rapid catalyst deactivation. In contrast, the DTG curve of the spent Co·Fe·DL-Pya·DL-HMOR (0.8) shows only two small weight loss peaks above 250 °C, a smaller peak at 430 °C caused by pyrazole combustion and a larger peak at 580 °C caused by hard carbon combustion, and the combustion weight loss peak of soft carbon is almost invisible [16]. The less-soft and hard carbon-generated spent Co·Fe·DL-Pya·DL-HMOR (0.8) is attributed to the shielding of BAS in the 12 MR channel by pyridine following Pya·DL ion exchange modification. In summary, the introduction of Pya·DL into the 12 MR channel of HMOR effectively shields BAS, inhibiting carbon accumulation and enhancing carbonylation reaction stability.

3. Materials and Methods

3.1. Materials

A specific type of ammonia-treated mercerized zeolite with a silica–aluminum ratio of 15, designated as NH_4MOR, was obtained from Wuhan Zhizhen Molecular Sieve Company (Wuhan, China). All chemicals and reagents, including $Co(NO_3)_2·6H_2O$, $Fe(NO_3)_3·9H_2O$, $C_4H_6O_6$, and $C_3H_4N_2$, are commercially available and were used directly as received.

3.2. Preparation of the Catalyst

The NH_4MOR was heated in a muffle furnace at a rate of 3 °C min^{-1} and calcined at a temperature of 500 °C for 3 h in air. The product was hydrogen-treated mercerized zeolite, denoted as HMOR.

Firstly, 1.164 g $Co(NO_3)_2·6H_2O$ and 1.616 g $Fe(NO_3)_3·9H_2O$ were weighed and dissolved in 40 mL deionized water and stirred until the metal salt was completely dissolved. The obtained solution was a cobalt–iron bimetallic salt aqueous solution with a concentration of 0.2 mol/L and a molar ratio of cobalt to iron of 1:1. Afterward, under stirring,

0.008 moles of tartaric acid (DL) were added into 40 mL at a 0.2 mol·L^{-1} concentration of cobalt–iron bimetallic salt aqueous solution (cobalt–iron molar ratio = 1:1) to obtain DL-complexed cobalt–iron bimetallic salt aqueous solution. Next, 2 g of NH$_4$MOR was added to the bimetallic salt aqueous solution, which was stirred evenly. The obtained solution was then subjected to ion exchange at 80 °C in a water bath. After filtration, the resulting material was washed with deionized water 3–5 times, dried at 120 °C overnight, and calcined in air at 500 °C for 3 h. The final product was DL-complexed cobalt–iron modified HMOR, denoted as Co·Fe·DL-HMOR.

Pyrazole was added to DL to prepare a pyrazole tartrate solution (Pya·DL) with a 1:1 molar ratio of Pya to DL. Subsequently, 2 g of Co·Fe·DL-HMOR was immersed in 40 mL of the Pya·DL solution with concentrations of 0.4, 0.6, 0.8, and 1.0 mol·L^{-1}. The mixtures were thoroughly stirred, and ion exchange was conducted at 80 °C. After filtration, washing, and drying overnight at 120 °C, Co·Fe·DL-Pya·DL-HMOR (x) was obtained. The value x represents the molar concentration of Pya·DL (x = 0.4, 0.6, 0.8, 1.0) during the ion exchange process.

3.3. Characterization

The XRD patterns of the samples were recorded using a Bruker D8 Advance X-ray diffractometer with Cu Kα radiation (λ = 0.154 nm), operating at a current of 40 mA and a voltage of 40 kV. The scanning range was set between 5 and 50°. Before the test, 50 mg powder samples were smeared uniformly onto a sample holder to ensure a flat upper surface.

Nitrogen adsorption–desorption was conducted on the ASAP 2020 fully automatic physical adsorption instrument manufactured by the Micromeritics Company in the United States. The nitrogen adsorption–desorption process was executed at −196 °C. Before testing, the samples underwent degassing and pretreatment at 220 °C for 6 h. The specific surface area was determined using the BET method, while the micropore volume was calculated using the t-plot method.

The ammonia temperature-programmed desorption (NH$_3$-TPD) test was carried out using the AutoChem II 2920 instrument manufactured by the Micromeritics Company in the Norcross, GA, USA, and TCD was used as the detector. A sample weighing 100 mg was placed in the heating zone of a quartz tube, purged with 30 mL·min^{-1} of helium, and heated to 210 °C. After constant-temperature water removal for 1 h, the temperature was lowered below 100 °C. Subsequently, NH$_3$ was introduced at a flow rate of 30 mL·min^{-1} and maintained for 30 min to saturate the sample with NH$_3$ adsorption. Following this process, helium was purged at 373 °C for 1 h. When the baseline signal corresponding to the mass spectrum stabilizes, the temperature is ramped from room temperature to 700 °C at a heating rate of 10 °C·min^{-1}. The signal of NH$_3$ desorbed on the catalyst during this process is detected, and, finally, the NH$_3$ temperature-programmed desorption curve is obtained.

In the pyridine adsorption infrared (Py-IR) characterization test, pyridine was employed as the probe molecule, and the Vector 33-IR model Fourier-transform infrared spectrometer from Bruker, Ettlingen, Germany, was used to assess the acid amount and acid type of the sample. In general, a sample of about 15 mg was weighed, finely ground with an agate mortar, and compressed into cohesive flakes. The compacted sheet was inserted into an in situ cell capable of both heating and evacuation and equipped with CaF$_2$ windows. Spectral analysis was performed on the sample using an MCT detector within the wavenumber range of 4000–1000 cm^{-1}. Before pyridine adsorption, the sample was degassed at 400 °C for 1 h to purify the catalyst surface. Subsequently, a background scan was conducted when the temperature decreased to 150 °C. Pyridine was introduced into the inlet by employing an injector under N$_2$ carrier gas for 0.5 h and was evacuated for 0.5 h, and then the sample was scanned, and its spectrum was recorded.

The FT-IR experiments were carried out on a Vertex 33-IR infrared spectrometer from Bruker, Germany. The samples were self-supported, and the samples were mixed with

KBr at a mass ratio of 1:10 and fully ground three times, and, then, the test samples were pressed at 15 MPa to obtain homogeneous semi-transparent films, which were dried at 120 °C for 20 min. In total, 32 scans were used for the tests, with a resolution of 4 cm^{-1} and a scanning range of 4000~400 cm^{-1}.

A German NETZSCH thermogravimetric analyzer (TG) was employed to assess carbon deposits and other organic matter in the samples. Approximately 8 mg of the sample was accurately weighed and placed in an Al$_2$O$_3$ ceramic crucible. Subsequently, under an airflow of 20 mL·min^{-1}, the temperature was incrementally increased from 40 °C to 850 °C at a heating rate of 10 °C·min^{-1}, and the mass change curve of the sample was recorded.

3.4. DME Carbonylation Reaction

The core reaction equation of the carbonylation reaction of DME is as follows:

$$CH_3OCH_3 + CO \xrightarrow{cata/1.5\ MPa/215\ °C} CH_3COOCH_3 \tag{1}$$

The schematic diagram of the catalyst testing system is presented in Figure S3 as supporting information. The 0.25 g catalyst with a 40–60 mesh size was loaded into a stainless steel reactor with an inner diameter of 6 mm. Before the reaction, the catalyst was dried at 240 °C under a nitrogen flow of 20 mL·min^{-1}. After the catalyst bed cooled to 215 °C, the reactants (4% DME, 76% CO, and 20% N$_2$) were introduced into the reactor at a gas hourly space velocity of 4800 mL·g^{-1}·h^{-1}. The reaction pressure was then increased to 1.5 MPa. The effluents from the reactor were analyzed using an online Agilent 4890 gas chromatograph equipped with an FID detector and a capillary column (APPARATUS 0807242514). The conversion of DME (X$_{DME}$) and the selectivity of each component (S$_i$) were calculated based on the carbon balance principle and the corrected area normalization method.

$$X_{DME} = \frac{\sum_{k=2}^{5} A_k \cdot f_{M(k/DME)} + \sum A_{C_nH_m}}{\sum_{k=1}^{5} A_k \cdot f_{M(k/DME)} + \sum A_{C_nH_m}} \times 100\% \tag{2}$$

$$S_i = \frac{A_i \cdot f_{M(i/DME)}}{\sum_{k=2}^{5} A_k \cdot f_{M(k/DME)} + \sum A_{C_nH_m}} \times 100\% \tag{3}$$

In the formula, A$_i$ is the chromatographic peak area of DME, methanol, ethanol, MA, and ethyl acetate components (i = 1, 2, 3, 4, 5), f$_{(M(i/DME))}$ is the molar correction factor of component i relative to that of DME, and C$_n$H$_m$ is the hydrocarbon by-product.

4. Conclusions

In conclusion, a Pya·DL and DL complex cobalt–iron bimetallic modified HMOR catalyst with superior DME carbonylation activity and stability was successfully prepared using the ion exchange method in this study. Through the modification of the DL complexed cobalt–iron bimetal, the dispersion of cobalt–iron was greatly improved, and new metal Lewis acidic sites (LAS) were formed; thus, the activity of the catalyst significantly improved. Furthermore, the ion exchange of Pya·DL effectively removed non-skeletal aluminum in HMOR, resulting in an enlarged pore diameter and enhanced mesopore formation, which facilitated carbon deposition diffusion and prevented pore blockage. Simultaneously, the shielding of BAS by replacing equilibrium charge H$^+$ in the 12 MR pore with larger pyrazole ions also inhibited carbon accumulation on the 12 MR and significantly enhanced the stability of the DME carbonylation reaction.

Supplementary Materials: The following supporting information can be downloaded at https://www.mdpi.com/article/10.3390/molecules29071510/s1, Figure S1: XRD spectrum of fresh and spent Co·Fe·DL-Pya·DL-HMOR (0.8) catalyst; Figure S2: N$_2$ adsorption–desorption isotherm of HMOR, Co·Fe·DL-HMOR and Co·Fe·DL-Pya·DL-HMOR (x) (x = 0.4, 0.6, 0.8, 1.0); Figure S3: The schematic diagram of the catalyst testing system; Table S1: Comparison of the DME carbonylation performance of HMOR modified by selective shielding and removal of BAS within 12 MR in recent years. Refs. [42–45] are cited in the Supplementary Materials.

Author Contributions: Methodology, G.F. and X.D.; formal analysis, G.F. and X.D.; resources, G.F.; data curation, G.F.; writing—original draft preparation, G.F.; writing—review and editing, G.F. and X.D.; investigation, G.F.; supervision, X.D.; funding acquisition, X.D. All authors have read and agreed to the published version of the manuscript.

Funding: This work was financially supported by the National Natural Science Foundation of China (No. 21978098).

Institutional Review Board Statement: Not applicable.

Informed Consent Statement: Not applicable.

Data Availability Statement: The datasets generated and/or analyzed during the current study are available from the corresponding author upon reasonable request.

Conflicts of Interest: The authors declare no conflicts of interest.

References

1. Luk, H.T.; Mondelli, C.; Ferré, D.C.; Stewart, J.A.; Pérez-Ramírez, J. Status and Prospects in Higher Alcohols Synthesis from Syngas. *Chem. Soc. Rev.* **2017**, *46*, 1358–1426. [CrossRef]
2. Cheung, P.; Bhan, A.; Sunley, G.; Law, D.; Iglesia, E. Site Requirements and Elementary Steps in Dimethyl Ether Carbonylation Catalyzed by Acidic Zeolites. *J. Catal.* **2007**, *245*, 110–123. [CrossRef]
3. Blasco, T.; Boronat, M.; Concepción, P.; Corma, A.; Law, D.; Vidal-Moya, J.A. Carbonylation of Methanol on Metal–Acid Zeolites: Evidence for a Mechanism Involving a Multisite Active Center. *Angew. Chem. Int. Ed.* **2007**, *46*, 3938–3941. [CrossRef] [PubMed]
4. He, T.; Ren, P.; Liu, X.; Xu, S.; Han, X.; Bao, X. Direct Observation of DME Carbonylation in the Different Channels of H-MOR Zeolite by Continuous-Flow Solid-State NMR Spectroscopy. *Chem. Commun.* **2015**, *51*, 16868–16870. [CrossRef]
5. Yang, G.; San, X.; Jiang, N.; Tanaka, Y.; Li, X.; Jin, Q.; Tao, K.; Meng, F.; Tsubaki, N. A New Method of Ethanol Synthesis from Dimethyl Ether and Syngas in a Sequential Dual Bed Reactor with the Modified Zeolite and Cu/ZnO Catalysts. *Catal. Today* **2011**, *164*, 425–428. [CrossRef]
6. Li, X.; San, X.; Zhang, Y.; Ichii, T.; Meng, M.; Tan, Y.; Tsubaki, N. Direct Synthesis of Ethanol from Dimethyl Ether and Syngas over Combined H-Mordenite and Cu/ZnO Catalysts. *ChemSusChem* **2010**, *3*, 1192–1199. [CrossRef]
7. Wang, D.; Yang, G.; Ma, Q.; Yoneyama, Y.; Tan, Y.; Han, Y.; Tsubaki, N. Facile Solid-State Synthesis of Cu–Zn–O Catalysts for Novel Ethanol Synthesis from Dimethyl Ether (DME) and Syngas (CO+H_2). *Fuel* **2013**, *109*, 54–60. [CrossRef]
8. Lu, P.; Yang, G.; Tanaka, Y.; Tsubaki, N. Ethanol Direct Synthesis from Dimethyl Ether and Syngas on the Combination of Noble Metal Impregnated Zeolite with Cu/ZnO Catalyst. *Catal. Today* **2014**, *232*, 22–26. [CrossRef]
9. San, X.; Zhang, Y.; Shen, W.; Tsubaki, N. New Synthesis Method of Ethanol from Dimethyl Ether with a Synergic Effect between the Zeolite Catalyst and Metallic Catalyst. *Energy Fuels* **2009**, *23*, 2843–2844. [CrossRef]
10. Cheung, P.; Bhan, A.; Sunley, G.J.; Iglesia, E. Selective Carbonylation of Dimethyl Ether to Methyl Acetate Catalyzed by Acidic Zeolites. *Angew. Chem. Int. Ed.* **2006**, *45*, 1617–1620. [CrossRef]
11. Huo, H.; Peng, L.; Gan, Z.; Grey, C.P. Solid-State MAS NMR Studies of Brønsted Acid Sites in Zeolite H-Mordenite. *J. Am. Chem. Soc.* **2012**, *134*, 9708–9720. [CrossRef] [PubMed]
12. Yang, Y.; Ding, J.; Xu, C.; Zhu, W.; Wu, P. An Insight into Crystal Morphology-Dependent Catalytic Properties of MOR-Type Titanosilicate in Liquid-Phase Selective Oxidation. *J. Catal.* **2015**, *325*, 101–110. [CrossRef]
13. Bhan, A.; Iglesia, E. A Link between Reactivity and Local Structure in Acid Catalysis on Zeolites. *Acc. Chem. Res.* **2008**, *41*, 559–567. [CrossRef] [PubMed]
14. Li, Y.; Huang, S.; Cheng, Z.; Wang, S.; Ge, Q.; Ma, X. Synergy between Cu and Brønsted Acid Sites in Carbonylation of Dimethyl Ether over Cu/H-MOR. *J. Catal.* **2018**, *365*, 440–449. [CrossRef]
15. Wang, S.; Guo, W.; Zhu, L.; Wang, H.; Qiu, K.; Cen, K. Methyl Acetate Synthesis from Dimethyl Ether Carbonylation over Mordenite Modified by Cation Exchange. *J. Phys. Chem. C* **2015**, *119*, 524–533. [CrossRef]
16. Liu, S.; Liu, H.; Ma, X.; Liu, Y.; Zhu, W.; Liu, Z. Identifying and Controlling the Acid Site Distributions in Mordenite Zeolite for Dimethyl Ether Carbonylation Reaction by Means of Selective Ion-Exchange. *Catal. Sci. Technol.* **2020**, *10*, 4663–4672. [CrossRef]
17. Liu, S.; Fang, X.; Liu, Y.; Liu, H.; Ma, X.; Zhu, W.; Liu, Z. Dimethyl Ether Carbonylation over Mordenite Zeolite Modified by Alkyimidazolium Ions. *Catal. Commun.* **2020**, *147*, 106161. [CrossRef]
18. Ma, M.; Zhan, E.; Huang, X.; Ta, N.; Xiong, Z.; Bai, L.; Shen, W. Carbonylation of Dimethyl Ether over Co-HMOR. *Catal. Sci. Technol.* **2018**, *8*, 2124–2130. [CrossRef]
19. Zhou, H.; Zhu, W.; Shi, L.; Liu, H.; Liu, S.; Xu, S.; Ni, Y.; Liu, Y.; Li, L.; Liu, Z. Promotion Effect of Fe in Mordenite Zeolite on Carbonylation of Dimethyl Ether to Methyl Acetate. *Catal. Sci. Technol.* **2015**, *5*, 1961–1968. [CrossRef]
20. Liu, Y.; Shen, Y.; Geng, J.; Dong, X. Enhancing the Dimethyl Ether Carbonylation Performance over Hydrogen-Type Mordenites Modified by Pyrazole Hydrochloride. *RSC Adv.* **2022**, *12*, 123–128. [CrossRef]

21. Reule, A.A.C.; Prasad, V.; Semagina, N. Effect of Cu and Zn Ion-Exchange Locations on Mordenite Performance in Dimethyl Ether Carbonylation. *Microporous Mesoporous Mater.* **2018**, *263*, 220–230. [CrossRef]
22. Zhang, L.-Y.; Feng, X.-B.; He, Z.-M.; Chen, F.; Su, C.; Zhao, X.-Y.; Cao, J.-P.; He, Y.-R. Enhancing the Stability of Dimethyl Ether Carbonylation over Fe-Doped MOR Zeolites with Tunable 8-MR Acidity. *Chem. Eng. Sci.* **2022**, *256*, 117671. [CrossRef]
23. Liu, R.; Zeng, S.; Sun, T.; Xu, S.; Yu, Z.; Wei, Y.; Liu, Z. Selective Removal of Acid Sites in Mordenite Zeolite by Trimethylchlorosilane Silylation to Improve Dimethyl Ether Carbonylation Stability. *ACS Catal.* **2022**, *12*, 4491–4500. [CrossRef]
24. Reule, A.A.C.; Semagina, N. Zinc Hinders Deactivation of Copper-Mordenite: Dimethyl Ether Carbonylation. *ACS Catal.* **2016**, *6*, 4972–4975. [CrossRef]
25. Ban, S.; van Laak, A.N.C.; Landers, J.; Neimark, A.V.; de Jongh, P.E.; de Jong, K.P.; Vlugt, T.J.H. Insight into the Effect of Dealumination on Mordenite Using Experimentally Validated Simulations. *J. Phys. Chem. C* **2010**, *114*, 2056–2065. [CrossRef]
26. Reule, A.A.C.; Sawada, J.A.; Semagina, N. Effect of Selective 4-Membered Ring Dealumination on Mordenite-Catalyzed Dimethyl Ether Carbonylation. *J. Catal.* **2017**, *349*, 98–109. [CrossRef]
27. Chen, N.; Zhang, J.; Gu, Y.; Zhang, W.; Cao, K.; Cui, W.; Xu, S.; Fan, D.; Tian, P.; Liu, Z. Designed Synthesis of MOR Zeolites Using Gemini-Type Bis(Methylpyrrolidinium) Dications as Structure Directing Agents and Their DME Carbonylation Performance. *J. Mater. Chem. A* **2022**, *10*, 8334–8343. [CrossRef]
28. Wang, M.; Huang, S.; Lü, J.; Cheng, Z.; Li, Y.; Wang, S.; Ma, X. Modifying the Acidity of H-MOR and Its Catalytic Carbonylation of Dimethyl Ether. *Chin. J. Catal.* **2016**, *37*, 1530–1537. [CrossRef]
29. Zhao, P.; Qian, W.; Ma, H.; Sheng, H.; Zhang, H.; Ying, W. Effect of Zr Incorporation on Mordenite Catalyzed Dimethyl Ether Carbonylation. *Catal. Lett.* **2021**, *151*, 940–954. [CrossRef]
30. Zhao, N.; Cheng, Q.; Lyu, S.; Guo, L.; Tian, Y.; Ding, T.; Xu, J.; Ma, X.; Li, X. Promoting Dimethyl Ether Carbonylation over Hot-Water Pretreated H-Mordenite. *Catal. Today* **2020**, *339*, 86–92. [CrossRef]
31. Liu, J.; Xue, H.; Huang, X.; Wu, P.-H.; Huang, S.-J.; Liu, S.-B.; Shen, W. Stability Enhancement of H-Mordenite in Dimethyl Ether Carbonylation to Methyl Acetate by Pre-Adsorption of Pyridine. *Chin. J. Catal.* **2010**, *31*, 729–738. [CrossRef]
32. Li, Y.; Huang, S.; Cheng, Z.; Cai, K.; Li, L.; Milan, E.; Lv, J.; Wang, Y.; Sun, Q.; Ma, X. Promoting the Activity of Ce-Incorporated MOR in Dimethyl Ether Carbonylation through Tailoring the Distribution of Brønsted Acids. *Appl. Catal. B Environ.* **2019**, *256*, 117777. [CrossRef]
33. Xia, Y.; Li, Z.; Li, Y.; Cai, K.; Liu, Y.; Lv, J.; Huang, S.; Ma, X. Promotion Effect and Mechanism of Ga Modification on Dimethyl Ether Carbonylation Catalyzed by Mordenite. *Catal. Today* **2022**, *405–406*, 152–158. [CrossRef]
34. Chen, J.G.; Basu, P.; Ballinger, T.H.; Yates, J.T. A Transmission Infrared Spectroscopic Investigation of the Reaction of Dimethyl Ether with Alumina Surfaces. *Langmuir* **1989**, *5*, 352–356. [CrossRef]
35. Wei, Y.; Zhang, D.; Liu, Z.; Su, B. Highly Efficient Catalytic Conversion of Chloromethane to Light Olefins over HSAPO-34 as Studied by Catalytic Testing and In Situ FTIR. *J. Catal.* **2006**, *238*, 46–57. [CrossRef]
36. Bhan, A.; Allian, A.D.; Sunley, G.J.; Law, D.J.; Iglesia, E. Specificity of Sites within Eight-Membered Ring Zeolite Channels for Carbonylation of Methyls to Acetyls. *J. Am. Chem. Soc.* **2007**, *129*, 4919–4924. [CrossRef] [PubMed]
37. Deng, F.; Du, Y.; Ye, C.; Wang, J.; Ding, T.; Li, H. Acid Sites and Hydration Behavior of Dealuminated Zeolite HZSM-5: A High-Resolution Solid State NMR Study. *J. Phys. Chem.* **1995**, *99*, 15208–15214. [CrossRef]
38. Hayashi, S.; Kojima, N. Acid Properties of H-Type Mordenite Studied by Solid-State NMR. *Microporous Mesoporous Mater.* **2011**, *141*, 49–55. [CrossRef]
39. Boronat, M.; Martínez-Sánchez, C.; Law, D.; Corma, A. Enzyme-like Specificity in Zeolites: A Unique Site Position in Mordenite for Selective Carbonylation of Methanol and Dimethyl Ether with CO. *J. Am. Chem. Soc.* **2008**, *130*, 16316–16323. [CrossRef]
40. He, T.; Liu, X.; Xu, S.; Han, X.; Pan, X.; Hou, G.; Bao, X. Role of 12-Ring Channels of Mordenite in DME Carbonylation Investigated by Solid-State NMR. *J. Phys. Chem. C* **2016**, *120*, 22526–22531. [CrossRef]
41. Liu, Z.; Yi, X.; Wang, G.; Tang, X.; Li, G.; Huang, L.; Zheng, A. Roles of 8-Ring and 12-Ring Channels in Mordenite for Carbonylation Reaction: From the Perspective of Molecular Adsorption and Diffusion. *J. Catal.* **2019**, *369*, 335–344. [CrossRef]
42. Li, Y.; Sun, Q.; Huang, S.; Cheng, Z.; Cai, K.; Lv, J.; Ma, X. Dimethyl Ether Carbonylation over Pyridine-Modified MOR: Enhanced Stability Influenced by Acidity. *Catal. Today* **2018**, *311*, 81–88. [CrossRef]
43. Cao, K.; Fan, D.; Li, L.; Fan, B.; Wang, L.; Zhu, D.; Wang, Q.; Tian, P.; Liu, Z. Insights into the Pyridine-Modified MOR Zeolite Catalysts for DME Carbonylation. *ACS Catal.* **2020**, *10*, 3372–3380. [CrossRef]
44. Zhao, N.; Tian, Y.; Zhang, L.; Cheng, Q.; Lyu, S.; Ding, T.; Hu, Z.; Ma, X.; Li, X. Spacial Hindrance Induced Recovery of Over-Poisoned Active Acid Sites in Pyridine-Modified H-Mordenite for Dimethyl Ether Carbonylation. *Chin. J. Catal.* **2019**, *40*, 895–904. [CrossRef]
45. Xue, H.; Huang, X.; Zhan, E.; Ma, M.; Shen, W. Selective Dealumination of Mordenite for Enhancing Its Stability in Dimethyl Ether Carbonylation. *Catal. Commun.* **2013**, *37*, 75–79. [CrossRef]

Disclaimer/Publisher's Note: The statements, opinions and data contained in all publications are solely those of the individual author(s) and contributor(s) and not of MDPI and/or the editor(s). MDPI and/or the editor(s) disclaim responsibility for any injury to people or property resulting from any ideas, methods, instructions or products referred to in the content.

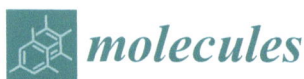

Article

$[BMP]^+[BF_4]^-$-Modified $CsPbI_{1.2}Br_{1.8}$ Solar Cells with Improved Efficiency and Suppressed Photoinduced Phase Segregation

Haixia Xie [1,2,*], Lei Li [3], Jiawei Zhang [3], Yihao Zhang [1], Yong Pan [1], Jie Xu [1], Xingtian Yin [3,*] and Wenxiu Que [3]

[1] School of Science, Xi'an University of Architecture and Technology, Xi'an 710055, China; hao@xauat.edu.cn (Y.Z.); panyong@xauat.edu.cn (Y.P.); jiexu@xauat.edu.cn (J.X.)
[2] State Key Laboratory for Strength and Vibration of Mechanical Structures, School of Aerospace Engineering, Xi'an Jiaotong University, Xi'an 710049, China
[3] Electronic Materials Research Laboratory, Key Laboratory of the Ministry of Education, International Center for Dielectric Research, Shaanxi Engineering Research Center of Advanced Energy Materials and Devices, School of Electronic Science and Engineering, Xi'an Jiaotong University, Xi'an 710049, China; xjtu_li@stu.xjtu.edu.cn (L.L.); zjw3026@stu.xjtu.edu.cn (J.Z.); wxque@xjtu.edu.cn (W.Q.)
* Correspondence: xiehaixia@xauat.edu.cn (H.X.); xt_yin@xjtu.edu.cn (X.Y.)

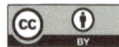

Citation: Xie, H.; Li, L.; Zhang, J.; Zhang, Y.; Pan, Y.; Xu, J.; Yin, X.; Que, W. $[BMP]^+[BF_4]^-$-Modified $CsPbI_{1.2}Br_{1.8}$ Solar Cells with Improved Efficiency and Suppressed Photoinduced Phase Segregation. *Molecules* **2024**, *29*, 1476. https://doi.org/10.3390/molecules29071476

Academic Editor: Qingguo Shao

Received: 31 January 2024
Revised: 21 March 2024
Accepted: 22 March 2024
Published: 26 March 2024

Copyright: © 2024 by the authors. Licensee MDPI, Basel, Switzerland. This article is an open access article distributed under the terms and conditions of the Creative Commons Attribution (CC BY) license (https://creativecommons.org/licenses/by/4.0/).

Abstract: With the rapid progress in a power conversion efficiency reaching up to 26.1%, which is among the highest efficiency for single-junction solar cells, organic–inorganic hybrid perovskite solar cells have become a research focus in photovoltaic technology all over the world, while the instability of these perovskite solar cells, due to the decomposition of its unstable organic components, has restricted the development of all-inorganic perovskite solar cells. In recent years, Br-mixed halogen all-inorganic perovskites ($CsPbI_3-xBr_x$) have aroused great interests due to their ability to balance the band gap and phase stability of pure $CsPbX_3$. However, the photoinduced phase segregation in lead mixed halide perovskites is still a big burden on their practical industrial production and commercialization. Here, we demonstrate inhibited photoinduced phase segregation all-inorganic $CsPbI_{1.2}Br_{1.8}$ films and their corresponding perovskite solar cells by incorporating a 1-butyl-1-methylpiperidinium tetrafluoroborate ($[BMP]^+[BF4]^-$) compound into the $CsPbI_{1.2}Br_{1.8}$ films. Then, its effect on the perovskite films and the corresponding hole transport layer-free $CsPbI_{1.2}Br_{1.8}$ solar cells with carbon electrodes under light is investigated. With a prolonged time added to the reduced phase segregation terminal, this additive shows an inhibitory effect on the photoinduced phase segregation phenomenon for perovskite films and devices with enhanced cell efficiency. Our study reveals an efficient and simple route that suppresses photoinduced phase segregation in cesium lead mixed halide perovskite solar cells with enhanced efficiency.

Keywords: $CsPbI_{1.2}Br_{1.8}$; phase segregation; Br-mixed halogen perovskites; perovskite solar cell; stability

1. Introduction

Organic–inorganic hybrid perovskite solar cells have gained significant attention due to their exceptional performance, tunable bandgap, high light-absorption coefficient, low cost and versatile applications, making them highly valuable for commercial use. The certified power conversion efficiency (PCE) of perovskite solar cells has rocketed up to 26.1% at a lab-scale at present, from 3.8% in 2009, which is comparable to that of well-developed single-junction silicon solar cells [1–5]. Currently, most of the perovskite solar cells with high PCEs over 20% are constructed from organic–inorganic hybrid perovskite materials listed as ABX_3, where usually A is one or more monovalent methylamine ions such as methylamine ions ($CH_3NH_3^+$, referred to as MA^+), ethylamine ions ($CH_3CH_2NH_3^+$, referred to as EA^+), formamidine cations ($NH = CHNH_3^+$, referred to as FA^+), etc. B is one or more of a divalent metal cation of a carbon family such as lead (Pb^{2+}), tin (Sn^{2+}), germanium (Ge^{2+}) cations), etc. And X is one or more of the halogen ions such as Cl^-, Br^-, and I^- [3,6–8]. However, the long-term stability issues of organic–inorganic hybrid perovskite materials under moisture, oxygen, thermal external force and even persistent light are still big burdens for their future application. These issues are caused by the inevitable phase segregation, ion migration, and crystal decomposition in the volatile nature of the organic components [9–13].

To address the issue of instability, it is suggested that the organic cations be replaced with all inorganic Cs^+ to create $CsPbX_3$ (X = I^-, Br^-, Cl^- or their mixtures) [14–18]. $CsPbX_3$ typically has four types of crystal structures, including the cubic structure (α-, Pm3m), the tetragonal structure (β-, P4/mbm), the orthorhombic structure (γ-, Pbnm), and a non-perovskite structure (δ-, Pnma) [19]. Research into $CsPbX_3$ perovskite solar cells started in 2014, when Choi et al. attempted to improve the performance of perovskite solar cells by removing MA^+ from $Cs_xMA_{1-x}PbI_3$ solar cells. All inorganic δ-$CsPbI_3$ (E_g = 2.82 eV) perovskite solar cells showed a PCE of only 0.09% [20]. In 2015, Gary Hodes et al. first fully investigated whether the organic cation was necessary to obtain devices with high photovoltaic performance. They found that the fabricated inorganic $CsPbBr_3$ perovskite solar cells, which performed equally as well as the organic ones, were much more temperature stable than the hybrid analogues. This study conducted useful comparative studies between hybrid organic–inorganic and all-inorganic perovskite materials [21]. Shortly thereafter, Snaith et al. reported on inorganic $CsPbI_3$ (E_g = 1.73 eV) perovskite solar cells. The current density–voltage (J-V) curve showed an efficiency of up to 2.9%, which was more stable than that of the hybrid organic–inorganic perovskite solar cells [22]. In 2017, Snaith's group used vacuum-based vapor deposition for alternating very thin layers of CsI and PbI_2 and obtained a stabilized PCE of 7.8%, compared to the 4.3% for spin-coated $CsPbI_3$ solar cells. The main improvement in vapor-deposited perovskite films was attributed to the much longer carrier lifetimes (>10 μs) compared to the spin-coated ones and their presumed lower trap densities [23]. $CsPbX_3$ perovskite solar cells then entered a period of rapid development through various optimization strategies such as additive engineering, interfacial engineering and precursor solution engineering. Cs-based perovskite solar cells have achieved a high PCE of approximately 21% with a high stability against humidity and heat [24]. From this progress, $CsPbX_3$ materials are emerging as a new research area and will play a significant role in the photovoltaic field in the near future.

Within the $CsPbX_3$ family, $CsPbBr_3$ exhibits exceptional moisture and thermal stability. However, due to its large band gap of approximately 2.3 eV, it can only absorb light from the UV region [25]. Compared to other $CsPbX_3$ compounds, cubic $CsPbI_3$ has the narrowest band gap of 1.73 eV, which allows for a wider range of light absorption. However, its application is limited due to the phase instability caused by transitions between the desirable photoactive perovskite black phase (α-$CsPbI_3$, cubic Pm3m) and the undesirable non-perovskite yellow phase (δ-$CsPbI_3$, orthorhombic Pnma), although the transition to the yellow phase is reversible [26,27]. Br-mixed halogen perovskites ($CsPbI_{3-x}Br_x$) are of great interest due to their ability to balance the band gap and phase stability of $CsPbX_3$. Additionally, the band gap of $CsPbI_{3-x}Br_x$ can be precisely tuned from ~1.2 to 2.4 eV by adjusting the value of x. This is because the changes in the Br^- and Cl^- ratio can monotonically shift the absorption onset and lead to lattice transitions for perovskite, resulting an alteration in the photonic bandgaps and, thus, making them promising candidates for the sub-cells of tandem solar cells [17,28–30].

Unexpectedly, some researchers have found that mixed halide perovskites suffer from intrinsic photoinduced halide segregation, with more bromide replacing iodide ions [31–34]. And, numerous studies have demonstrated that the phenomenon of photoinduced phase segregation decreases the V_{oc} of the device and significantly impacts its photoelectric performance [35,36]. Eric T. Hoke et al. are the pioneers who discovered the photoinduced phase segregation in mixed halide perovskite films in 2015. They found that when 0.2 < x < 1, the photoluminescence (PL) spectra of the $MAPb(Br_xI_{1-x})_3$ films formed a new emission peak at 1.68 eV and a redshift phenomenon occurred, indicating photoinduced phase segregation. Surprisingly, these changes in photoinduced phase segregation were completely reversible by switching between light and dark [31]. In 2017, Yi-Bing Cheng et al. observed iodide-rich phase segregation near grain boundaries in nanoscale all-inorganic $CsPbIBr_2$ films. The authors found that iodide segregation can occur due to the immiscibility between iodine and bromine, which exacerbates ion migration and hysteresis, thereby affecting the photoelectric performance of the corresponding devices [32]. However, the exact mechanism by which the photoinduced phase segregation phenomenon affects the V_{oc} of the devices is not clear. In addition, since the photoinduced phase segregation phenomenon destabilizes the perovskite solar cells, leading to a decrease in the PCE and V_{oc} of the devices, researchers have done a great deal of research work to inhibit and mitigate the occurrence of the photoinduced phase segregation phenomenon in perovskite solar cell devices. For example, Yue Hao et al. proposed a simple and effective strategy to inhibit the photoinduced phase segregation in $CsPbIBr_2$ films by modifying their crystalline grains with poly(methyl methacrylate) (PMMA). As a result, the carbon electrode-based $CsPbIBr_2$ PSC exhibited a more suppressed photocurrent hysteresis, coupled with an excellent PCE of 9.21% and a high V_{oc} of 1.307 V. Their work not only provided a new avenue to address the general halide phase segregation issue of $CsPbIBr_2$ materials, but also provided guidance to achieve the superior performance of opto-electronic devices [37]. Very recently, Wei Li et al. unveiled the impact of phase segregation in $Cs_{0.17}FA_{0.83}Pb(I_{0.80}Br_{0.20})_3$ films with a bandgap of 1.67 eV through a photoconductive atomic force microscopy. By testing the I-V curves at both grain boundaries and grain interiors with nanoscopic resolution, they identified that iodide-rich phases primarily segregated at defect-enriched grain boundaries under continuous illumination, causing a more significant local open-circuit voltage (V_{OC}) decrease than that occurring at grain interiors [38].

In this work, all inorganic $CsPbI_{1.2}Br_{1.8}$ perovskite films with inhibited photoinduced phase segregation are modified by adding different amounts of 1-butyl-1-methylpiperidinium tetrafluoroborate ($[BMP]^+[BF_4]^-$) (0.5, 1, 2 and 3 mg mL^{-1}) to the $CsPbI_{1.2}Br_{1.8}$ precursor solution, and then its effect on the photovoltaic performance of the corresponding devices and perovskite films under light is investigated. The PCE of hole transport layer-free carbon-based perovskite solar cell is improved from 7.13% for a device with a pristine perovskite film to the highest amount of 8.44% for a device with 1 mg mL^{-1} of $[BMP]^+[BF_4]^-$-modified perovskite film. And the PCE of the device increases first with the increase in the doping concentration of $[BMP]^+[BF_4]$ in the perovskite film, but then decreases gradually, and the stability under light is also increased. The modified $CsPbI_{1.2}Br_{1.8}$ perovskite film also shows an inhibitory effect on the photoinduced phase segregation phenomenon when compared with the pristine one, with a prolonged time attributed to the reduced phase segregation terminal (pristine: 30.42%@7 min, while the modified: 24.29%@30 min), and the reduced phase segregation rate remaining constant (pristine: k_s = 1.53×10^{-2} s^{-1}, while modified one: k_s = 1.83×10^{-3} s^{-1}).

2. Experimental Section

2.1. Chemicals

Cesium iodide (CsI, $\geq$99.9%) powder was purchased from Sigma-Aldrich (Shanghai) Trading Co. (Shanghai, China). Lead iodide (PbI_2, $\geq$99.99%) and lead bromide ($PbBr_2$, $\geq$99.99%) were purchased from Xi'an Yuri Solar Co., Ltd. (Xi'an, China). A tin (IV) oxide colloidal dispersion (SnO_2, 15 wt% in H_2O) and dimethyl sulfoxide (DMSO) solution were obtained from Alfa Aesar (China) Chemical Co. (Shanghai, China). Conductive carbon paste was obtained from Shanghai MaterWin New Materials Co., Ltd. (Shanghai, China). Deionized water (DI water) with a resistivity of 18.3 MΩ cm was used in all the preparations. ITO substrates with a sheet resistance of ~15 $\Omega\ \square^{-1}$ were purchased from Yingkou OPV tech new energy Co., Ltd. (Yingkou, China). The 1-butyl-1-methylpiperidinium tetrafluoroborate ($[BMP]^+[BF_4]^-$, $C_{10}H_{22}BF_4N$, 99%) was supported by Aladdin Scientific Corp. (Riverside, CA, USA). All of these were used as received unless otherwise specified.

2.2. Preparation of SnO$_2$ Precursor

The purchased SnO$_2$ colloidal dispersion was diluted with DI water in a mass ratio of 1:5, followed by ultrasonic dispersing for over 3 h before use.

2.3. Preparation of Perovskite Precursor

A total of 259.8 mg of CsI, 46.1 mg of PbI$_2$ and 330.3 mg of PbBr$_2$ (in a molar ratio of 1:0.1:0.9) were dissolved in 1 mL of DMSO. The mixture was then placed on a stirrer and stirred continuously overnight at room temperature. Before use, the resulting transparent yellow solution was filtered through a polytetrafluoroethylene (PTFE) filter with a pore size of 0.45 μm.

2.4. Preparation of Perovskite Precursors with Different Mass Concentrations of [BMP]$^+$[BF$_4$]$^-$

Various amounts of [BMP]$^+$[BF$_4$]$^-$ powder were added directly to the perovskite precursors with mass concentrations of 0.5, 1, 2, and 3 mg mL^{-1}. The mixtures were subsequently dispersed using ultrasonic waves for a duration of over 3 h. Before use, the solutions underwent filtration through a polytetrafluoroethylene (PTFE) filter with a pore size of 0.45 μm.

2.5. Device Fabrication

The ITO substrates were carefully cleaned using a foamless eradicator and then ultrasonically cleaned with DI water, acetone and ethanol for 15 min in sequence. Before the deposition of the electron transport layers, they were all dried with high-pressure nitrogen gas and then exposed to a UV/ozone cleaner for 15 min. SnO$_2$ electron transport layers were then spin-coated onto the ITO substrates from a SnO$_2$ precursor solution. The preparation process of the SnO$_2$ precursor solution was listed as follows: After cooling, the samples were transferred to a nitrogen-filled glove box to deposit the perovskite layers using a spin-coating method. Briefly, 100 μL of the perovskite precursor without (pristine) or with different mass concentrations of [BMP]$^+$[BF$_4$]$^-$ (0.5, 1, 2 or 3 mg mL^{-1}) was dropped onto the SnO$_2$ layer and then spin-coated first at a low speed of 1500 rpm for 20 s and then at a high speed of 5000 rpm for 60 s. The wet perovskite films were then annealed at 35 °C for 15 s and then at 280 °C for 10 min. Finally, compact layers of carbon electrodes were screen printed onto the perovskite films in air, followed by annealing at 120 °C for 15 min on a hot plate. The active area of each electrode was fixed at 0.07 cm^{-2} via screen printing.

2.6. Characterization

The top view and cross-sectional morphologies of the samples were characterized using a Quanta 250FEG (FEI Co., Tokyo, Japan) scanning electron microscope (SEM). The crystalline properties of the perovskite films were characterized by an X-ray diffractometer (XRD, SmartLab, Rigaku, Japan) using Cu K$_\alpha$ radiation (40 kV, 30 mA). The scanning speed was 5° per minute at a step of 0.02°. Absorption spectra were obtained using a JASCOV-570 (JASCO., Tokyo, Japan) UV/VIS/NIR spectrometer. J-V curves were measured in air using a Keithley 2400 source meter (Keithley Instruments, Inc., Solon, OH, USA) under simulated AM 1.5 G irradiation (100 mA cm^{-2}), with the illumination source pre-calibrated using a Si reference cell system (91150V, Newport) (Newport Corporation, Irvine, CA, USA). The scan was performed in 0.02 V steps from 1.2 to −0.1 V (reverse scan) with a 0.1 s time delay between each point.

3. Results and Discussion

In terms of film morphology, CsPbI$_x$Br$_{3-x}$ is sensitive to deposition methods, doping and processing conditions such as the spinning speed, environmental temperature and annealing temperature, etc. Figure 1 shows the top view SEM images of the pristine CsPbI$_{1.2}$Br$_{1.8}$ and CsPbI$_{1.2}$Br$_{1.8}$ films doped with different mass concentrations (0.5, 1, 2 and 3 mg mL^{-1}) of [BMP]$^+$[BF$_4$]$^-$. It is evident that the surface morphologies of the

$CsPbI_{1.2}Br_{1.8}$ films doped with different concentrations of $[BMP]^+[BF_4]^-$ do not differ significantly from the undoped film. All films have a flat surface without any pinholes.

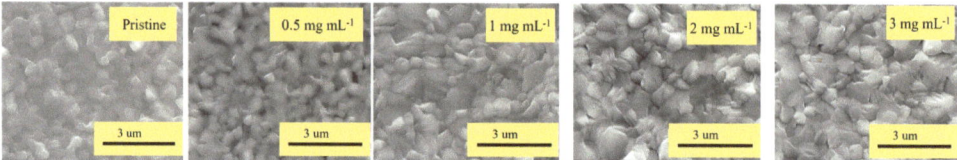

Figure 1. Top view SEM images of pristine $CsPbI_{1.2}Br_{1.8}$ and $CsPbI_{1.2}Br_{1.8}$ films doped with different mass concentrations (0.5, 1, 2 and 3 mg mL^{-1}) of $[BMP]^+[BF_4]^-$.

To establish the impact of the $[BMP]^+[BF_4]^-$ additive on the crystallinity and photon absorption of the perovskite thin films, an X-ray diffractometer and UV/VIS spectrometer characterization of the pristine and $[BMP]^+[BF_4]^-$-modified thin films is carried out. The XRD patterns of the pristine and $[BMP]^+[BF_4]^-$-modified films all exhibit typical perovskite peaks at 2θ = 15.45°, 20.41° and 30.63°, which are assigned to the (100), (110), and (200) lattice planes of the $CsPbI_{1.2}Br_{1.8}$ perovskite crystal, respectively [39], as shown Figure 2a. And there are no impurity phases in any of the films. However, the normalized XRD spectra in Figure S1 (Supporting Information) show that the crystalline grains in the $[BMP]^+[BF_4]^-$-modified $CsPbI_{1.2}Br_{1.8}$ film all have a much more preferred (100) orientation. It is speculated that the (100) orientation of the $CsPbI_{1.2}Br_{1.8}$ grains is preferentially perpendicular to that of the ITO/SnO$_2$ substrate. This orientation is highly advantageous for effective carrier transport and injection in the corresponding devices. Furthermore, the peak intensity of the perovskite film decreases as the mass concentration of the $[BMP]^+[BF_4]^-$ increases to 3 mg mL^{-1}. This suggests that higher mass concentrations may weaken the crystallinity of the modified films with increased scattering from grain boundaries or intragranular defects, which is not beneficial for the photovoltaic performance of the final devices [40].

The absorption spectra in Figure 2b indicate that the control film and the $[BMP]^+[BF_4]^-$-modified $CsPbI_{1.2}Br_{1.8}$ films process a similar sharp-cutting absorption edge at ~605 nm corresponding to a bandgap of ~2.05 eV, which is consistent with the values reported in the literature [39,41]. However, this increase in mass concentration leads to a slight decrease in the absorption intensity in the 500–580 nm absorption region, mainly due to the addition of $[BMP]^+[BF_4]^-$ in the perovskite films.

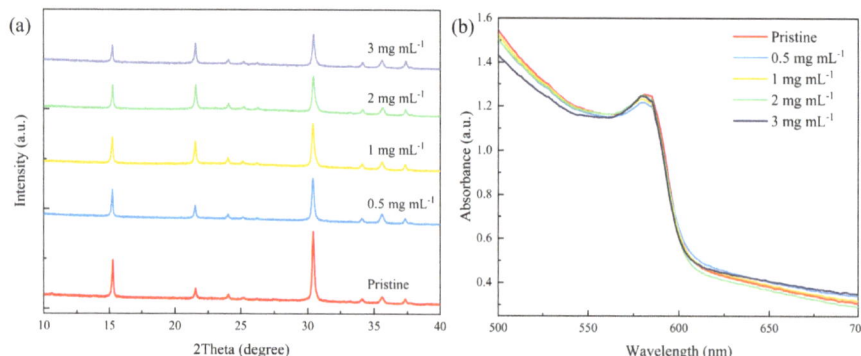

Figure 2. (a) XRD pattern and (b) absorption spectrum for pristine $CsPbI_{1.2}Br_{1.8}$ and $CsPbI_{1.2}Br_{1.8}$ films doped with different mass concentrations (0.5, 1, 2 and 3 mg mL^{-1}) of $[BMP]^+[BF_4]^-$.

The effect of the $[BMP]^+[BF_4]^-$ additive on the performance of $CsPbI_{1.2}Br_{1.8}$ solar cell devices are also investigated. Therefore, we depict the all-inorganic device with a hole transport layer-free architecture (Figure 3a), where SnO_2 and carbon are used as the electron transport layer and counter electrode, respectively. The cross-sectional SEM image for a representative cell based on 1 mg mL^{-1} of a [BMP]$^+$[BF$_4$]$^-$ (see Figure 3b for the chemical structure)-modified $CsPbI_{1.2}Br_{1.8}$ film is shown in Figure 3c (note that the SnO_2 is too thin to be observed). For comparison, we also prepare pristine and 0.5, 2 and 3 mg mL^{-1} of [BMP]$^+$[BF$_4$]$^-$ -modified $CsPbI_{1.2}Br_{1.8}$ perovskite solar cells, of which the typical J-V curves and corresponding parameters for the best-performing target devices are shown in Figure 3d and Table 1, respectively. As we can see, the pristine device exhibited an open circuit voltage (V_{OC}) of 1.14 V, a short circuit current density (J_{SC}) of 12.06 mA cm^{-2} and a fill factor (FF) of 0.52, resulting in a PCE of 7.13%. With the increase in the doping concentration of [BMP]$^+$[BF$_4$]$^-$ in the perovskite film, the PCE increases first and then decreases gradually. When the doping concentration of the [BMP]$^+$[BF$_4$]$^-$ reaches 1 mg mL^{-1}, the corresponding $CsPbI_{1.2}Br_{1.8}$ device exhibits the highest PCE, that of 8.44%, with a V_{OC} of 1.21 V, a J_{SC} of 12.32 mA cm^{-2} and an FF of 0.57. In addition, the additions of [BMP]$^+$[BF$_4$]$^-$ to the perovskite light absorber all provide a higher performance compared to that of the pristine one, mainly in terms of the increase in the V_{OC} and FF. The optimized addition mass concentration of the [BMP]$^+$[BF$_4$]$^-$ can be determined to be 1 mg mL^{-1}.

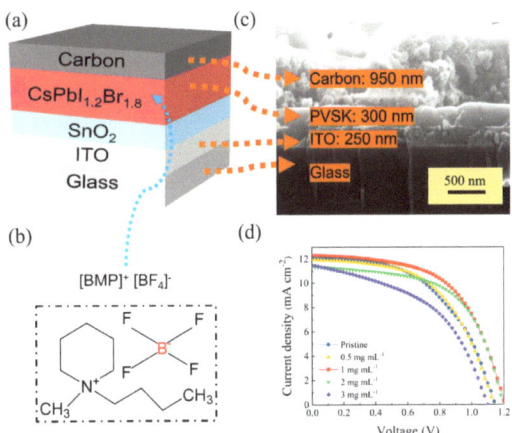

Figure 3. Perovskite solar cell characterization. (**a**) Schematic of the carbon-based all-inorganic perovskite solar cell, (**b**) the chemical structure of [BMP]$^+$[BF$_4$]$^-$, (**c**) cross-sectional SEM image of the full device stack made from $CsPbI_{1.2}Br_{1.8}$ with 1 mg mL^{-1} of [BMP]$^+$[BF$_4$]$^-$ as the additive in the perovskite precursor, (**d**) J-V characteristics of the representative pristine and 0.5, 1, 2 and 3 mg mL^{-1} of [BMP]$^+$[BF$_4$]$^-$-modified $CsPbI_{1.2}Br_{1.8}$ devices with the best-performing targets.

Table 1. J-V parameters of the representative devices according to Figure 3d.

Devices	V_{OC}/V	J_{SC}/mA cm^{-2}	FF	PCE/%
Pristine	1.14	12.06	0.52	7.13
0.5 mg mL^{-1}	1.13	11.97	0.54	7.36
1 mg mL^{-1}	1.21	12.32	0.57	8.44
2 mg mL^{-1}	1.19	11.39	0.59	8.03
3 mg mL^{-1}	1.20	11.58	0.58	8.02

To further understand the effect of [BMP]$^+$[BF$_4$]$^-$ additives on the performance of $CsPbI_{1.2}Br_{1.8}$ perovskite solar cells, the J-V curves of the pristine and 1 mg mL^{-1} of [BMP]$^+$[BF$_4$]$^-$-modified perovskite solar cells were tested after exposure to different light durations. Figure 4a–d shows the variations in the four normalized photovoltaic parameters (V_{OC}, J_{SC}, FF and PCE) of the different devices with respect to the light duration. It can be seen that the four parameters of the pristine device show a significant decrease with the increase in light exposure time, whereas the decrease for that of the 1 mg mL^{-1} [BMP]$^+$[BF$_4$]$^-$-modified device is significantly slower. For example, the PCE of the untreated device gradually decreased from an initial 6.99% to 4.04% after 30 min of light exposure, with a decrease of about 42%, while the PCE of the [BMP]$^+$[BF$_4$]$^-$-treated device gradually decreased from an initial 7.39% to 6.95%, with a decrease of only about 6%. It can be speculated that due to the suppressive effect of the [BMP]$^+$[BF$_4$]$^-$ additive on the photoinduced phase segregation phenomenon of the CsPbI$_{1.2}$Br$_{1.8}$ films, the stability of the perovskite solar cells under light is increased.

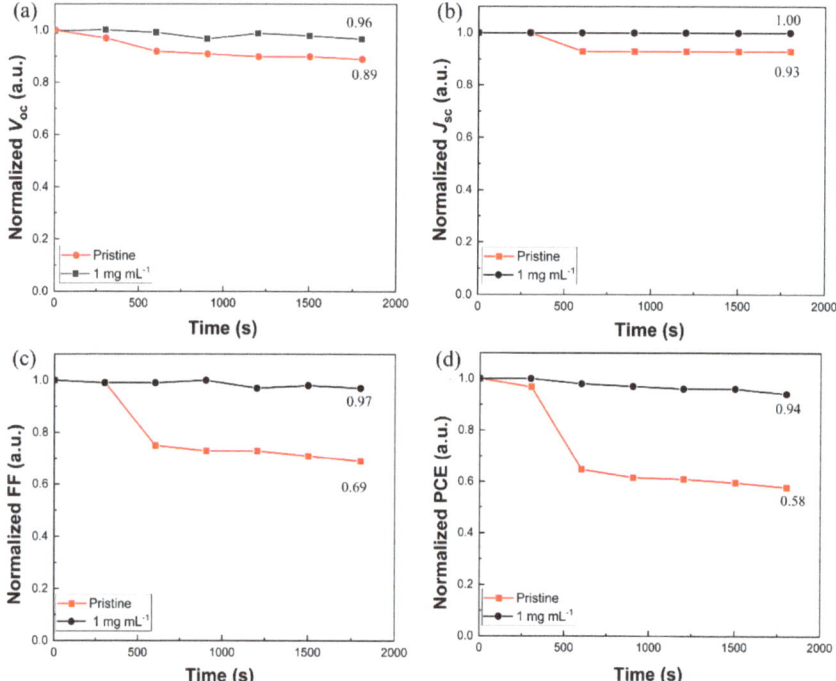

Figure 4. Evolution of the four normalized parameters obtained from the J-V curves for the representative pristine and 1 mg mL^{-1} of [BMP]$^+$[BF$_4$]$^-$-modified CsPbI$_{1.2}$Br$_{1.8}$ perovskite solar cells after exposure to different light durations, aged under a simulated air mass and 1.5 sunlight (400 mW cm^{-2}) at room temperature in ambient air: (**a**) V_{OC}, (**b**) J_{SC}, (**c**) FF and (**d**) PCE.

Upon irradiation, Br-mixed halogen perovskites will undergo the internal segregation of halogen ions, resulting in the formation of structural domains that are enriched in either bromides or iodides. To investigate the photoinduced phase separation phenomenon of CsPbI$_{1.2}$Br$_{1.8}$ thin films, we prepared pristine and 1 mg mL^{-1} of [BMP]$^+$[BF$_4$]$^-$-modified CsPbI$_{1.2}$Br$_{1.8}$ perovskite films. Both films were then subjected to UV-Vis absorption spectroscopy after irradiation for different times using simulated sunlight at 400 mW cm^{-2} AM1.5G. Under this continuous irradiation, the temperature of the films is approximately 40 °C. From the UV-Vis absorption spectra (Figure 5a) of the pristine perovskite film, it can be found that when the light duration was between 0 and 7 min, the intensity of the absorption peak at the wavelength of 584 nm gradually weakened with the increase in light duration, indicating a decrease in the mixed halide content in the perovskite films. The intensities of the absorption peaks at 560 and 620 nm gradually increase, indicating the formation of Br-rich and I-rich phases. As the illumination time is further increased (10 min and 15 min), the intensity of the absorption peaks at 584 nm gradually increases, while the intensity of the absorption peaks at 560 and 620 nm gradually decreases (Figure 5a). This suggests that after the film reaches the phase segregation terminal (30.42%@7 min, Figure 5b,e), the continued strong illumination leads to the phase recovery phenomenon of the perovskite film portion, i.e., the light-induced self-healing phenomenon, which is consistent with a previous report [17]. Similarly, from Figure 5c–e, it can be seen that under continuous light irradiation, the CsPbI$_{1.2}$Br$_{1.8}$ (treated with 1 mg mL^{-1} of [BMP]$^+$[BF$_4$]$^-$) film initially showed a photoinduced phase segregation phenomenon, and the continuous light irradiation led to a photoinduced self-healing phenomenon when the duration time exceeded the limit of the phase segregation terminal (24.29%@30 min, Figure 3d,e). In addition, the curves representing the phase segregation rates were analyzed using a monoexponential decay function, as shown in Figure 5f. The phase segregation rate constant k_s of the [BMP]$^+$[BF$_4$]$^-$-modified CsPbI$_{1.2}$Br$_{1.8}$ is 1.83×10^{-3} s^{-1}, while that of the pristine one is 1.53×10^{-2} s^{-1}. There is an order of magnitude difference between the former and the latter, suggesting that the addition of [BMP]$^+$[BF$_4$]$^-$ could reduce the rate of phase segregation. Thus, we can conclude that under continuous light irradiation, the CsPbI$_{1.2}$Br$_{1.8}$ films will undergo photoinduced phase separation followed by the light-induced self-healing phenomenon upon reaching the limit of the phase separation. And, the addition of [BMP]$^+$[BF$_4$]$^-$ can inhibit the photoinduced phase separation of CsPbI$_{1.2}$Br$_{1.8}$ films.

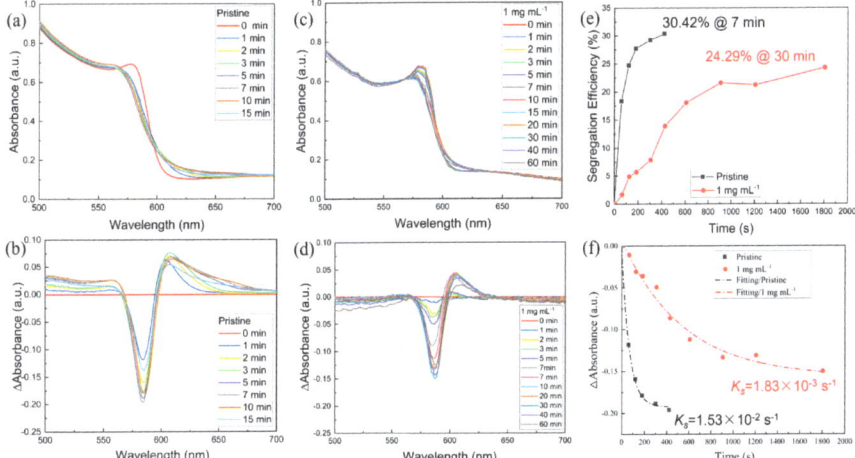

Figure 5. UV-Vis absorption spectra of (**a**) pristine and (**c**) 1 mg mL^{-1} of [BMP]$^+$[BF$_4$]$^-$-modified CsPbI$_{1.2}$Br$_{1.8}$ perovskite films recorded after different light exposure duration times (AM 1.5G 400 mW cm^{-2}). (**b,d**) Spectra of ΔA values obtained from (**a,c**), respectively. (**e**) The phase segregation terminal and (**f**) spectra of ΔA values as a function of the light exposure duration curves obtained from (**a,c**). The dashed, doted lines in (**f**) are linear fits to the data using monoexponential decay.

4. Conclusions

Our study mainly focuses on the effect of [BMP]$^+$[BF$_4$]$^-$ additives on the performance of CsPbI$_{1.2}$Br$_{1.8}$ solar cells and their impact on the phenomenon of the photoinduced phase segregation of CsPbI$_{1.2}$Br$_{1.8}$ thin films, paving the way for their use as efficient and light irradiation stable photovoltaic devices. The effects of [BMP]$^+$[BF$_4$]$^-$ additives on the photovoltaic properties and stability of the devices were investigated by preparing hole transport layer-free carbon-based perovskite solar cells, with pristine or 0.5, 1, 2 and 3 mg mL^{-1} of [BMP]$^+$[BF$_4$]$^-$-modified CsPbI$_{1.2}$Br$_{1.8}$ films as the light harvester layers for each device.

The results showed that the PCE of the device increases first with the increase in the doping concentration of [BMP]$^+$[BF$_4$] in the perovskite film, but then it decreases gradually. The device without the addition of [BMP]$^+$[BF$_4$]$^-$ additives in the perovskite shows a PCE of 7.13%, while the device shows the highest PCE of 8.44% with the doping concentration of [BMP]$^+$[BF$_4$]$^-$ reaching 1 mg mL^{-1}, and its stability under light increases substantially, which may be related to the significant inhibition of the photoinduced phase segregation process. The impact of the [BMP]$^+$[BF$_4$]$^-$ additive on the photoinduced phase separation of CsPbI$_{1.2}$Br$_{1.8}$ films is investigated using UV-Vis absorption spectra and the corresponding difference in absorption spectra as a function of the light exposure time at room temperature. The photoinduced phase segregation limit time of the CsPbI$_{1.2}$Br$_{1.8}$ films increased from 7 to 30 min after the addition of 1 mg mL^{-1} of the [BMP]$^+$[BF$_4$]$^-$ additive. This indicates that the [BMP]$^+$[BF$_4$]$^-$ additive could effectively reduce the phase segregation phenomenon of the CsPbI$_{1.2}$Br$_{1.8}$ films. The photoinduced phase segregation phenomenon of CsPbI$_{1.2}$Br$_{1.8}$ films is suppressed by the [BMP]$^+$[BF$_4$]$^-$ additive.

Supplementary Materials: The following supporting information can be downloaded at: https://www.mdpi.com/article/10.3390/molecules29071476/s1, Figure S1. Normalized XRD patterns of pristine CsPbI1.2Br1.8 and CsPbI1.2Br1.8 films doped with different mass concentrations (0.5, 1, 2 and 3 mg mL-1) of [BMP]+[BF4]-.

Author Contributions: Conceptualization, H.X. and L.L.; methodology, H.X. and J.Z.; validation, H.X.; investigation, Y.Z. and Y.P.; resources, J.X.; data curation, H.X. and L.L.; writing—original draft preparation, H.X.; writing—review and editing, X.Y.; supervision, W.Q.; project administration, H.X.; funding acquisition, Y.P., J.X. and X.Y. All authors have read and agreed to the published version of the manuscript.

Funding: This research was funded by the Fundamental Research Funds for the Central Universities (xzy 012022090), the National Natural Science Foundation of China (62305262) and the Natural Science Basic Research Plan in the Shaanxi Province of China (2023-JC-QN-0693). SEM work was conducted at the International Center for Dielectric Research at Xi'an Jiaotong University.

Institutional Review Board Statement: Not applicable.

Informed Consent Statement: Not applicable.

Data Availability Statement: Data are contained within the article and Supplementary Materials.

Conflicts of Interest: The authors declare no conflicts of interest.

References

1. Kojima, A.; Teshima, K.; Shirai, Y.; Miyasaka, T. Organometal halide perovskites as visible-light sensitizers for photovoltaic cells. *J. Am. Chem. Soc.* **2009**, *131*, 6050–6051. [CrossRef] [PubMed]
2. Yin, X.; Guo, Y.; Xie, H.; Que, W.; Kong, L.B. Nickel oxide as efficient hole transport materials for perovskite solar cells. *Sol. RRL* **2019**, *3*, 1900001. [CrossRef]
3. Min, H.; Lee, D.Y.; Kim, J.; Kim, G.; Lee, K.S.; Kim, J.; Paik, M.J.; Kim, Y.K.; Kim, K.S.; Kim, M.G.; et al. Perovskite solar cells with atomically coherent interlayers on SnO$_2$ electrodes. *Nature* **2021**, *598*, 444–450. [CrossRef]
4. Laboratory, N.R.E. National Renewable Energy Laboratory, Best Research-Cell Efficiency Chart. Available online: https://www.nrel.gov/pv/national-center-for-photovoltaics.html (accessed on 17 January 2024).
5. Sun, Z.; Chen, X.; He, Y.; Li, J.; Wang, J.; Yan, H.; Zhang, Y. Toward efficiency limits of crystalline silicon solar cells: Recent progress in high-efficiency silicon heterojunction solar cells. *Adv. Energy Mater.* **2022**, *12*, 2200015. [CrossRef]
6. Kajal, S.; Jeong, J.; Seo, J.; Anand, R.; Kim, Y.; Bhaskararao, B.; Beom Park, C.; Yeop, J.; Hagdfeldt, A.; Young Kim, J.; et al. Coordination modulated passivation for stable organic-inorganic perovskite solar cells. *Chem. Eng. J.* **2023**, *451*, 138740. [CrossRef]
7. Zhao, Y.; Ma, F.; Qu, Z.; Yu, S.; Shen, T.; Deng, H.-X.; Chu, X.; Peng, X.; Yuan, Y.; Zhang, X. Inactive (PbI$_2$)$_2$RbCl stabilizes perovskite films for efficient solar cells. *Science* **2022**, *377*, 531–534. [CrossRef] [PubMed]
8. Wang, K.; Wu, C.; Hou, Y.; Yang, D.; Ye, T.; Yoon, J.; Sanghadasa, M.; Priya, S. Isothermally crystallized perovskites at room-temperature. *Energy Environ. Sci.* **2020**, *13*, 3412–3422. [CrossRef]
9. Ardimas; Pakornchote, T.; Sukmas, W.; Chatraphorn, S.; Clark, S.J.; Bovornratanaraks, T. Phase transformations and vibrational properties of hybrid organic-inorganic perovskite MAPbI$_3$ bulk at high pressure. *Sci. Rep.* **2023**, *13*, 16854. [CrossRef] [PubMed]
10. Yang, J.; Sheng, W.; Li, R.; Gong, L.; Li, Y.; Tan, L.; Lin, Q.; Chen, Y. Uncovering the mechanism of poly(ionic-liquid)s multiple inhibition of ion migration for efficient and stable perovskite solar cells. *Adv. Energy Mater.* **2022**, *12*, 2103652. [CrossRef]

11. Zhang, H.; Pfeifer, L.; Zakeeruddin, S.M.; Chu, J.; Grätzel, M. Tailoring passivators for highly efficient and stable perovskite solar cells. *Nat. Rev. Chem.* **2023**, *7*, 632–652. [CrossRef]
12. Zhu, H.; Teale, S.; Lintangpradipto, M.N.; Mahesh, S.; Chen, B.; McGehee, M.D.; Sargent, E.H.; Bakr, O.M. Long-term operating stability in perovskite photovoltaics. *Nat. Rev. Mater.* **2023**, *8*, 569–586. [CrossRef]
13. Park, S.M.; Wei, M.; Xu, J.; Atapattu, H.R.; Eickemeyer, F.T.; Darabi, K.; Grater, L.; Yang, Y.; Liu, C.; Teale, S.; et al. Engineering ligand reactivity enables high-temperature operation of stable perovskite solar cells. *Science* **2023**, *381*, 209–215. [CrossRef]
14. Abate, S.Y.; Qi, Y.; Zhang, Q.; Jha, S.; Zhang, H.; Ma, G.; Gu, X.; Wang, K.; Patton, D.; Dai, Q. Eco-friendly solvent engineered CsPbI$_{2.77}$Br$_{0.23}$ ink for large-area and scalable high performance perovskite solar cells. *Adv. Mater.* **2023**, *36*, 2310279. [CrossRef] [PubMed]
15. Ma, S.; Xue, X.; Wang, K.; Wen, Q.; Han, Y.; Wang, J.; Yao, H.; Lu, H.; Cui, L.; Ma, J.; et al. Intermediate phase modification enables high-performance iodine-rich inorganic perovskite solar cells with 3000-hour stability. *Adv. Energy Mater.* **2023**, *14*, 2303193. [CrossRef]
16. Yue, Y.; Yang, R.; Zhang, W.; Cheng, Q.; Zhou, H.; Zhang, Y. Cesium cyclopropane acid-aided crystal growth enables efficient inorganic perovskite solar cells with a high moisture tolerance. *Angew. Chem. Int. Ed.* **2023**, *63*, e202315717. [CrossRef] [PubMed]
17. Guo, Y.; Yin, X.; Liu, D.; Liu, J.; Zhang, C.; Xie, H.; Yang, Y.; Que, W. Photoinduced self-healing of halide segregation in mixed-halide perovskites. *ACS Energy Lett.* **2021**, *6*, 2502–2511. [CrossRef]
18. Guo, Y.; Yin, X.; Que, M.; Zhang, J.; Wen, S.; Liu, D.; Xie, H.; Que, W. Quantum dot-modified CsPbIBr$_2$ perovskite absorber for efficient and stable photovoltaics. *Org. Electron.* **2020**, *86*, 105917. [CrossRef]
19. Zhang, J.; Hodes, G.; Jin, Z.; Liu, S. All-Inorganic CsPbX$_3$ perovskite solar cells: Progress and prospects. *Angew. Chem. Int. Ed.* **2019**, *58*, 15596–15618. [CrossRef]
20. Choi, H.; Jeong, J.; Kim, H.-B.; Kim, S.; Walker, B.; Kim, G.-H.; Kim, J.Y. Cesium-doped methylammonium lead iodide perovskite light absorber for hybrid solar cells. *Nano Energy* **2014**, *7*, 80–85. [CrossRef]
21. Kulbak, M.; Cahen, D.; Hodes, G. How important is the organic part of lead halide perovskite photovoltaic cells? Efficient CsPbBr$_3$ cells. *J. Phys. Chem. Lett.* **2015**, *6*, 2452–2456. [CrossRef]
22. Eperon, G.E.; Paternò, G.M.; Sutton, R.J.; Zampetti, A.; Haghighirad, A.A.; Cacialli, F.; Snaith, H.J. Inorganic caesium lead iodide perovskite solar cells. *J. Mater. Chem. A* **2015**, *3*, 19688–19695. [CrossRef]
23. Hutter, E.M.; Sutton, R.J.; Chandrashekar, S.; Abdi-Jalebi, M.; Stranks, S.D.; Snaith, H.J.; Savenije, T.J. Vapour-deposited cesium lead iodide perovskites: Microsecond charge carrier lifetimes and enhanced photovoltaic performance. *ACS Energy Lett.* **2017**, *2*, 1901–1908. [CrossRef] [PubMed]
24. Gu, X.; Xiang, W.; Tian, Q.; Liu, S. Rational surface-defect control via designed passivation for high-efficiency inorganic perovskite solar cells. *Angew. Chem. Int. Ed.* **2021**, *60*, 23164–23170. [CrossRef] [PubMed]
25. Zhu, J.; He, B.; Zhang, W.; Tui, R.; Chen, H.; Duan, Y.; Huang, H.; Duan, J.; Tang, Q. Defect-dependent crystal plane control on inorganic CsPbBr$_3$ film by selectively anchoring (pseudo-) halide anions for 1.650 V voltage perovskite solar cells. *Adv. Funct. Mater.* **2022**, *32*, 2206838. [CrossRef]
26. Ho-Baillie, A.; Zhang, M.; Lau, C.F.J.; Ma, F.-J.; Huang, S. Untapped potentials of inorganic metal halide perovskite solar cells. *Joule* **2019**, *3*, 938–955. [CrossRef]
27. Yao, Z.; Zhao, W.; Liu, S. Stability of the CsPbI$_3$ perovskite: From fundamentals to improvements. *J. Mater. Chem. A* **2021**, *9*, 11124–11144. [CrossRef]
28. Yang, S.; Duan, Y.; Liu, Z.; Liu, S. Recent advances in CsPbX$_3$ perovskite solar cells: Focus on crystallization characteristics and controlling strategies. *Adv. Energy Mater.* **2023**, *13*, 2201733. [CrossRef]
29. Sutter-Fella, C.M.; Li, Y.; Amani, M.; Ager, J.W., III; Toma, F.M.; Yablonovitch, E.; Sharp, I.D.; Javey, A. High photoluminescence quantum yield in band gap tunable bromide containing mixed halide perovskites. *Nano Lett.* **2016**, *16*, 800–806. [CrossRef]
30. Beal, R.E.; Slotcavage, D.J.; Leijtens, T.; Bowring, A.R.; Belisle, R.A.; Nguyen, W.H.; Burkhard, G.F.; Hoke, E.T.; McGehee, M.D. Cesium Lead Halide Perovskites with Improved Stability for Tandem Solar Cells. *J. Phys. Chem. Lett.* **2016**, *7*, 746–751. [CrossRef]
31. Hoke, E.T.; Slotcavage, D.J.; Dohner, E.R.; Bowring, A.R.; Karunadasa, H.I.; McGehee, M.D. Reversible photo-induced trap formation in mixed-halide hybrid perovskites for photovoltaics. *Chem. Sci.* **2015**, *6*, 613–617. [CrossRef]
32. Li, W.; Rothmann, M.U.; Liu, A.; Wang, Z.; Zhang, Y.; Pascoe, A.R.; Lu, J.; Jiang, L.; Chen, Y.; Huang, F.; et al. Phase segregation enhanced ion movement in efficient inorganic CsPbIBr$_2$ solar cells. *Adv. Energy Mater.* **2017**, *7*, 1700946. [CrossRef]
33. Rehman, W.; Milot, R.L.; Eperon, G.E.; Wehrenfennig, C.; Boland, J.L.; Snaith, H.J.; Johnston, M.B.; Herz, L.M. Charge-carrier dynamics and mobilities in formamidinium lead mixed-halide perovskites. *Adv. Mater.* **2015**, *27*, 7938–7944. [CrossRef] [PubMed]
34. Wang, H.; Yang, M.; Cai, W.; Zang, Z. Suppressing phase segregation in CsPbIBr$_2$ films via anchoring halide ions toward underwater solar cells. *Nano Lett.* **2023**, *23*, 4479–4486. [CrossRef] [PubMed]
35. Guo, Z.; Teo, S.; Xu, Z.; Zhang, C.; Kamata, Y.; Hayase, S.; Ma, T. Achievable high V_{oc} of carbon based all-inorganic CsPbIBr$_2$ perovskite solar cells through interface engineering. *J. Mater. Chem. A* **2019**, *7*, 1227–1232. [CrossRef]
36. An, Y.; Zhang, N.; Zeng, Z.; Cai, Y.; Jiang, W.; Qi, F.; Ke, L.; Lin, F.R.; Tsang, S.W.; Shi, T. Optimizing crystallization in wide-bandgap mixed halide perovskites for high-efficiency solar cells. *Adv. Mater.* **2023**, 2306568. [CrossRef] [PubMed]
37. Chai, W.; Ma, J.; Zhu, W.; Chen, D.; Xi, H.; Zhang, J.; Zhang, C.; Hao, Y. Suppressing halide phase segregation in CsPbIBr$_2$ Films by polymer modification for hysteresis-less all-inorganic perovskite solar cells. *ACS Appl. Mater. Interfaces* **2021**, *13*, 2868–2878. [CrossRef] [PubMed]

38. Tao, Z.-W.; Lu, T.; Gao, X.; Rothmann, M.U.; Jiang, Y.; Qiang, Z.-Y.; Du, H.-Q.; Guo, C.; Yang, L.-H.; Wang, C.-X.; et al. Heterogeneity of light-induced open-circuit voltage loss in perovskite/si tandem solar cells. *ACS Energy Lett.* **2024**, *9*, 1455–1465. [CrossRef]
39. Liu, D.; Guo, Y.; Yin, X.; Yang, Y.; Que, W. Nucleation Regulation and Anchoring of Halide Ions in All-Inorganic Perovskite Solar Cells Assisted by $CuInSe_2$ Quantum Dots. *Adv. Funct. Mater.* **2023**, *33*, 2210754. [CrossRef]
40. Zhu, W.; Zhang, Q.; Chen, D.; Zhang, Z.; Lin, Z.; Chang, J.; Zhang, J.; Zhang, C.; Hao, Y. Intermolecular exchange boosts efficiency of air-stable, carbon-based all-inorganic planar $CsPbIBr_2$ perovskite solar cells to over 9%. *Adv. Energy Mater.* **2018**, *8*, 1802080. [CrossRef]
41. Sanchez, S.; Christoph, N.; Grobety, B.; Phung, N.; Steiner, U.; Saliba, M.; Abate, A. Efficient and stable inorganic perovskite solar cells manufactured by pulsed flash infrared annealing. *Adv. Energy Mater.* **2018**, *8*, 1802060. [CrossRef]

Disclaimer/Publisher's Note: The statements, opinions and data contained in all publications are solely those of the individual author(s) and contributor(s) and not of MDPI and/or the editor(s). MDPI and/or the editor(s) disclaim responsibility for any injury to people or property resulting from any ideas, methods, instructions or products referred to in the content.

Article

Mechanism of Phosphate Desorption from Activated Red Mud Particle Adsorbents

Zhiwen Yang [1,2,3], Longjiang Li [1,2,3,*] and Yalan Wang [1,2,3]

- [1] Mining College, Guizhou University, Guiyang 550025, China; yzwyy1011@163.com (Z.Y.); 15809275281@163.com (Y.W.)
- [2] National & Local Joint Laboratory of Engineering for Effective Utilization of Regional Mineral Resources from Karst Areas, Guiyang 550025, China
- [3] Guizhou Key Laboratory of Comprehensive Utilization of Nonmetallic Mineral Resources, Guiyang 550025, China
- * Correspondence: mnlljiang@163.com

Abstract: Herein, activated red mud particles are used as adsorbents for phosphorus adsorption. HCl solutions with different concentrations and deionized water are employed for desorption tests, and the desorption mechanism under the following optimal conditions is investigated: HCl concentration = 0.2 mol/L, desorbent dosage = 0.15 L/g, desorption temperature = 35 °C, and desorption time = 12 h. Under these conditions, the phosphate desorption rate and amount reach 99.11% and 11.29 mg/g, respectively. Notably, the Langmuir isothermal and pseudo-second-order kinetic linear models exhibit consistent results: monomolecular-layer surface desorption is dominant, and chemical desorption limits the rate of surface desorption. Thermodynamic analysis indicates that phosphorus desorption by the desorbents is spontaneous and that high temperatures promote such desorption. Moreover, an intraparticle diffusion model demonstrates that the removal of phosphorus in the form of precipitation from the surface of an activated hematite particle adsorbent primarily occurs via a chemical reaction, and surface micromorphological analysis indicates that desorption is primarily accompanied by Ca dissolution, followed by Al and Fe dissolutions. The desorbents react with the active elements in red mud, and the vibrations of the $[SiO_4]^{4-}$ functional groups of calcium–iron garnet and calcite or aragonite disappear. Further, in Fourier-transform infrared spectra, the intensities of the peaks corresponding to the PO_4^{3-} group considerably decrease. Thus, desorption primarily involves monomolecular-layer chemical desorption.

Keywords: red mud; granular adsorbent; desorption mechanism; regeneration

1. Introduction

Red mud is a porous, alkaline solid material synthesized during alumina production; it exhibits a satisfactory particle size distribution, an average particle size of <0.1 mm, and a specific surface area of ~10–25 m^2/g [1]. Red mud has satisfactory adsorption characteristics; in particular, it exhibits excellent phosphate adsorption characteristics [2,3]. However, red mud has not been industrially employed for phosphorus adsorption from water, primarily owing to the difficulty involved in phosphorus desorption from red mud particle adsorbents (hereinafter called "red mud adsorbents"), hindering the regeneration and subsequent reuse of the adsorbents. Notably, besides regenerating red mud adsorbents, desorption can also be used for recycling phosphorus resources. Phosphate desorption generally involves using acid, alkali, and salt leaching for phosphate recovery. Simple low-cost salts, such as NaCl and KCl, can be only employed to desorb phosphate from adsorbents exhibiting weak adsorption strengths and nonspecific adsorption [4,5]. High concentrations of such salts generally result in effective desorption [6]; owing to the risk of high salinity, this approach can be problematic if the desorbed phosphate is to be used in crop fertilization and irrigation [5]. Simple salts are ineffective in desorbing phosphate from adsorbents that strongly adsorb phosphate through specific adsorption mechanisms (e.g., ligand exchange and inner-sphere complexation) [7].

As phosphorus adsorption occurs at pH values below 3–4 and above 8–10, acids and bases can be used to specifically and nonspecifically desorb the adsorbed phosphate [8]. At pH values below 3–4, the phosphate adsorption capacity of an adsorbent is low because, at low pH values, phosphate primarily exists as H_3PO_4, which is very weakly adsorbed. At pH values above 8–10, adsorbents and the phosphate species in the considered solutions carry highly negative charges (HPO_4^{2-} and PO_4^{3-}), providing unfavorable adsorption conditions. In addition, the increase in the concentration of OH^- with increasing pH increases the competition between phosphate and OH^- for adsorption, reducing the phosphate adsorption capacity. If phosphate removal occurs through precipitation at high pH values, as when using Ca and Mg carbonates, then high-pH bases may not desorb phosphate [7,9]. Urano et al. [10] employed activated alumina and $Al_2(SO_4)_3$ as adsorbents to remove phosphate from water; the adsorbed phosphate was desorbed using NaOH. NaOH treatment resulted in some sulfate desorption and some aluminum dissolution. Therefore, the desorbed adsorbents could not be reused and had to be regenerated by recirculating a solution of $Al_2(SO_4)_3$ and hydrochloric acid. After alkaline-NaCl treatment, Kuzawa et al. [11–14] regenerated the adsorbent using 25% (wt%) $MgCl_2$ to rebuild the adsorbent structure and restore the adsorption capacity.

In mechanistic studies on phosphorus desorption from red mud adsorbents, acids desorbed phosphorus and concomitantly degraded the adsorbent surface structure, bases reduced the adsorbent adsorption capacity, and salts desorbed phosphate through ion exchange [15–17]. Commonly used salts for phosphorus desorption include sodium and potassium chlorides; however, special salts (e.g., NaCl) are sometimes employed to restore the adsorbent structure degraded during desorption. Yaqin et al. [12] studied phosphorus desorption from calcined red mud and reported that the calcination temperature does not substantially affect phosphate desorption. In addition, they reported that the efficiency of phosphorus desorption from the red mud particles was lower in NaOH solutions than in HCl solutions because desorption causes no notable mass loss in the case of alkaline desorbents. However, this mass loss is slightly higher than in the case of deionized water. This is because when using deionized water, compared to physical adsorption, <1% basic desorption occurs and, presumably, because of the involved reverse process of phosphate adsorption [18,19]. For phosphorus adsorption, Mingyang prepared microwave-roasted red mud–fly ash–cement composite granules (85:10:5 mass ratio) using an HCl solution under the following conditions: microwave power = 700 W, roasting duration = 15 min, and roasting temperature = 800 °C. Moreover, they employed a low-concentration NaOH solution for subsequent desorption. Notably, a low-concentration HCl solution is considered a better desorbent, as acids result in the unclogging of adsorbent particles, exposing the effective particle sites for better resorption [20].

Although both acids and alkalis are good desorption agents, the final comprehensive applicability of the employed adsorbent (i.e., after desorption) must be considered to maximize material usage. The results of the present study indicate that, because red mud is alkaline, its desorption using a base increases the risk of introducing high alkalinity in the downstream industrial applications of red mud adsorbents that require a low pH, especially concrete processes. Meanwhile, red mud adsorbents desorbed using acids reduce the adsorbent alkalinity, thus minimally impacting concrete processes. With regard to engineering applications, HCl exhibits good phosphorus desorption from red mud adsorbents; however, the involved desorption mechanism has been little studied. Moreover, if hydrochloric acid is to be used in substantial quantities for such desorption, the involved hydrochloric acid–adsorbent surface interactions and desorption mechanism need to be clarified. Further, the conditions required for optimal desorption (including the hydrochloric acid concentration) must be investigated. The present study is an attempt to address these issues.

Herein, red mud is employed as the primary raw material, sintering-modified charcoal powder is employed as a pore-making agent, and silica sol is employed as a bonding agent. Sintering is used to modify red mud, and static adsorption and desorption tests with HCl solutions of varying concentrations and deionized water are conducted. Finally, surface micromorphological analysis, energy-dispersive X-ray spectroscopy (EDS), mineral composition analysis, Fourier-transform infrared spectroscopy, and fittings of desorption kinetics and thermodynamics are performed to determine the desorption mechanism.

2. Results and Discussion

2.1. Influence of Different Desorbents on Phosphorus Desorption

Alkali (NaOH), acid (HCl), salt (NaCl), and deionized water were used to investigate the influence of different adsorbents on phosphorus desorption at a liquid–solid ratio of 0.15 L/g at 35 °C for 18 h. Figure 1 shows phosphorus desorption from activated red mud particles after adsorption. The results indicate that, after 3 h of desorption in deionized water and a NaCl solution, the desorption rate of phosphorus is <10%, which is much lower than those for HCl and NaOH solutions under the same desorption conditions. The phosphorus desorption rate is in the following order: HCl solution > NaOH solution > NaCl solution > deionized water. However, the desorption of the 1.0 mol/L NaOH solution is inconsiderable, which may be due to the insufficient desorption time or desorbent concentration.

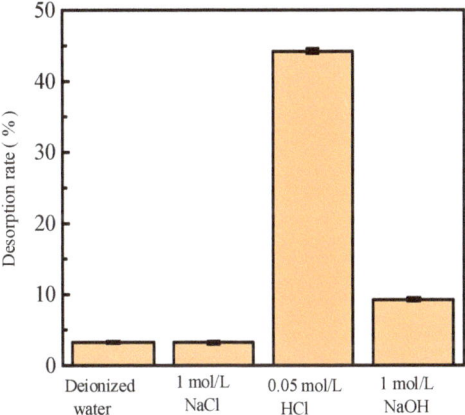

Figure 1. The desorption of phosphorus by alkali (NaOH), acid (HCl), salt (NaCl), and deionized water solutions.

2.2. Readsorption Performance of Activated Red Mud Adsorbents

The activated red mud adsorbents after phosphorus desorption were used to readsorb phosphorus. Notably, 25 g/L of activated red mud adsorbents were injected into a 40 mL conical flask in a phosphorus-containing 300 mg/L solution at a constant temperature of 35 °C to undergo static adsorption for 1, 2, 3, 6, 12, 18, and 24 h. The concentration of phosphorus contained in the solution supernatant was determined through inductively coupled plasma (ICP) emission spectrometry. Figure 2 shows phosphorus resorption by the adsorbent after desorption. The resorption performances for deionized water and 0.2 and 0.5 mol/L HCl solutions are considerably better than those for a low-concentration HCl solution and any concentration of a NaOH solution. Figure 2 shows that 0.2–0.5 mol/L HCl does not destroy the particle structure and even dredges the particle pores, thereby exposing the effective sites inside the particles. This explains why the 0.2–0.5 mol/L HCl solution is better than deionized water. By combining desorption–readsorption and the loss of particles, a 0.2 mol/L HCl solution can serve as a desorbent for desorption and subsequent phosphorus readsorption studies of activated red mud adsorbents.

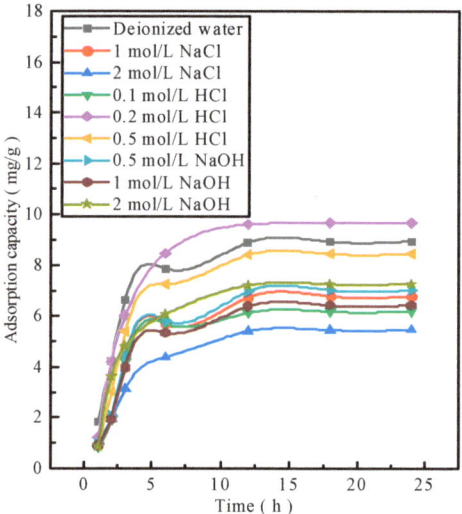

Figure 2. Adsorbent resorption performance.

2.3. Effect of Desorbent Dosage on Phosphorus Desorption

With the HCl desorbent concentration of 0.2 mol/L, phosphorus-containing wastewater at an initial concentration of 300 mg/L was adsorbed by the activated red mud adsorbents, which were then dried at 105 °C for 2 h. The liquid-to-solid ratios of the adsorbents were 0.05, 0.1, 0.15, 0.2, 0.25, 0.3, 0.35, and 0.4 L/g, and static desorption was performed at 35 °C for 12 h. The test was performed at the same time in a conical flask with a liquid-to-solid ratio 1:3 of the adsorbent. The phosphorus concentration in the supernatant of the solution was determined via ICP after the test, and the results were expressed in terms of the amount and rate of phosphorus desorption (Figure 3). The desorption rate and amount of the resorbent leveled off after the liquid–solid ratio exceeded 0.15 L/g. The desorption rate increased to 94.54%, and the desorption amount increased to 11.29 mg/g. The optimal desorbent dosage (0.15 L/g) was employed for phosphorous desorption.

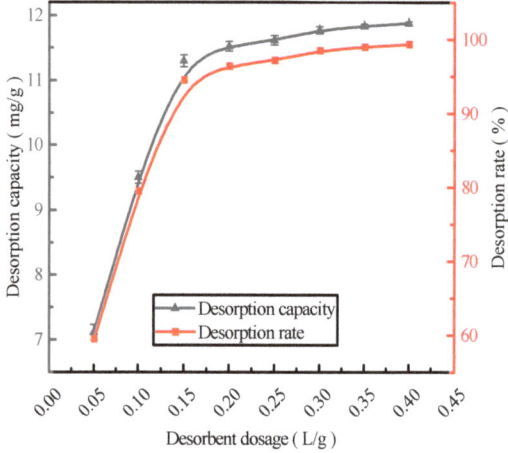

Figure 3. The effect of the desorbent dosage on the phosphorus desorption capacity.

2.4. Effect of Initial Adsorption on Phosphorus Desorption

Here, we discuss the adsorption at the initial concentrations of 200, 250, 300, 400, 500, 600, 700, 900, and 1200 mg/L of activated red mud adsorbents (105 °C for 2 h) and the static desorption of 0.2 mol/L HCl with a desorbent and adsorbent liquid–solid ratio of 0.15 L/g (35 °C in a conical flask for 12 h). Once the phosphorous concentration in the solution supernatant is determined through ICP, the results are based on the amount of desorbed phosphorus. After the test, the phosphorus concentration in the solution supernatant was determined via ICP; the results are expressed in terms of the amount of phosphorus desorbed and the desorption rate in Figure 4. With increasing initial phosphorus concentration, the desorption of the desorbent for the phosphorus adsorbed by the adsorbents increased. The phosphorus desorption was 7.98 mg/g for an initial concentration of 200 mg/L, with a desorption rate of 99.57%, which was primarily attributed to the high adsorption rate. The main reason for this result is that high adsorption rates drove the desorption of the desorbent to the adsorbent, increasing the number of adsorption sites used on the particle surfaces and leading to better desorption. The desorption rate decreased with increasing initial phosphorus concentration, which was consistent with adsorption. The particles presented in Figure 4 show that the desorption rate of phosphorus adsorbed by the adsorbents exceeded 99% when the initial concentration was <300 mg/L. Thus, high-efficiency phosphorus removal was realized.

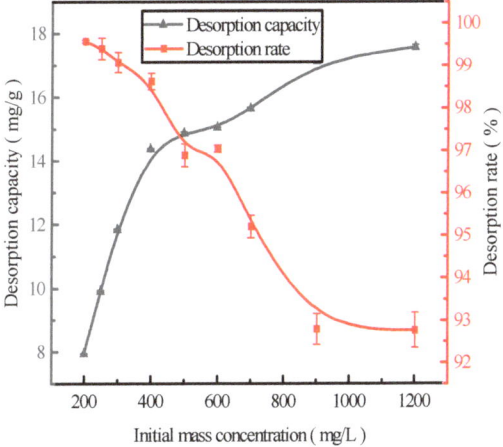

Figure 4. The effect of the initial adsorption on phosphorus desorption.

2.5. Effect of the Reaction Time on Phosphorous Desorption

The reaction time is also an important factor affecting the desorption effect of the desorbent on pollutants. We use activated red mud adsorbent for adsorption at 105 °C (drying for 2 h), a desorbent and adsorbent liquid–solid ratio of 0.15 L/g, and the initial concentrations of 200, 300, and 500 mg/L of the desorbent solution at 35 °C in a conical flask to conduct static desorption for 1, 2, 3, 6, 12, 18, and 24 h. The tests were performed via ICP to determine the effect of phosphorus desorption. After each test, the phosphorus concentration in the supernatant of the solution was determined via ICP, with the results expressed in terms of the amount of phosphorus desorbed (Figure 5).

The trend of the desorption amount of phosphorus adsorbed by the desorbent for the activated red mud adsorbent remained consistent for different initial phosphorus concentrations, and the increase in the desorption amount of the desorbent for an initial solution of 200 mg/L was considerably less than that for the initial concentrations of 300 and 500 mg/L for the first 12 h of the reaction. This result is attributable to the low concentration of phosphorus in the initial phosphorus solution of 200 mg/L, which resulted in less phosphorus adsorbed by the activated red mud adsorbent, in turn increasing the desorption rate. The desorption was lower when phosphorus was adsorbed by the adsorbent and desorbed after 12 h of the reaction under the condition of a low concentration.

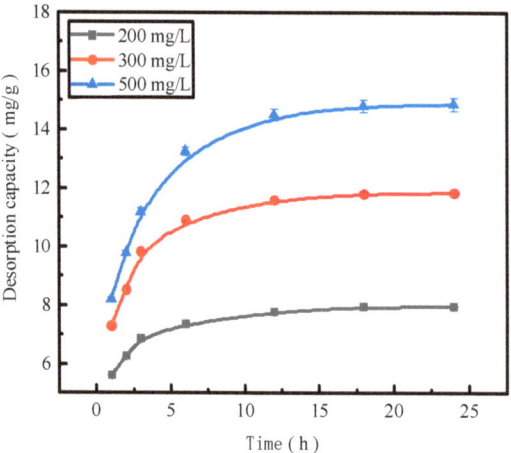

Figure 5. The phosphorus desorption capacity as a function of time.

2.6. Effect of the Reaction Temperature on Phosphorous Desorption

The reaction temperature is also an important factor affecting the desorption effect of the desorbent on pollutants. Figure 6 presents the results in terms of the phosphorus desorption rate. The desorption rate and the amount of desorbent desorbed for a liquid–solid ratio of 0.15 L/g, the initial concentration of 300 mg/L of a 150 mL desorbent solution at 15 °C, 20 °C, 25 °C, 30 °C, and 35 °C for static desorption, and the static desorption in a conical flask for 12 h were determined by employing ICP to obtain the concentration of phosphorus in the solution supernatant. The phosphorus desorption rate increased with increasing reaction temperatures. At 35 °C, the phosphorus desorption rate was 99.11%, and the desorption rate stabilized above 25 °C, indicating that desorption was heat absorbing. The increase in temperature accelerated the intermolecular thermal motion and the diffusion of phosphorus because adsorption and desorption are constantly converted for the reaction to occur. Moreover, desorption is a chemical reaction process in which HCl and the adsorbent surface of phosphate dissolve the other ions while sparing the HCl action channel. This increases the contact area of the reaction and temperature, elevating the chemical reaction rate and, thus, the desorption rate. In addition, according to the previous adsorption behavior study, phosphorus adsorbed on the adsorbent of red mud particles is an attached state, with only hydrogen bonding forces and van der Waals forces acting on it. Consequently, the rate at which phosphate escapes the system will increase as a result of the temperature increase intensifying the molecular movement.

2.7. Desorption Isotherm

Adsorption by activated red mud adsorbent was conducted for the initial concentrations of 200, 250, 300, 400, 500, 600, 700, 900, and 1200 mg/L, and adsorption after drying at 105 °C for 2 h and the desorption of a 0.2 mol/L HCl desorbent were performed at a desorbent and adsorbent solid–liquid ratio of 0.15 L/g and constant temperatures of 15 °C, 25 °C, and 35 °C. Static desorption was performed in a conical flask for 18 h. The desorption effect of the desorbent on phosphorus was investigated at different ambient temperatures, with the results expressed as the desorption rate of phosphorus (Figure 7). The experimental results fit with Langmuir and Freundlich isotherms and a D–R model, and the results of the fits are presented in Figure 8 and Table 1. The Freundlich model explains multimolecular-layer surface desorption, and the Langmuir model describes homogeneous desorption, wherein pollutants are desorbed as a monomolecular layer with homogeneous active sites on the desorbent surface [21].

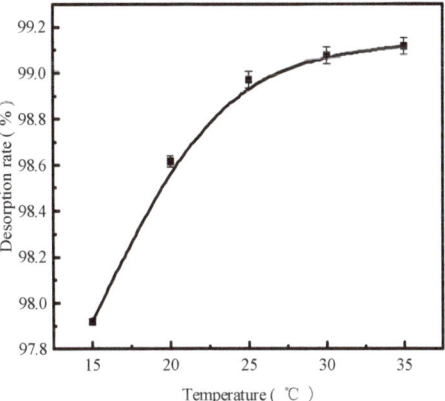

Figure 6. The phosphorous desorption rate as a function of time.

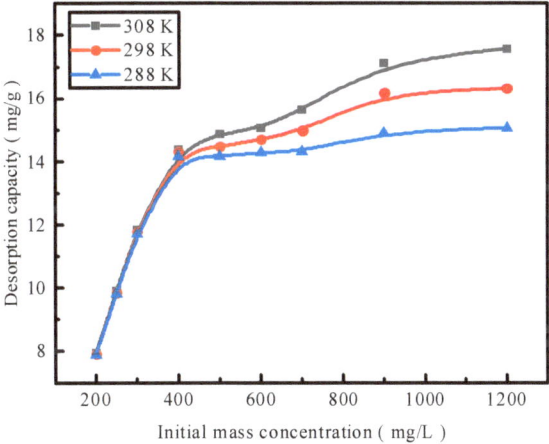

Figure 7. The effect of the reaction temperature on phosphate desorption.

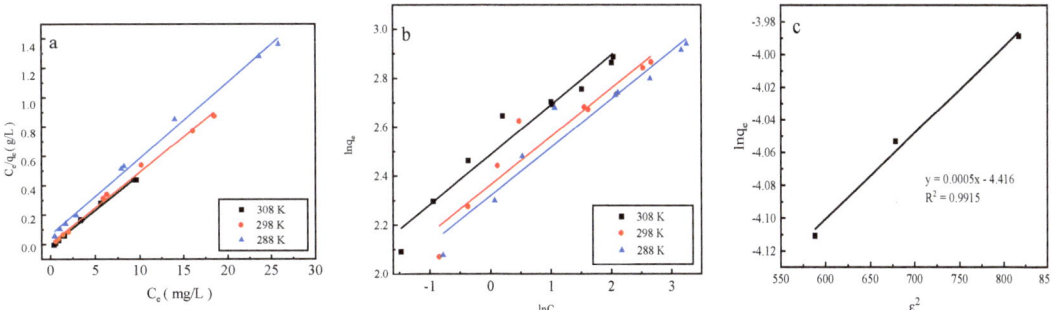

Figure 8. The fits of three desorption isotherm models: (**a**) the Langmuir model, (**b**) the Freundlich model, and (**c**) the D–R model.

Table 1. Desorption isotherm parameters.

Desorption Isotherm	Constants		
	308 K	298 K	288 K
Langmuir	R = 0.9947 a (mg/g) = 19.4175 b (L/mg) = 1.8392	R = 0.9946 a (mg/g) = 19.3798 b (L/mg) = 1.0639	R = 0.9950 a (mg/g) = 19.3050 b (L/mg) = 0.7674
Freundlich	R = 0.9400 N = 4.7393 K_F (mg^{1-n}/g L^n) = 12.0637	R = 0.9118 n = 4.8852 K_F/(mg^{1-n}/g L^n) = 10.8038	R = 0.9438 n = 5.0684 K_F/(mg^{1-n}/g L^n) = 10.1808
D–R	R = 0.9916 q_m (mmol/L) = 0.03255 k (mol^2/kJ^2) = 0.0005 E (kJ/mol) = −31.6228		

Desorption is primarily affected by the Langmuir adsorption isotherm model, indicating that monomolecular-layer phosphorus desorption occurs on the surfaces of the red mud particles activated by HCl. The average adsorption free energy |E| obtained using the D–R model is 31.62 kJ/mol, which exceeds 16 kJ/mol, indicating that desorption is chemical.

2.8. Desorption Thermodynamic Analysis

To further investigate the effect of temperature on phosphorus desorption, thermodynamic parameters were utilized to reflect the desorption characteristics. The desorption thermodynamic curves of lnK_d versus $\frac{1}{T}$ were numerically fitted using Equations (9)–(12) (Figure 9 and Table 2).

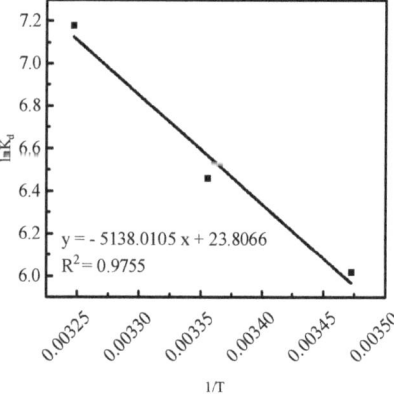

Figure 9. The thermodynamic curves of phosphorus desorption from activated red mud particle sorbents.

Table 2. The thermodynamic parameters of phosphorus desorption from activated red mud particle sorbents.

T (K)	ΔG^θ (kJ/mol)	ΔH^θ (kJ/mol)	ΔS^θ (J/(mol·K))	R^2
288	−14.4085			
298	−16.0027	42.7173	197.9314	0.9755
308	−18.3846			

In Table 2, ΔG^θ is <0, indicating that hydrochloric acid is favorable for phosphorus desorption and desorption is spontaneous. Moreover, ΔH^θ is >0, indicating that phosphorus desorption using hydrochloric acid is a heat-absorbing reaction, suggesting that high temperatures are favorable for desorption. Further, ΔS^θ is >0, suggesting that the solid–liquid interface degree of freedom of desorption increases.

Notably, ΔG^θ is −400−−80 kJ/mol for chemical desorption and −20–0 kJ/mol for physical desorption, with ΔH^θ being >40 kJ/mol for chemical desorption and <40 kJ/mol for physical desorption. In the above three temperature conditions, the effects of hydrochloric acid on phosphorus desorption, the ΔG^θ of physical adsorption, and the ΔH^θ of chemical adsorption indicate that there is a chemical desorption of the desorption agent on the phosphorus of chemical and physical desorptions.

2.9. Desorption Kinetics

This study employs a pseudo-first-order kinetic linear model, a pseudo-second-order kinetic linear model, and an intraparticle diffusion model to fit the phosphorus kinetic properties of adsorption by the desorbent desorption of activated red mud adsorbents. After adsorption with the different initial concentrations of 200, 300, and 500 mg/L, the activated red mud adsorbents were dried at 105 °C for 2 h. The desorbent was 0.2 mol/L HCl, and the desorbent and adsorbent solid–liquid ratio was 0.15 L/g. Static desorption was conducted at a constant temperature of 35 °C in conical flasks for 1, 2, 3, 6, 12, 18, and 24 h. The fitting results are presented in Figure 10 and Table 3.

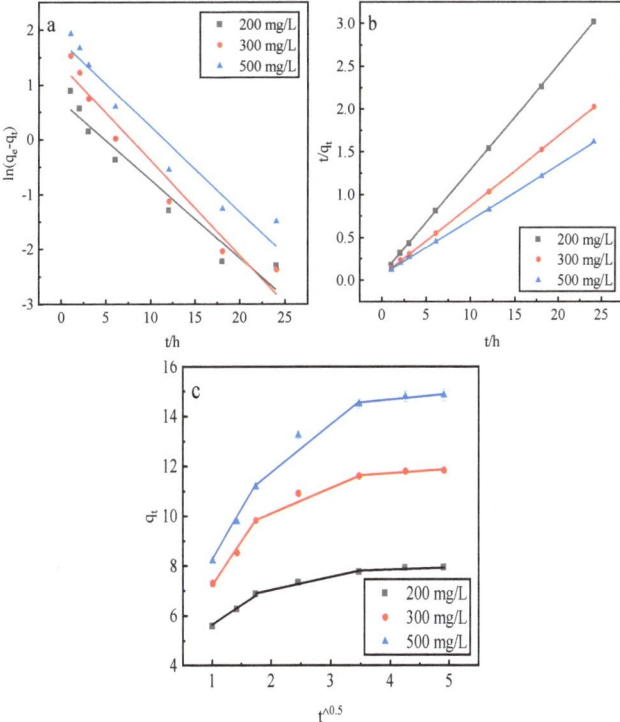

Figure 10. The fits of three desorption kinetic models: (**a**) the pseudo-first-order model, (**b**) the pseudo-second-order model, and (**c**) the intraparticle diffusion model.

Based on the correlation coefficient R^2, the pseudo-second-order kinetic model exhibited better fitting for the phosphorus adsorption kinetics than the pseudo-first-order kinetic model, and the theoretical equilibrium detachment amounts were 15.073 mg/g at a concentration of 500 mg/L, 11.898 mg/g at a concentration of 300 mg/L, and 8.102 mg/g at a concentration of 200 mg/L. The theoretical equilibrium detachment amounts obtained are close to the experimental result q_e, indicating that the chemical reaction limits the rate of surface desorption. The calculated q_e is greater than the actual desorption maximum, which is also related to precipitation arising from the chemical reaction on the red mud surface. According to the intraparticle diffusion model, three main stages are observed: the first stage is the rapid desorption stage, which is primarily manifested in the form of the chemical precipitation of metal ions and phosphorus and the reaction occurring in the desorption agent. The second stage is slower and primarily involves the activation of the well-developed pore structure of the red mud to perform desorption. In the third stage, which is the slowest desorption, a relative equilibrium is gradually achieved. Because the internal diffusion curve of the particles does not pass through the origin of the coordinates, a high-concentration results in a greater deviation of the curve from the origin, indicating that internal diffusion is not the main mechanism of phosphorus desorption. Rather, desorption is dominated by the chemical reaction, in which phosphorus is removed through precipitation on the adsorbent surface of the activated red mud particles.

Table 3. Desorption kinetic parameters.

Adsorption Kinetics		Constant	500 mg/L	300 mg/L	200 mg/L
Pseudo-first-order dynamic linear model		q_e (mg/g) k_1 (1/h) R^2	5.9817 0.1554 0.9438	3.8551 0.1734 0.9537	2.0100 0.1427 0.9433
Pseudo-second-order dynamic linear model		q_e (mg/g) k_2 (1/h) R^2	15.5763 0.0613 0.9998	12.2549 0.1102 0.9999	8.1499 0.2221 0.9999
Intraparticle diffusion model	Phase I	k_i (mg/g·h$^{1/2}$) C (mg/g) R^2	3.9826 4.2189 0.9978	1.7320 3.8600 0.9984	3.2657 4.0257 0.9929
	Phase II	k_i (mg/g·h$^{1/2}$) C (mg/g) R^2	1.9701 7.9605 0.9462	0.5040 6.0442 0.9889	1.0750 8.0460 0.9525
	Phase III	k_i (mg/g·h$^{1/2}$) C (mg/g) R^2	0.2629 13.6168 0.9138	0.1053 7.4382 0.8535	0.1749 11.0230 0.9120

2.10. Surface Morphology Analysis after Desorption

Scanning electron microscopy (SEM) was used to observe the surface morphology of the activated particle adsorbents before (Figure 11a) and after (Figure 11b) desorption at 10,000× magnification and as well as before (Figure 11c) and after (Figure 11d) desorption at 25,000× magnification. The pores on the surface of the activated red mud adsorbent before desorption are covered by the precipitate, showing crystallization, multilayer adsorption on the surface of the activated red mud adsorbent, and precipitation products covering the material surface. The surface of the adsorbent after the desorption of the red mud adsorbent revealed notable corrosion after the destruction of the particle structure. To a certain extent, owing to the acid making the particles sparse in the pores, the effective points inside the particle pores were exposed. Figure 11c,d shows that the surface after desorption by the desorbent exhibits a laminated structure, which indicates surface disintegration, suggesting that the desorption of phosphorus is primarily caused by the particles disintegrating easily under the strong acid conditions of the desorbent.

Comparing the EDS measurements before and after the desorption of the activated red mud adsorbents reveals that the desorbent may have led to the disintegration of the adsorbent, as observed through SEM imaging. To explore the changes of the surface elements, EDS analyses were performed before and after desorption of the activated red mud adsorbents, and the surface of the particulate adsorbent before and after desorption was subjected to a narrow sweep of elements such as O, Ca, Al, Na, Si, Fe, and P (Figure 12).

Figure 12a presents the narrow sweep of EDS before desorption, and Figure 12b shows this after desorption.

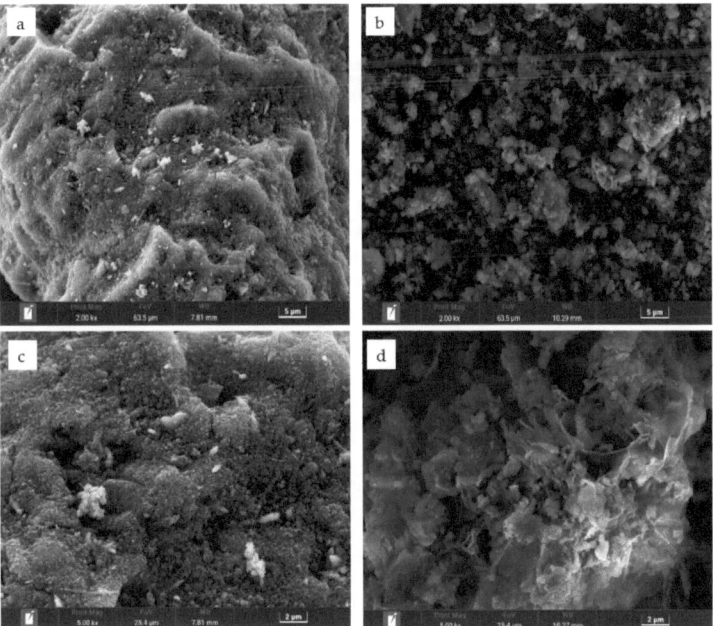

Figure 11. Scanning electron micrographs of the surface of activated red mud adsorbents before and after desorption. (**a,b**) Before and after desorption at 5 µm, respectively. (**c,d**) Before and after desorption at 2 µm, respectively.

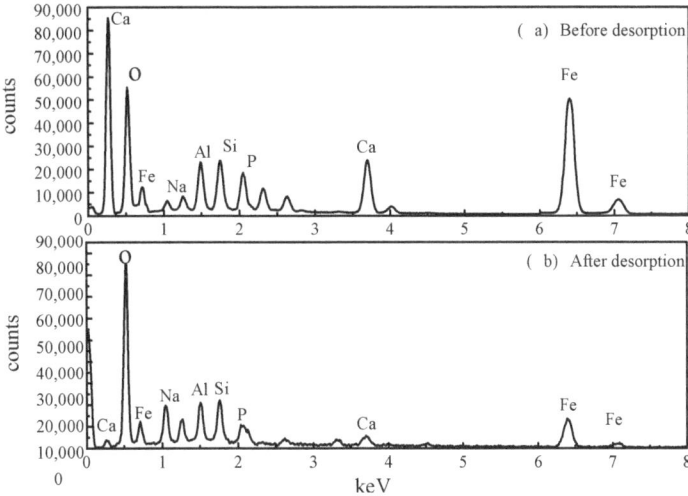

Figure 12. The narrow sweep of EDS before and after the desorption of activated red mud adsorbents.

A comparison between Figure 12a,b and Table 4 shows that the elemental phosphorus on the surface of the adsorbent decreases after desorption, which is consistent with the SEM surface images presented in Figure 11. Less elemental calcium appeared on the surface of the granular adsorbents after desorption than before desorption, indicating that the dissolution of Ca in the activated red mud adsorbents under acidic conditions was linked to the reaction between the desorbent and the $(Ca)_3(PO_4)_2$ precipitation on the adsorbent surface, causing certain phosphorus desorption. In addition, the specific surface elements before and after the desorption of phosphorus from the adsorbent were measured, with the results expressed in terms of elemental mass. The phosphorus adsorbed by the adsorbent on activated red mud particles after desorption decreased from 4.84% to 0.84%, Ca decreased from 15.54% to 8.97%, Al decreased from 6.47% to 5.48%, and Fe decreased from 13.65% to 12.65%, which also demonstrated that the desorbent reacted with the reactive elements in the red mud to cause the adsorption of the adsorbent on the surface by the active elements on the adsorbent surface. This result indicated that the desorbent reacted with the active elements in red mud, removing phosphorus originally adsorbed on the adsorbent surface. This was especially the case for the considerable reduction in Ca, which may react with the Cl^- in the desorbent to form water-soluble $CaCl_2$. The corrosive effect caused these elements to detach from the surface of the activated red mud particles dissolved in the water and accompanied by phosphorus desorption.

Table 4. The elemental composition mass fraction (%) of activated red mud adsorbents before and after desorption.

Element	Before Desorption (%)	After Desorption (%)
O	51.04	61.03
Na	2.21	3.84
Al	6.47	5.48
Si	6.25	7.22
P	4.84	0.84
Ca	15.54	8.97
Fe	13.65	12.62
Total	100.00	100.00

2.11. Analysis of Morphological Changes

Figure 13 shows the mineral composition of the activated red mud adsorbent before and after desorption. With desorption, the intensities of the characteristic peaks of the chalcopyrite, calcium chalcopyrite, and calcium–iron garnet considerably decreased. This result is related to the disintegration and dissolution of elements such as Ca, Fe, and Si during phosphorus desorption in water. Variations in the crystal type and mineral composition are inconsiderable, indicating that the activated red mud adsorbents can continue to adsorb phosphorus after desorption. Thus, the adsorbents may be reused.

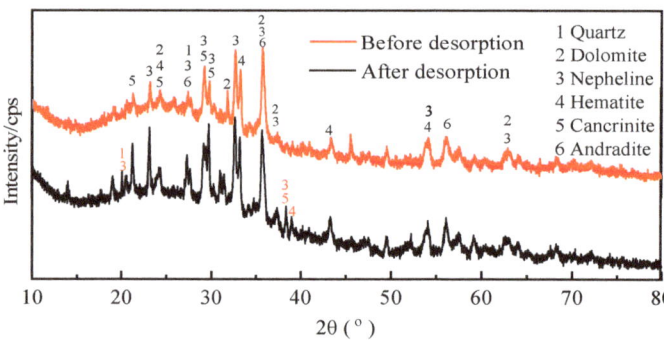

Figure 13. The XRD patterns of the activated red mud particles before and after desorption.

2.12. Fourier-Transform Infrared Spectroscopy Analysis

Fourier-transform infrared spectroscopy was conducted to examine the changes in the structure and chemical groups of the activated red mud adsorbent with desorption. The goal was to verify the phosphorus fugacity state on the activated hematite particulate adsorbent from 400 to 1500 cm^{-1}. Figure 14 presents the spectral maps before and after desorption. After desorption, the peaks at 992 cm^{-1} were considerably strengthened primarily by the Si(AlIV)–O telescopic vibration as shelly silicate or chalcocite, which was consistent with the increase in the Si content (EDS results). The peaks at 814, 874.76, and 1463 cm^{-1} disappeared, the main desorption agent led to the dissociation of Ca and Fe, and the vibrations of the $[SiO_4]^{4-}$ functional groups of the calcium–iron garnet and calcite or aragonite basically disappeared. The peaks at 3600–3000 cm^{-1} were due to water crystallization, indicating that desorption was accompanied by water desorption. Overall, the material changes before and after desorption were clearer than before desorption, especially for Ca and Fe compounds. After desorption, the intensities of the strong peaks for PO_4^{3-} groups at 1087.03 and 572 cm^{-1} substantially decreased [22], indicating that the desorption of phosphorus from the activated red mud adsorbents was accompanied by a chemical reaction.

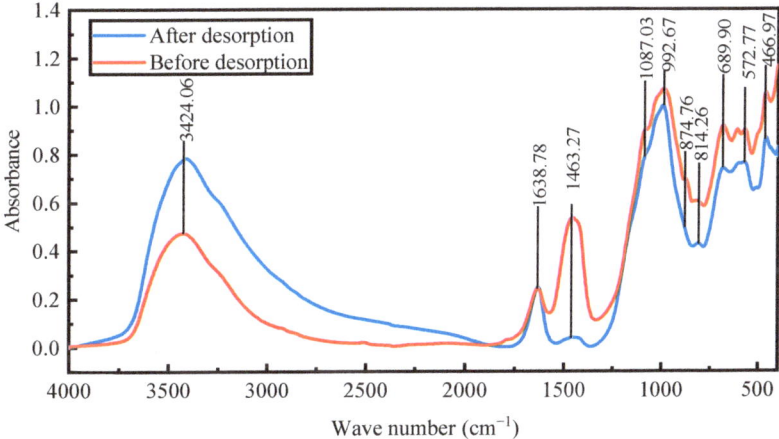

Figure 14. The Fourier-transform infrared spectra of activated red mud adsorbents before and after desorption.

3. Materials and Methods

3.1. Materials

The raw materials for preparing modified red mud adsorbents primarily included red mud, charcoal powder, and silica sol. Red mud was procured from Guizhou Huajin Aluminum Co., Ltd., Guiyang, China, with the water content being 30%. It was dried at 50 °C for 12 h and then passed through a 0.075 mm sieve after grinding in a ball mill. Charcoal powder was procured from Henan Xingnuo Environmental Protection Materials Co., Ltd. (Changge, China), and silica sol was purchased from Wuhan Jiye Sheng Chemical Co. (Wuhan, China). The chemical components of the red mud were Fe_2O_3 (21.94%), Al_2O_3 (21.04%), SiO_2 (19.05%), CaO (17.95%), Na_2O (8.96%), and others (11.06%). The used phosphorus-containing wastewater was return water from a phosphorous-ore-dressing plant in Guizhou, China, and contained flotation tailings. Red mud particles were activated for use as adsorbents by mixing red mud, charcoal powder, and silica sol in a preset mass ratio of 92:5:3 by employing a disk granulator for granulation; the water–ash ratio was 1:2. These particles of 1–2 mm diameter were sintered in a muffle furnace at 700 °C for 30 min. The primary elements in the wastewater were P (1278.0 mg/L), Ca (213.15 mg/L),

Mg (401.40 mg/L), Al (0.25 mg/L), Fe (0.02 mg/L), Cr (0.04 mg/L), K (66.35 mg/L), and Na (0.25 mg/L). The wastewater was weakly acidic (pH = 3–4); phosphorus was primarily present in the form of $H_2PO_4^{2-}$, which could be diluted to the required concentration by adding deionized water.

3.2. Test Methods for Phosphorus Adsorption and Desorption Using and from, Respectively, Activated Red Mud Particles

The initial pH was 4. The effects of the operating and environmental conditions on the adsorption of the adsorbents were investigated as functions of the adsorbent dosage, adsorption time, and adsorption temperature to obtain the optimal adsorption conditions.

The initial phosphorus concentrations were 200, 250, 300, 400, 500, 600, 700, 900, and 1200 mg/L, the adsorption temperatures were 15 °C, 20 °C, 25 °C, 30 °C, and 35 °C, and the adsorption times were 1, 2, 3, 6, 12, 18, and 24 h. Further, 40 mL of phosphorus-containing wastewater was poured into a conical flask, and 0.8, 1, 1.2, 1.4, 1.6, 1.8, 2, 2.2, and 2.4 g of granular adsorbents were added for static adsorption. The test was conducted thrice using a model ICP-7400 inductively coupled plasma emission spectrometer and a yttrium internal standard to measure the contents of phosphorus and other ions in the supernatant. The phosphorus removal rate (η%) and the amount of phosphorus adsorbed per unit adsorbent mass (Q, mg/g) were calculated as follows [23]:

$$\eta = \frac{(C_0 - C_e)}{C_0} \times 100\%, \quad (1)$$

$$Q = \frac{V(C_o - C_e)}{m} \times 100\%, \quad (2)$$

where C_o (mg/L) and C_e (mg/L) are the concentrations of phosphorus in the used solution before and after adsorption, respectively, V is the solution volume (L), and M is the mass of the adsorbent after drying (g).

Phosphorus desorption test. Activated red mud adsorbents were removed and dried and then added into different types of desorbents. Acid: 0.2, 0.1, and 0.05 mol/L HCl; alkali: 0.5, 1, and 2 mol/L NaOH; and salt: 1 and 2 mol/L NaCl. The desorption temperatures were 15 °C, 20 °C, 25 °C, 30 °C, and 35 °C, and the desorption times were 1, 2, 3, 6, 12, 18, and 24 h. The concentration of phosphorus desorbed from the solution was determined at the end of the test. The amount of phosphorus desorbed per unit adsorbent mass after adsorption (Y, mg/g) and the phosphorus desorption rate (y, %) were calculated using Equations (4) and (5) [24]:

$$q_e = (C_0 - C_e)\frac{V_1}{m_1}, \quad (3)$$

$$Y = C_p \frac{V_2}{m_2}, \quad (4)$$

$$y = \frac{Y}{q_e} \times 100\%, \quad (5)$$

where q_e is the amount of phosphorus adsorbed per unit adsorbent mass (mg/g), C_0(mg/L) and C_e (mg/L) are the concentrations of phosphate in the adsorption solution before and after the test, respectively, V_1 is the adsorption solution volume (L), m_1 is the added adsorbent mass (g), C_p is the concentration of phosphorus in the desorption solution (mg/L), V_2 is the volume of the desorption solution (L), and m_2 is the dry weight of the adsorbents after adsorption (g).

Phosphorus adsorption test. After desorption, the activated red mud adsorbents were first rinsed with deionized water and then dried to be used again for phosphorus adsorption. To obtain the optimal adsorption conditions for any other pharmaceutical compound, the steps are the same as those for the activated red mud adsorbents.

3.3. Characterization and Analysis Methods

The specific surface area and porosity were determined using a specific surface area and porosity analyzer model (Micromeritics APSP 2460, Norcross, GA, USA), with a degassing temperature of 200 °C, a degassing time of 8 h, and nitrogen adsorption gas. The specific surface area and pore volume of the red mud samples were calculated before and after activation using the Brunauer–Emmett–Teller (BET) and Barrett–Joyner–Halenda (BJH) models.

The elemental content and composition of red mud before and after the test were analyzed using an ARL PERFORM'X X-ray (Basel, Switzerland) fluorescence spectrometer. The red mud to be tested was dried, ground, and filtered using a 200 mesh; 4 g of the sample was weighed and analyzed in a vacuum.

Thermogravimetric analysis was performed using synchronous PE thermogravimetry–differential scanning calorimetry to determine the activation temperature by analyzing the changes in the masses of the charcoal powder and red mud as functions of temperature. The heating rate was 10 °C/min, the temperature range was 30 °C–1000 °C, and the atmosphere was nitrogen.

Surface micromorphological analysis and energy spectroscopy were performed using a TESCAN MIRA LMS scanning electron microscope (Brno, Czech Republic) to image and analyze the surface configuration of the red mud adsorbents. The morphology was enlarged to 2–5 μm, and the particle surfaces were scanned through EDS in the spectral spot scanning mode to analyze the relative contents of phosphorus and other elements on the sample surface.

Mineral composition analysis was performed using an X-ray diffractometer model (XPert PRO MPD, Almelo, The Netherlands) to determine the mineral composition of the samples through powder X-ray diffraction (operating parameters: Cu Kα line; 40 kV and 40 mA; scanning speed = 2°/s; and scanning range = 10°–80°).

The surface functional groups were analyzed using a Fourier infrared spectrometer model (Nicolet 670, Waltham, MA, USA). The position and intensity of the Fourier infrared absorption peaks reflect the characteristics of the molecular structure and serve to identify the structural composition of the unknown substance or to determine its chemical composition. For infrared analysis of the bulk, a small amount of the dried sample was mixed with potassium bromide powder that was ground and pressed in a vacuum. The functional groups were then identified via infrared spectral scanning from 400 to 4000 cm^{-1}.

3.4. Kinetic and Thermodynamic Methods

3.4.1. Desorption Isotherm Analysis

Desorption curves at different temperatures are nonlinear and can, therefore, be fitted using the Freundlich and Langmuir adsorption isotherm equations [25]. The isotherms reveal the interaction between (i) the adsorbent and desorbent and (ii) the adsorbate at the interface of the two phases to obtain the desorption properties and mechanism [26]. The D–R model provides the ideal state, assuming that the adsorbent pore space is filled with solute. The Freundlich adsorption isotherm model (Equation (6)) and the Langmuir adsorption isotherm model (Equation (7)) were employed to analyze the adsorption isotherms.

$$q_e = KC_e^{1/n}, \tag{6}$$

$$q_e = \frac{abC_e}{1+bC_e}, \tag{7}$$

$$ln q_e = ln q_m - k\varepsilon^2, \tag{8}$$

where K is the Freundlich constant of adsorption and desorption, the exponent $1/n$ is the Freundlich affinity coefficient for the adsorption–desorption intensity, a and b are the Langmuir adsorption–desorption capacity and binding strength, respectively, C_e is the phosphate concentration at adsorption–desorption equilibrium, q_e is the equilibrium adsorption amount (mmol/g), q_m is the theoretical maximum adsorption amount (mmol/g), k and ε are constants, and $E = -1/(2k)^{0.5}$.

3.4.2. Desorption Thermodynamic Analysis

Thermodynamics is employed from the energy point of view to explain a possible desorption mechanism, explore the energy conversion law, and use thermodynamic parameters to understand the characteristics of the following thermodynamic equations [27]:

$$K_d = q_e/C_e, \tag{9}$$

$$\Delta G^\theta = -RT \ln K_d, \tag{10}$$

$$\Delta G^\theta = \Delta H^\theta - T\Delta S^\theta, \tag{11}$$

where ΔG^θ is the change in the Gibbs free energy, K_d is a thermodynamic constant, ΔH^θ is the change in enthalpy, ΔS^θ is the change in entropy, R is the universal gas constant, and T is the absolute temperature. Combining Equations (10) and (11) results in the following equation:

$$\ln K_d = \frac{\Delta S^\theta}{R} - \frac{\Delta H^\theta}{RT}. \tag{12}$$

3.4.3. Analysis of Desorption Kinetics

Desorption kinetic models were employed to evaluate the adsorption–desorption behavior of red mud for phosphate as a function of the reaction time [28]. Ruthven used an adsorption dynamics model to calculate and investigate the relation between desorption and adsorption penetration curves, indicating the difference between the two based on the equilibrium theory applied to desorption [29]. The kinetic models used in this study are based on a pseudo-first-order kinetic linear model (Equation (13)) [29], a pseudo-second-order kinetic linear model (Equation (14)) [30], and an intraparticle diffusion model (Equation (15)) [31,32] to fit the following kinetics of phosphate adsorption by activated red mud adsorbent:

$$q_t = q_e - (q_e \times 10^{\frac{-k_1 t}{2.303}}), \tag{13}$$

$$\frac{t}{q_t} = \frac{1}{k_2 q_e^2} + \frac{t}{q_e}, \tag{14}$$

$$q_t = k_i t^{1/2} + C, \tag{15}$$

where k_1 and k_2 are the rate constants of the pseudo-first-order and pseudo-second-order kinetic linear models, respectively, k_i is the intraparticle diffusion constant, q_t is the amount of phosphate desorbed by the adsorbent in the desorption time (h), and C is the amount of diffusion.

4. Conclusions

(1) For static desorption, the comprehensive desorption effect may be ranked as HCl > NaOH > NaCl > deionized water. The higher the desorbent concentration, the greater the desorption and the better the desorption of 0.2 mol/L of HCl in resorption. Regeneration improves owing to acids, which clean the pores of red mud particles, thereby exposing the effective sites inside the pores.
(2) The desorption thermodynamics and kinetics show that desorption conforms to the average-adsorption-free-energy reaction obtained by the D–R model. The desorption isotherm correlates well with the Langmuir model, indicating that desorption is dominated by monomolecular-layer surface desorption. The thermodynamics show

(3) The kinetics indicate that desorption conforms to the pseudo-second-order kinetic linear simulation, indicating that chemical desorption restricts the desorption rate. The intraparticle diffusion model indicates that the desorbent removes phosphorus in the form of precipitation from the surface of the activated red mud adsorbent primarily through a chemical reaction.

(4) Microanalysis before and after the desorption of the desorbent and surface elemental analysis demonstrate that P is removed and that Ca is dissolved the most, followed by Al and Fe, indicating that the desorbents react with the active elements in red mud. The corrosive effect leads to the disintegration and dissolution of the elements at the surfaces of the activated red mud adsorbents in water. This is accompanied by phosphorus desorption; hence, the characteristic peak intensities of chalcopyrite, calcite chalcopyrite, and calcite garnet decrease more than that of the activated red mud adsorbents. After desorption, the mineral composition remains similar because adsorbent reuse has a negligible impact on adsorption. The vibrations of the $[SiO_4]^{4-}$ functional groups of calcium–iron garnet and calcite or aragonite disappear, the PO_4^{3-} group peak intensities substantially decrease, and the desorption of phosphorus is accompanied by a chemical reaction.

Author Contributions: L.L.: Supervision, Project administration, Data curation, Writing—review and editing. Z.Y.: Methodology, Investigation, Data curation, Formal analysis, Writing—original draft. Y.W.: Investigation, Data curation, Formal analysis, Writing—review and editing. All authors have read and agreed to the published version of the manuscript.

Funding: This research was funded by the National Natural Science Foundation of China under grant number 51964010.

Institutional Review Board Statement: The study was conducted in accordance with the Declaration of Helsinki and approved by the Institutional Review Board (or Ethics Committee) of NAME OF 106 INSTITUTE. Moreover, it did not involve humans or animals.

Informed Consent Statement: Not applicable.

Data Availability Statement: Data are contained within the article.

Acknowledgments: The authors thank Mining College, Guizhou University of China as well as acknowledge the use of the Large Analysis and Testing Instrument Sharing Platform of Guizhou University.

Conflicts of Interest: The authors declare no conflict of interest.

References

1. Chen, W. Exploratory study on the preparation of modified red mud porous material and wastewater treatment. *J. China Univ. Geosci.* **2010**, *20*, 5–14.
2. Wang, Y.B.; Zhu, X.F.; Zhang, X.L. Removal of high concentration phosphorus wastewater by red mud. *Chem. Eng. Prog.* **2010**, *29*, 1771–1774.
3. Azizian, S. Kinetic models of sorption: A theoretical analysis. *J. Colloid Interf. Sci.* **2004**, *276*, 47–52. [CrossRef] [PubMed]
4. Xing, X.; Gao, B.; Yue, Q.; Zhong, Q. Sorption of phosphate onto giant reed based adsorbent: FTIR, Raman spectrum analysis and dynamic sorption/desorption properties in filter bed. *Bioresour. Technol.* **2011**, *102*, 5278–5282.
5. Johir, M.A.H.; George, J.; Vigneswaran, S.; Kandasamy, J.; Grasmick, A. Removal and recovery of nutrients by ion exchange from high rate membrane bio-reactor (MBR) effluent. *Desalination* **2011**, *275*, 197–202. [CrossRef]
6. Park, K.Y.; Song, J.H.; Lee, S.H.; Kim, H.S. Utilization of a selective adsorbent for phosphorus removal from wastewaters. *Environ. Eng. Sci.* **2010**, *27*, 805–810. [CrossRef]
7. Cheng, X.; Huang, X.; Wang, X.; Zhao, B.; Chen, A.; Sun, D. Phosphate adsorption from sewage sludge filtrate using zinc–aluminum layered double hydroxides. *J. Hazard. Mater.* **2009**, *169*, 958–964. [CrossRef] [PubMed]
8. Urano, K.; Tachikawa, H. Process development for removal and recovery of phosphorus from wastewater by a new adsorbent. 1. Preparation method and adsorption capability of a new adsorbent. *Ind. Eng. Chem. Res.* **1991**, *30*, 1897–1899. [CrossRef]

9. Delaney, P.; McManamon, C.; Hanrahan, J.P.; Copley, M.P.; Holmes, J.D.; Morris, M.A. Development of chemically engineered porous metal oxides for phosphate removal. *J. Hazard. Mater.* **2011**, *185*, 382–391. [CrossRef]
10. Urano, K.; Tachikawa, H. Process development for removal and recovery of phosphorus from wastewater by a new adsorbent. 3. Desorption of phosphate and regeneration of adsorbent. *Ind. Eng. Chem. Res.* **1992**, *31*, 1510–1513. [CrossRef]
11. Ye, J.; Cong, X.; Zhang, P.; Zeng, G.; Hoffmann, E.; Liu, Y.; Hahn, H.H. Application of acid-activated Bauxsol for wastewater treatment with high phosphate concentration: Characterization, adsorption optimization, and desorption behaviors. *J. Environ. Manag.* **2016**, *167*, 1–7. [CrossRef]
12. Zhao, Y.; Yue, Q.; Li, Q.; Gao, B.; Han, S.; Yu, H. The regeneration characteristics of various red mud granular adsorbents (RMGA) for phosphate removal using different desorption reagents. *J. Hazard. Mater.* **2010**, *182*, 309–316. [CrossRef]
13. Zhang, G.; Liu, H.; Liu, R.; Qu, J. Removal of phosphate from water by a Fe–Mn binary oxide adsorbent. *J. Colloid Interf. Sci.* **2009**, *335*, 168–174. [CrossRef]
14. Zeng, L.; Li, X.; Liu, J. Adsorptive removal of phosphate from aqueous solutions using iron oxide tailings. *Water Res.* **2004**, *38*, 1318–1326. [CrossRef] [PubMed]
15. Ajmal, Z.; Muhmood, A.; Usman, M.; Kizito, S.; Lu, J.; Dong, R.; Wu, S. Phosphate removal from aqueous solution using iron oxides: Adsorption, desorption and regeneration characteristics. *J. Colloid Interf. Sci.* **2018**, *528*, 145–155. [CrossRef] [PubMed]
16. Xie, W.M.; Zhou, F.P.; Bi, X.L.; Chen, D.D.; Li, J.; Sun, S.Y.; Liu, J.-Y.; Chen, X.-Q. Accelerated crystallization of magnetic 4A-zeolite synthesized from red mud for application in removal of mixed heavy metal ions. *J. Hazard. Mater.* **2018**, *358*, 441–449. [CrossRef] [PubMed]
17. Kuzawa, K.; Jung, Y.J.; Kiso, Y.; Yamada, T.; Nagai, M.; Lee, T.G. Phosphate removal and recovery with a synthetic hydrotalcite as an adsorbent. *Chemosphere* **2006**, *62*, 45–52. [CrossRef] [PubMed]
18. Li, Y.; Liu, C.; Luan, Z.; Peng, X.; Zhu, C.; Chen, Z.; Zhang, Z.; Fan, J.; Jia, Z. Phosphate removal from aqueous solutions using raw and activated red mud and fly ash. *J. Hazard. Mater.* **2006**, *137*, 374–383. [CrossRef] [PubMed]
19. Zhao, Y.Q. *Preparation and Characterisation of New Red Mud Particle Adsorbent Material and Its Performance on Phosphorus Removal from Water Body*; Shandong University: Jinan, China, 2013.
20. Xu, M.Y. *Preparation, Characterisation and Properties of Red Mud-Based Granular Phosphorus Removal Materials*; China University of Mining and Technology: Xuzhou, China, 2020. [CrossRef]
21. Wu, H.L.; Wei, S.N.; Cui, S.L. Introduction and application of adsorption isotherms. *Dye. Finish. Technol.* **2006**, *35*, 12–14.
22. Pepper, R.-A.; Couperthwaite, S.-J.; Millar, G.-J. Re-use of waste red mud: Production of a functional iron oxide adsorbent for removal of phosphorous. *J. Water Process Eng.* **2018**, *25*, 138–148. [CrossRef]
23. Huang, Q.B. *Research on the Removal of Nitrate and Phosphate in Water by Adsorption of Organically Modified Aluminium-Manganese Composite Oxides*; Xi'an University of Architecture and Technology: Xi'an, China, 2018. [CrossRef]
24. Wu, J. *Preparation of Red Mud Base Polymer Porous Material and Its Adsorption Performance*; Guangxi University: Nanning, China, 2016. [CrossRef]
25. Jiang, Y.; Ma, X.L.; Guo, Y.X.; Sun, F.Y.; Sun, J.; He, X.Y. Adsorption and desorption characteristics of zinc in different layered soils. *J. Northeast. Univ.* **2021**, *49*, 99–107.
26. Deihimi, N.; Irannajad, M.; Rezai, B. Equilibrium and kinetic studies of ferricyanide adsorption from aqueous solution by activated red mud. *J. Environ. Manag.* **2018**, *227*, 277–285. [CrossRef]
27. Zhu, C.; Luan, Z.; Wang, Y.; Shan, X. Removal of cadmium from aqueous solutions by adsorption on granular red mud (GRM). *Sep. Purif. Technol.* **2007**, *57*, 161–169. [CrossRef]
28. Xia, L.Y. Effects of pH and organic matter on the adsorption-desorption characteristics of zinc in soil. *Energy Environ. Protection.* **2021**, *35*, 39–45.
29. Yao, H.Q.; Liu, X.Q.; Ma, Z.F. Kinetics of water desorption on zeolite. *J. Nanjing Univ.* **1990**, *56*, 6–11.
30. Ahmed, M.J.; Dhedan, S.K. Equilibrium isotherms and kinetics modeling of methylene blue adsorption on agricultural wastes-based activated carbons. *Fluid Phase Equilibria* **2012**, *317*, 9–14. [CrossRef]
31. Cheung, W.H.; Szeto, Y.S.; McKay, G. Intraparticle diffusion processes during acid dye adsorption onto chitosan. *Bioresour. Technol.* **2007**, *98*, 2897–2904. [CrossRef] [PubMed]
32. Weber, W.J.; Morris, J.C., Jr. Kinetics of adsorption on carbon from solution. *J. Sanit. Eng. Div.* **1963**, *89*, 31–59. [CrossRef]

Disclaimer/Publisher's Note: The statements, opinions and data contained in all publications are solely those of the individual author(s) and contributor(s) and not of MDPI and/or the editor(s). MDPI and/or the editor(s) disclaim responsibility for any injury to people or property resulting from any ideas, methods, instructions or products referred to in the content.

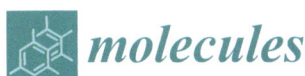

Article

Zwitterionic Tröger's Base Microfiltration Membrane Prepared via Vapor-Induced Phase Separation with Improved Demulsification and Antifouling Performance

Meng Wang, Tingting Huang, Meng Shan, Mei Sun, Shasha Liu * and Hai Tang *

School of Chemical and Environmental Engineering, Anhui Polytechnic University, Wuhu 241000, China; wm18855372043@163.com (M.W.); 18895367471@163.com (T.H.); 15551732072@163.com (M.S.); sunmei17855461938@163.com (M.S.)
* Correspondence: liushasha@ahpu.edu.cn (S.L.); tanghai@ahpu.edu.cn (H.T.)

Abstract: The fouling of separation membranes has consistently been a primary factor contributing to the decline in membrane performance. Enhancing the surface hydrophilicity of the membrane proves to be an effective strategy in mitigating membrane fouling in water treatment processes. Zwitterionic polymers (containing an equimolar number of homogeneously distributed anionic and cationic groups on the polymer chains) have been used extensively as one of the best antifouling materials for surface modification. The conventional application of zwitterionic compounds as surface modifiers is intricate and inefficient, adding complexity and length to the membrane preparation process, particularly on an industrial scale. To overcome these limitations, zwitterionic polymer, directly used as a main material, is an effective method. In this work, a novel zwitterionic polymer (TB)—zwitterionic Tröger's base (ZTB)—was synthesized by quaternizing Tröger's base (TB) with 1,3-propane sultone. The obtained ZTB is blended with TB to fabricate microfiltration (MF) membranes via the vapor-induced phase separation (VIPS) process, offering a strategic solution for separating emulsified oily wastewater. Atomic force microscopy (AFM), scanning electron microscopy (SEM), water contact angle, and zeta potential measurements were employed to characterize the surface of ZTB/TB blended membranes, assessing surface morphology, charge, and hydrophilic/hydrophobic properties. The impact of varying ZTB levels on membrane surface morphology, hydrophilicity, water flux, and rejection were investigated. The results showed that an increase in ZTB content improved hydrophilicity and surface roughness, consequently enhancing water permeability. Due to the attraction of water vapor, the enrichment of zwitterionic segments was enriched, and a stable hydration layer was formed on the membrane surface. The hydration layer formed by zwitterions endowed the membrane with good antifouling properties. The proposed mechanism elucidates the membrane's proficiency in demulsification and the reduction in irreversible fouling through the synergistic regulation of surface charge and hydrophilicity, facilitated by electrostatic repulsion and the formation of a hydration layer. The ZTB/TB blended membranes demonstrated superior efficiency in oil–water separation, achieving a maximum flux of 1897.63 LMH bar^{-1} and an oil rejection rate as high as 99% in the oil–water emulsion separation process. This study reveals the migration behavior of the zwitterionic polymer in the membrane during the VIPS process. It enhances our comprehension of the antifouling mechanism of zwitterionic membranes and provides guidance for designing novel materials for antifouling membranes.

Keywords: zwitterionic polymer; Tröger's base; antifouling; demulsification; microfiltration membrane

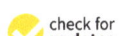

Citation: Wang, M.; Huang, T.; Shan, M.; Sun, M.; Liu, S.; Tang, H. Zwitterionic Tröger's Base Microfiltration Membrane Prepared via Vapor-Induced Phase Separation with Improved Demulsification and Antifouling Performance. *Molecules* **2024**, *29*, 1001. https://doi.org/10.3390/molecules29051001

Academic Editor: Qingguo Shao

Received: 29 January 2024
Revised: 19 February 2024
Accepted: 21 February 2024
Published: 25 February 2024

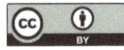

Copyright: © 2024 by the authors. Licensee MDPI, Basel, Switzerland. This article is an open access article distributed under the terms and conditions of the Creative Commons Attribution (CC BY) license (https://creativecommons.org/licenses/by/4.0/).

1. Introduction

In the past two decades, significant quantities of emulsified oily wastewater have been released from petrochemical, steel, and other industrial processes in China, which have caused severe environmental pollution in water ecosystems [1–3]. The conventional treatment technologies for emulsified oily wastewater include chemical demulsification, air flocculation, and biochemical treatment methods. Microfiltration (MF) membranes are commonly utilized for separating emulsified oily wastewater treatment due to their short separation time, low energy consumption, high efficiency, lack of additional chemicals, and convenient operation [4]. However, oil droplets frequently adhere to the hydrophobic membrane surface, exacerbating membrane fouling and increasing separation difficulty [5,6].

Several studies have shown that hydrophilic and charged MF membranes can effectively treat surfactant-stabilized emulsions (SSEs) [7–12]. Lin et al. [13] prepared a modified PEI electrospun fiber membrane, and the positive potential point generates electrostatic repulsion with the cationic surfactant molecules in the emulsion. The use of zwitterionic polymers reduces the adhesion of the surfactant to the membrane, resulting in decreased pollution and increased permeation flux. Zwitterionic polymers are also excellent materials for surface hydrophilization [14–17], and previous research has indicated that negatively charged zwitterionic-modified blended MF membranes show potential for treating SSE with excellent separation performance [8,18–20]. Maggay et al. [21] prepared zwitterionic PVDF membranes using a novel polymer made of styrene units and zwitterionic 4-vinylpyridine. The material exhibited exceptional anti-biofouling properties against various biofoulants. Zhu et al. [22] prepared a zwitterionic PTMAO-grafted PVDF membrane using the vapor-induced phase separation (VIPS) method. The results revealed that the presence of zwitterionic segments on the membrane surface attracted water vapor, resulting in a closely bound hydration layer on the membrane surface. This had led to strong oil repellency in water [23].

Recently, it has been shown that VIPS offers significant advantages in regulating membrane morphologies. This is due to the slower kinetics of the gaseous phase and non-solvency during the phase separation of the membrane [24,25]. This provides control over the phase separation process by adjusting the polymer concentration, vapor exposure time, and temperature [26–28]. Poly(vinylidene fluoride) (PVDF) has been widely used to prepare MFs for oil/water emulsions [29,30] due to its ability to achieve high porosity (>70%). For example, Chen et al. [31] reported a novel approach for regulating the pore structure of MF membranes via lowering the solution temperature. The results showed that elevating the temperature facilitated the formation of cell-like pores, resulting in an ultrahigh flux of 3028 LMH bar^{-1}. Nevertheless, the use of VIPS for MF membranes still presents practical challenges related to the regulation of pore structure, achieving optimal demulsification efficiency, and improving antifouling performance [27].

In our previous study, we regulated the structure and performance of a UF membrane derived from Tröger's base (TB) by blending different contents of zwitterionic TB (ZTB). The results suggested that the zwitterionic TB polymer enhanced the permeability and antifouling performance of the UF membrane [32]. This work investigated the potential applications of a TB polymer-based MF membrane via VIPS. This work explored the effects of the molar ratio of TB and ZTB, temperature, and vapor exposure time on the membrane's morphology, including porosity and pore size. The surface charge and hydrophilicity of the membrane surface were easily controlled. The hydrophilicity, surface roughness, and morphology of the membrane surface and cross-section were studied by using water contact angle (WCA), atomic force microscopy (AFM), and scanning electron microscopy (SEM). The performance of surfactant-stabilized emulsions, in terms of membrane permeability, rejection, and antifouling performance, were also analyzed. Additionally, the demulsification mechanism was examined. This work aims to enhance the demulsification and antifouling performance of MF membranes by blending TB and ZTB to fabricated zwitterionic MF membranes.

2. Results and Discussion

2.1. MF Membrane Morphology

In the VIPS method of preparation, it is notable that when the cast membrane is exposed to controlled humidity for a specific duration, the upper surface undergoes alteration due to the absorption of water vapor droplets, while the integrity of the majority of the polymeric cast film remains unaffected. Following precipitation in a coagulation nonsolvent bath, the changes observed extend throughout the entirety of the resulting membrane. Thus, the precise control of the conditions during the initial phase separation in the humid chamber impacts the formation pattern, surface pore size, and overall structure of the membrane. Water vapor droplets in a humid environment can leave distinct marks on soft membrane surfaces due to their high mobility and ability to deform the surface. The intensity of these marks can result in various morphologies depending on the specific conditions present. During VIPS membrane formation, due to the strong interactions between the solvent (NMP) and water vapor, when the water vapor enters the polymer solution, the surface layer of the membrane quickly precipitates. Either initial pores on the polymeric membrane or a coagulated surface could form. A thin layer of gel then forms, hindering the exchange of solvent and non-solvent, inhibiting the formation of macropores in the membrane and causing rough and uneven sponge-like holes to appear on the surface [31,33–35]. Similar results have been obtained in the preparation of high-strength PVDF porous membranes with a cellular structure via VIPS. The findings demonstrate that the membrane's pore size exhibits variability in response to exposure duration, temperature fluctuations, and additional environmental parameters [36]. The surface and cross-sectional SEM images of the M0–M7 membranes were observed and are shown in Figure 1, which shows that the cross-section of the final MF membranes has a sponge-like structure. The surface porosity (P_s), average surface pore size (r_s), maximum surface pore size (r_{max}), and top-layer thickness (T) of the membranes are summarized in Table 1. The P_s and r_s of M0 (pristine TB) are 1.2% and 0.178 µm, respectively.

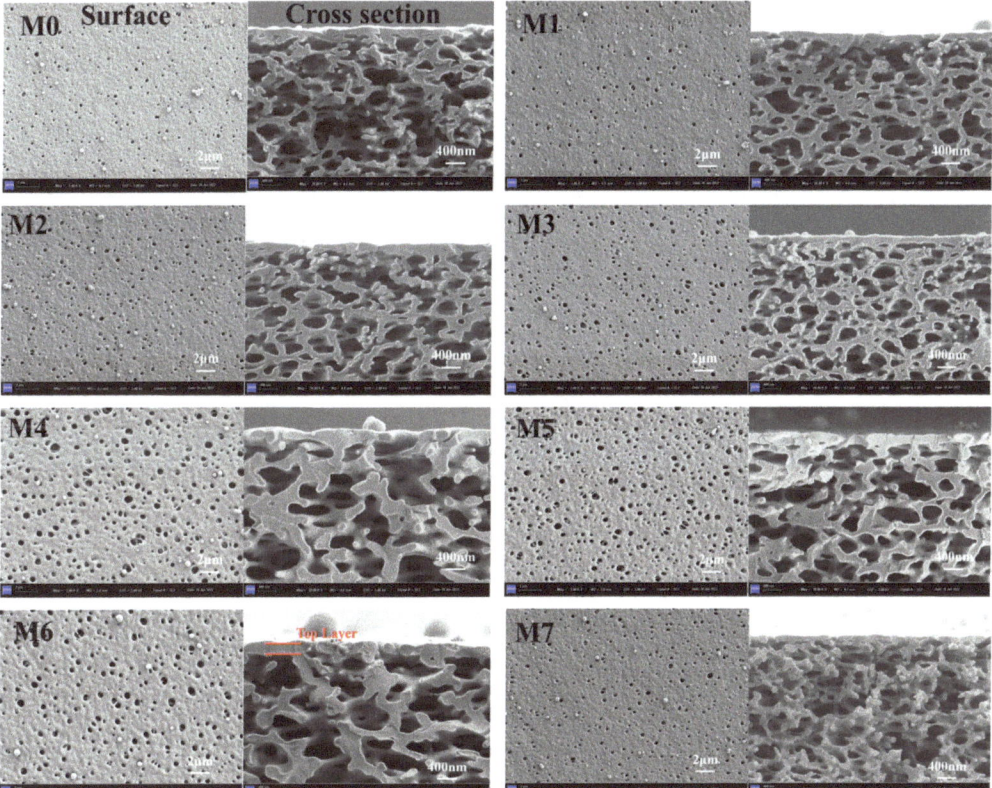

Figure 1. Surface and cross-sectional SEM images of membranes.

Table 1. The surface porosity (P_s), average surface pore size (r_s), maximum surface pore size (r_{max}), and top-layer thickness (T) of the membranes.

Membranes	P_s/%	r_s/μm	r_{max}/μm	T/μm
M0	1.2 ± 0.2	0.178 ± 0.002	0.462 ± 0.008	0.035 ± 0.004
M1	1.6 ± 0.1	0.203 ± 0.001	0.550 ± 0.039	0.030 ± 0.002
M2	2.9 ± 0.1	0.212 ± 0.008	0.660 ± 0.117	0.030 ± 0.005
M3	5.1 ± 0.1	0.247 ± 0.005	0.867 ± 0.070	0.025 ± 0.005
M4	3.9 ± 0.1	0.263 ± 0.006	0.963 ± 0.025	0.055 ± 0.011
M5	5.7 ± 0.4	0.278 ± 0.001	0.992 ± 0.209	0.036 ± 0.007
M6	4.0 ± 0.1	0.293 ± 0.001	1.311 ± 0.103	0.050 ± 0.012
M7	2.7 ± 0.1	0.214 ± 0.001	0.621 ± 0.035	0.021 ± 0.003

It was observed that the zwitterionic polymers significantly influenced the surface porosity. The surface porosity of the M0 membrane was 1.2 ± 0.2%, while that of the blended MF membranes gradually increased to 5.1 ± 0.1%, which was 1.4–4.4 times that of M0. The average surface pore size of M0 was 0.178 ± 0.002 μm, and the pore size in the blended MF membrane increased from 0.203 ± 0.001 μm to 0.247 ± 0.005 μm. This occurred because the phase separation rate of the blended membrane was slower and the hydrophilicity of the MF membrane gradually increased. As a result, more water vapor was required to permeate into the membrane [32,37], and the porosity increased. The different interactions of the hydrophilic ZTB and the hydrophobic Tröger's base polymer during the phase transformation led to a nanoscale microphase separation [38] and gave the MF membranes a relatively uniform size [39]. Furthermore, Figure 2 shows AFM images of the M0–M3 MF membrane surface, and Table 2 shows the average surface roughness (Ra) and root mean square roughness (Rq) of the membrane surface. Ra and Rq of the blended membranes increased with increasing numbers of ZTB polymers. Ra increased from 21.79 nm for M0 to 24.24 nm for M3, and Rq increased from 29.57 nm for M0 to 45.93 nm for M3, which was 1.6 times that of M0. This indicates that the surface roughness of the MF membrane gradually increased as the ZTB content increased. Previous studies have also shown that delayed phase separation allows sufficient time for the rich/poor polymer to grow before solidifying, resulting in a rough membrane surface [40] that improves membrane permeability [7].

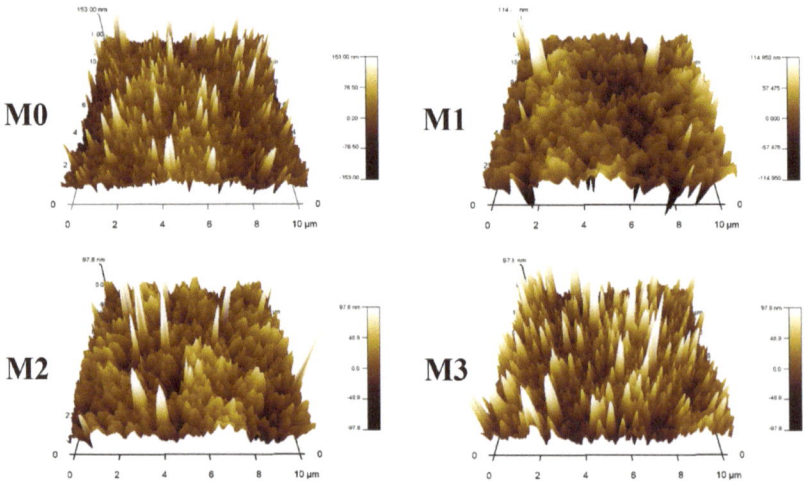

Figure 2. AFM images of membrane surfaces.

Table 2. Average surface roughness (Ra), root mean square roughness (Rq), and interfacial free energy ($-G_{ML}$).

Membranes	Ra (nm)	Rq (nm)	$-\Delta G_{ML}$ (mJ m^{-2})
M0	21.79 ± 2.22	29.57 ± 2.24	83.0
M1	22.38 ± 2.08	33.50 ± 3.34	95.9
M2	23.73 ± 3.35	34.76 ± 3.90	111.1
M3	24.24 ± 3.06	45.93 ± 1.25	118.1

Exposure time to solvent vapor has an important influence on membrane morphology [35], which was investigated by comparing M2, M4, and M5 membranes. As the t_e increased from 5 min to 10 min (M2), the amount of condensed water vapor on the membrane surface increased, which decreased the mass transfer resistance (concentration gradient) and the phase separation rate compared with the M4 membrane. Then, the pore size became smaller, and the pore size distribution was narrow [41]. When t_e continued to increase to 15 min (M5), the pores connected to each other to form larger pores. The slow penetration of the non-solvent may have caused this, with delayed phase separation controlling the lean phase of the polymer and contributing to the formation of highly porous membranes [9]. When exposed to humid air, the polymer membrane experienced water vapor condensation on its surface, resulting in slight phase separation. Subsequently, upon immersion in the coagulation bath, the top layer solidified rapidly, inhibiting the exchange of solvent and non-solvent, resulting in the disappearance of the dense top layer [25,37]. When t_e = 5 min (M4), there were insufficient condensed water droplets to form a gel layer, but the absorbed water served as the foundation for pore formation, thus promoting phase separation in the coagulation bath and the formation of macropores [42–44]. Prolonged exposure facilitated the crystallization process, which led to the development of a porous skin and particle morphology. This, in turn, enhanced the surface hydrophobicity [28].

M2, M6, and M7 MF membranes were compared to explore the effects of exposure temperature. A higher temperature shortened the polymer's gel time, preventing water vapor from infiltrating the solution [45]. At 30 °C (M6), the structure of finger and sponge pores underwent a phase transition, resulting in the formation of a thick surface layer and large cross-section pores due to the movement rate of the water molecules. Nevertheless, the rate of movement of the water vapor molecules accelerated when the temperature reached 50 °C. The formation of a gel layer on the membrane surface resulted in a decrease in the rate of phase separation. This, in turn, led to the formation of a thin epidermal layer and a reduction in the number of cross-section pores. At 80 °C (M7), the system's thermodynamic instability was worsened by higher temperatures, causing the phase transformation to accelerate more than the delayed phase separation effect of the ZTB polymer. The growth time of the polymer lean phase decreased, and the interaction time of the polymer chain also decreased. The structure of the MF membrane transitioned from a bicontinuous sponge-like structure to a sponge structure over time.

2.2. Hydrophilicity of MF Membrane

Previous studies have demonstrated that the hydrophilization and charge of the membrane surface can enhance the demulsification and antifouling performance of oil-in-water emulsions. This prevents foulants from adhering to the membrane due to significant steric hindrance [10,46]. Therefore, the wettability of membranes used for separating oil-in-water emulsions is a critical property [47]. The WCAs of membranes with different ZTB polymer contents are shown in Figure 3. The results show that the static WCA of the TB membrane (M0) was 81.1°, while that of membranes M1–M3 decreased to 69.72°, 54.81°, and 46.32°, respectively, upon increasing the ZTB polymer content from 1.0 wt% to 3.0 wt%. Similarly, $-\Delta G_{ML}$ (Table 2) increased from 83.0 mJ m^{-2} for M0 to 118.1 mJ m^{-2} for M3. Therefore, adding the ZTB polymer significantly improved the hydrophilicity of the MF membrane [32].

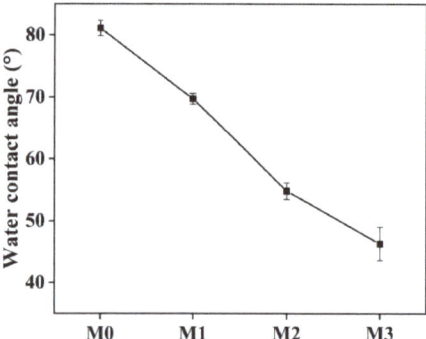

Figure 3. WCAs of membranes with different ZTB contents.

2.3. Zeta Potential of Oily Wastewater and MF Membrane

SDS is an anionic surfactant that exhibits a negative charge in PBS solution (pH 7.4), resulting in a zeta potential of −55.5 mV when added to emulsified oily wastewater. The zeta potential values of the M0–M3 MF membranes in the pH range of 3.0–10.0 are shown in Figure 4. The hydrophilic MF membrane with zwitterionic properties displayed varying surface zeta potential values. The M0 membrane surface exhibited a negative charge within the pH range of 4.0–10.0 with a zeta potential of −3.1 mV to −41.3 mV because of the protonation of the tertiary amine groups of TB under acidic conditions, which increased the positive charge density on the membrane surface [48]. After the addition of the ZTB polymer, the isoelectric point of the membrane gradually tended to electrical neutrality. –SO$_3$H remained uncharged, and the quaternary amine group showed a positive charge (–C–N$^+$) under acidic conditions. The –SO$_3$H group was negatively charged, and the quaternary amine group was neutral under alkaline conditions. The negatively charged membrane surface indicates that the introduction of a zwitterionic polymer weakened the electronegativity, in accordance with our previous report [14]. We also found that the zeta potential of the M3 membrane was slightly lower than that of the M2 membrane but still higher than that of the M0 membrane because the reaction consumed the tertiary amine groups on the membrane surface.

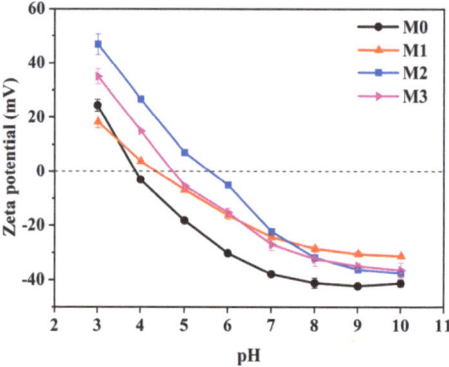

Figure 4. Zeta potential of M0–M3 MF membranes at pH 3–7.

2.4. Penetration and Rejection Performance

Three cycles of membrane performance measurement experiments were conducted using a cross-flow filtration system to assess the impact of ZTB addition, exposure time, and temperature on the permeability and rejection performance of the MF membranes. Figure 5 displays the flux and rejection rates of membranes fabricated using different parameters. The water flux of the M0 MF membrane reached 1634.34 LMH bar^{-1}, but after adding the ZTB polymer, the water flux gradually increased from 1703.44 LMH bar^{-1} for M1 to 1872.97 LMH bar^{-1} for M3. The membrane's surface porosity and pore size gradually increased, indicating that the ZTB polymer content could modulate the membrane's microstructure, which, in turn, altered its permeability. The rejection rate of M0 for SSE was 61.47%, while that of M1–M3 was 99.67%, 99.53%, and 87.19%, respectively. The blended MF membranes exhibited significantly improved rejection rates for emulsified oil wastewater while maintaining high penetration. Additionally, they effectively separated emulsified oil droplets from solutions containing surfactants.

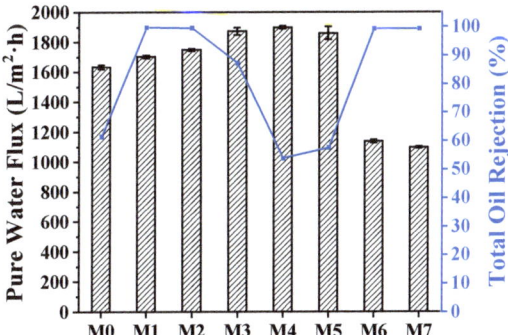

Figure 5. Flux and rejection rates of membranes fabricated using different parameters.

This study investigated the impact of exposure time and temperature on membrane performance. The flux of the UF membrane (t_e = 0 min) was significantly lower than that of the MF membrane. The fluxes of M4 (5 min) and M5 (15 min) were slightly higher than that of M2 (10 min), with rejection rates of emulsified oil droplets of 53.82%, 99.53%, and 57.55%, respectively. Different exposure times led to different membrane structures, and the pore size distribution ranges of the M4 and M5 blended MF membranes were larger than that of the M2, but the emulsified oil droplet particle size range was between 0.171 μm and 0.266 μm. Therefore, the oil droplets were able to pass through the membrane pores easily, resulting in a significant reduction in the rejection rate of emulsified oil. The fluxes of M2, M6, and M7 were 1138.76 LMH bar^{-1}, 1748.61 LMH bar^{-1}, and 1097.49 LMH bar^{-1}, respectively. The SSE rejection rates of all the membranes were above 99%. The fluxes of the M6 and M7 membranes were lower than that of the M2, which might be due to the higher membrane surface thickness (1.311 μm) and lower surface porosity. The water flow through the membrane was restricted due to the large hydraulic resistance.

2.5. Antifouling Performance of Membranes

The effectiveness of membranes in separating oil-in-water emulsions depends critically on their antifouling performance [49]. FRR, R_t, R_r, and R_{ir} are important indicators for judging the antifouling performance of a membrane. Figures 6 and 7 illustrate the pure water flux and antifouling performance of membranes when using emulsified oil, respectively. The FRR value of M0 was 57.5%, while the FRR values of the M1–M3 MF membranes exceeded that of M0. The FRR value of the M2 membrane was the highest (76.4%). The R_{ir} of the M1–M3 MF membranes slightly decreased upon increasing the ZTB content, and the R_{ir} of M2 reached the lowest value (23.6%). This demonstrates that adding the ZTB polymer improved the hydrophilicity of the membrane surface. Therefore, the FRR of the membrane rose significantly, and the antifouling performance was enhanced after washing with a NaOH solution (0.05 M) and distilled water. The FRR value of the M3 MF membrane decreased because it had the largest ZTB content, which may be due to the large increase in surface porosity and having the largest pore diameter on the membrane surface. During the cleaning process, it was difficult to remove blockages from the membrane surface due to the accumulation of large oil droplets that passed through the membrane pores. The FRR values of the M4 and M5 MF membranes were 69.32% and 65.86%, and their R_{ir} values were 30.68% and 34.14%, respectively. This confirmed that the antifouling performance of the membrane was directly related to the VIPS exposure time. At $t_e = 0$ min, the pore size of the membrane was smaller than the emulsified oil's particle size, resulting in the emulsified oil forming a filter cake layer on the membrane surface. This caused a sharp decrease in the membrane flux, an increase in irreversible fouling, and a decrease in reversible fouling. The M2 MF membrane exhibited mainly reversible fouling because of its small average pore size.

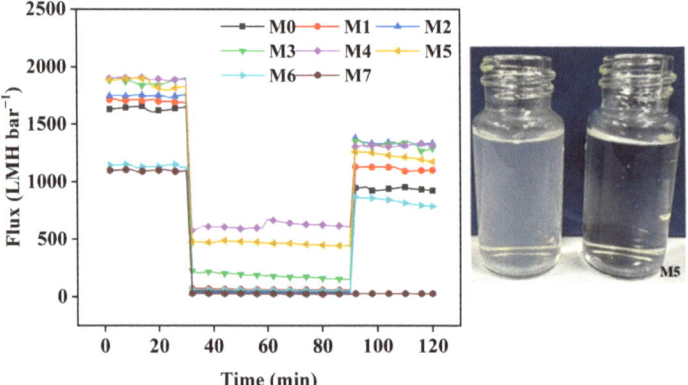

Figure 6. Pure water flux of the membrane using emulsified oil.

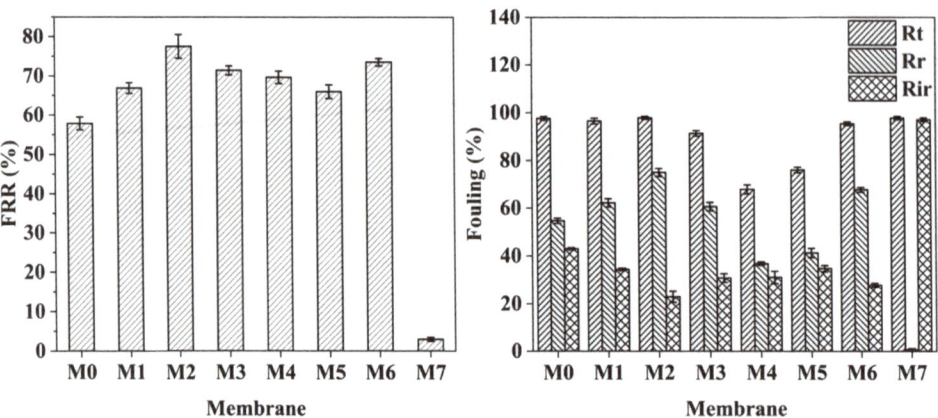

Figure 7. Antifouling performance of membranes fabricated using different parameters.

The antifouling performance of the M2, M6, and M7 MF membranes was analyzed to investigate the influence of exposure temperature. This study aimed to determine how exposure temperature affects the performance of the membranes. The FRR value of M6 was 73.0%, which was slightly lower than that of M2. The FRR value of M7 decreased to 2.6% due to a decrease in the resistance of water vapor diffusion into the film-forming solution when the temperature rose to 80 °C. The membranes that were prepared at higher temperatures formed cellular structures, while the polymers became denser and finer [33,40,50]. The oil particles in the wastewater were transported by external pressure and penetrated the support sublayer of the membrane through pores on its surface. This internal structure of the polymer was reached by the oil particles. They partially obstructed the spaces between polymer chains. Therefore, when cleaning the membrane, only oil particles on the surface layer of the membrane could be removed, while those between the deep layers of the polymer chains could not be removed. This ultimately made it difficult to continuously filter water, thus obtaining an extremely low FRR value and extremely high R_r value.

2.6. Possible Antifouling and Demulsification Mechanism

The previous literature on the permeate flux and oil rejection of oil–water separation membranes is summarized in Table 3. Generally, the pore size, surface wettability, surface charge, and membrane structure of membrane materials play a crucial role in selective separation and demulsification using membranes. The blended MF membranes containing ZTB demonstrated highly effective performance in demulsifying emulsified oily wastewater. The possible demulsification mechanism is suggested in Figure 8. The hydrophilic and charged membrane surface resulted in size screening and wetting coalescence effects, which contributed to the high separation and anti-fouling performance of the emulsified oily wastewater [4]. The zwitterionic polymer combined with water molecules to form a hydration layer by solvating ionic groups. As a result, the aqueous phase in the emulsified oil wastewater wets and spreads preferentially on the membrane's surface and pores. The hydration layer was established by the permeation of the interior, which enhanced the membrane's antifouling performance. Under pressure, the aqueous phase penetrated the membrane pores, while collisions and squeezing between oil droplets deformed them simultaneously [51]. Moreover, the zwitterionic polymer endowed the membranes with a surface charge that destabilized emulsified oil and prevented oil from adhering to the membrane surface due to electrostatic repulsion. The molecules of the emulsifier at the membrane interface were partially removed or rearranged due to electrostatic repulsion. This facilitated the coalescence of the oil droplets. The large oil droplets in the emulsion underwent demulsification due to a gradual change in particle size and formed free oil droplets.

Table 3. Previous literature on the permeate flux and oil rejection of oil–water separation membranes.

Membrane Material/Fabrication	Oil/Surfactant Content	Driving Force (bar)	Separation Efficiency (%)	Flux (LMH bar^{-1})	Flux Recovery Rate (%)	Refs
PVDF (VIPS + TIPS/VIPS + NIPS)	SDS:oil = 1:6 (w/w)	0.2	/	~3028	~77%	[31]
PSF(VISP)	SDS:oil = 1:99 (w/w)	0.2	~98.48	~501.89	~49.57%	[52]
PPSU/SPSf (V-LIPS)	Water:oil = 1:99 (w/w)	0.2	99.5–99.5	508.4~414.1	/	[53]
PVDF-co-HFP(VIPS)	oil/water = 1% (v/v)	1.0	99.5%	600	/	[54]
PVDF/PHEMA (VIPS)	20 mg SDS + 10 mL oil + 990 m water	1.0	99.1% (crude oil)	1866 ± 162 (pump oil)	/	[55]
zwitterionization PVDF(VIPS)	oil/water = 1:99 (w/w)	0.5	99.0%	180–240	/	[27]
tannic acid deposited onto PVDF MF membrane	Tween-80 + 2-dichloroethane/hexane/iso-octane and water ($v/v/v$ = 1:50:0.02)	0.8	98%	38 ± 13~401 ± 97	84	[56]
PMCSMA grafted PES MF membrane	Span-80 (4000 mg/L) + Kerosene (50 mg/L)	0.25	99.5%	43	/	[1]
Polydopamine/polyelectrolyte co-deposited onto PP MF membrane	SDS(1000 mg/L) + Oi/waterl ($v:v$ = 1:5/)	/	99%	0.65	/	[57]
Zwitterionic Tröger's base/VISP	SDS(50 mg/L) + Cutting oil(50 mg/L)	0.1	99%	1328	74%	This work

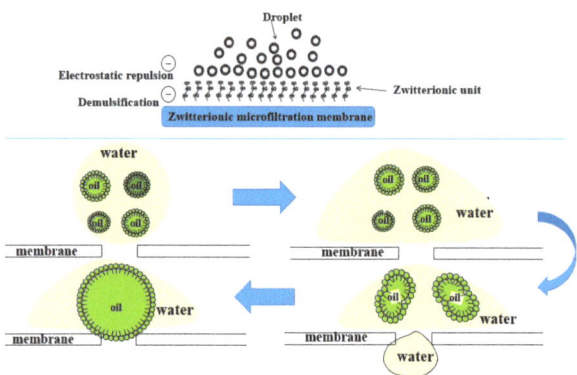

Figure 8. Demulsification mechanism of zwitterionic membranes.

3. Materials and Methods

3.1. Materials and Chemicals

Dimethoxymethane (98.0%), 3,3′-dimethylbiphenyl-4,4′-diamine (98.0%), o-xylidine (98.0%), N-methyl-2-pyrrolidone (NMP, >99.0%), trifluoroacetic acid (TFA, 99.0%), and 1,3-propane sulfonic acid lactone (99%) were obtained from Aladdin Industrial, Co. Methanol (CH_3OH, >99.7%), ammonia (NH_4OH, 25–28%), chloroform ($CHCl_3$, >99.0%), diethyl ether ($C_4H_{10}O$, >99.5%), sodium dodecyl sulfate (SDS), and sodium hydroxide (NaOH) were purchased from Chinese Medicine Co. (Shanghai, China) The chemicals were used in their original state without additional purification. The relative humidity (RH) during the VIPS process was achieved by adding water vapor to the membrane formation chamber.

3.2. Preparation of MF Membranes

The synthesis and characterization of ZTB is described in our previous work [32]. All MF membranes were prepared using the VIPS method. A typical preparation process is illustrated in Figure 9. The compositions and preparation conditions of the casting solution was listed in Table 4. Briefly, TB and ZTB polymers were added in a fixed molar ratio to 8.2 g NMP and stirred continuously at 25 °C for 12 h until dissolved completely. Then, they were defoamed in a vacuum-drying oven at 60 °C for 3 h to form a uniform casting solution. The obtained solution was poured onto a clean glass plate, and a scraper was used to generate a film with a thickness of 200 μm at a speed of 1.5 m min^{-1}. After exposure to humid air for 10 s, the film was transferred to a constant temperature and humidity chamber with a relative humidity (RH) of 90%. Then, it was placed into deionized water at 25 °C until completely exfoliated from the glass plate. Subsequently, the membrane was kept in deionized water for 48 h and it was replaced regularly to completely remove any NMP solvent remaining on the membrane.

Table 4. Compositions and preparation conditions of the casting solution (constant RH = 90%).

Membranes	Composition			Temperature of VIPS Chamber	Exposure Time
	TB (wt%)	ZTB (wt%)	NMP (wt%)	T_v (°C)	t_e (min)
M0	18	0	82	50	10
M1	17	1	82	50	10
M2	16	2	82	50	10
M3	15	3	82	50	10
M4	16	2	82	50	5
M5	16	2	82	50	15
M6	16	2	82	30	10
M7	16	2	82	80	10

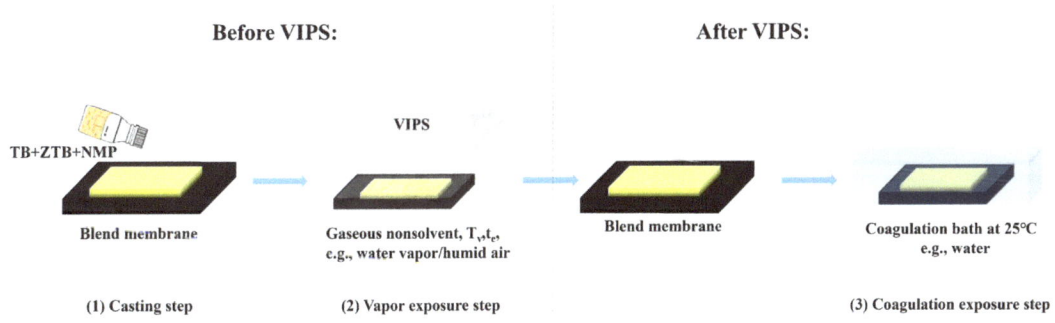

Figure 9. Illustration of the VIPS process used to prepare MF membranes.

3.3. Membrane Characterization

The hydrophilicity of the membrane surface was assessed according to its water contact angle (WCA; OSA60, Beijing Eastern-Dataphy Instruments Co.). At ambient temperature, 5 μL water droplets were dropped onto the membrane surface. After 10 s, images of the droplets were taken with a camera, and the WCA was calculated using imaging software. The average value was calculated by measuring five different positions on the membrane, and the membrane's liquid interface's free energy $-\Delta G_{ML}$ (mJ m^{-2}) was calculated using the modified Young–Dupré equation to measure its surface wettability [11,58], as shown in Formula (1).

$$\Delta G_{ML} = \gamma_L (1 + \frac{\cos\theta}{1 + SAD}) \quad (1)$$

where γ_L is the surface tension of water (72.8 mJ m^{-2}, 20 °C); θ is the average WCA; and $1 + SAD$ (a roughness area parameter) is the ratio of the actual area to the geometric area of the membrane surface.

Atomic force microscopy (AFM; Bruker Dimension Edge) was used to measure the surface roughness of the membrane. The average roughness (Ra) and root mean square roughness (Rq) of the membrane were measured from the AFM images of three different positions on the membrane surface using Gwyddion 2.48 software. The morphology and surface and cross-sectional structures of the membranes were observed by SEM (S-4800). Before observations, all membrane samples were sputtered with gold. The membrane samples were frozen and made brittle using liquid nitrogen to obtain a flat membrane cross-sectional structure. The average pore size and porosity of the membrane surface were quantitatively calculated using ImageJ v1.48 software.

3.4. Simulated Stabilized Oil-in-Water Emulsions

Cutting oil (0.05 g) and 0.05 g anionic surfactant sodium dodecyl sulfate (SDS) were added to a beaker and then ultrasonically mixed for 20 min. Then, the solution was stirred for 36 h at 500 rpm until a 0.05 g L^{-1} uniform yellow emulsion was obtained. To avoid suspension or separation of oil droplets during storage, the emulsions were configured 36 h before use. The size of the emulsified oil droplet was measured using a laser particle sizer (Master 2000). The results in Figure 10 and Table 5 show that the size distribution of the emulsified oil droplet was in the range of 0.171–0.266 μm, with a median average particle diameter D_{50} of 0.209 μm. This indicated that the particle size range of the prepared SSEW was narrow, and the overall oil droplet particle size was uniform.

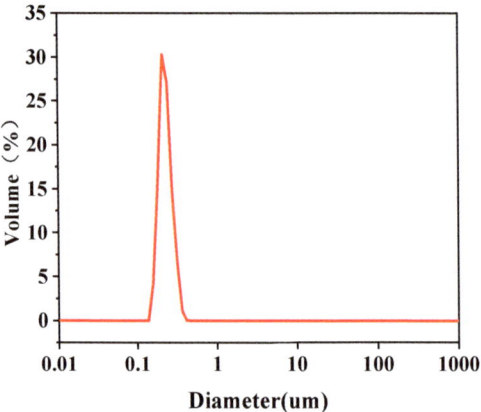

Figure 10. Particle size distribution of oil droplets in emulsions.

Table 5. Particle size distribution of emulsified oil droplets.

Emulsified Oil Droplet Size (µm)	D10	D50	D90	D(3,2)	D(4,3)
Feed liquid	0.171	0.209	0.266	0.208	0.214

3.5. Zeta Potential of the MF Membrane and Emulsified Oil

The zeta potential on the surface of the MF membrane was measured using a SurPASS solid surface zeta potential meter (Malvern Zetasizer Nano ZS90, Hefei, China). At ambient temperature, 1 mM KCl solution was employed as the electrolyte, and 5 mm HCl and NaOH solutions were used to adjust the pH in the range of 3–10. The test pressure was set to 30 kPa in terms of flowing current, and the two samples faced each other so that the slit spacing was controlled to 90–110 µm. Tests were repeated twice in the left and right directions. The zeta potential of emulsified oil wastewater was measured using a nanoparticle size analyzer (ZS-90, Malvern, UK). A certain content of samples was dispersed in deionized water (0.1 wt%), and ultrasonic oscillation was carried out for 20 min. The zeta potential was measured three times. All experiments were reported as the average values of three replicates.

3.6. Membrane Filtration and Antifouling Performance

The permeability, antifouling, and rejection performance of the MF membrane to the emulsified oil were measured using a cross-flow filtration device. The effective membrane area was 19 cm^2. The MF membrane was pre-pressed with deionized water for 30 min at a pressure of 0.15 MPa to obtain a stable pure water flux. Subsequently, the pressure was reduced to 0.1 MPa, and filtration was continued for 30 min to obtain the initial pure water flux of the membrane. Then, emulsified oil wastewater was treated as the feed liquid for 1.0 h. After that, the membrane was washed with 0.05 M NaOH solution for 5 min, and then deionized water for 25 min to remove residual NaOH. The membrane was filtered again with deionized water for 30 min to test the pure water flux recovered. The membrane flux J (LMH bar^{-1}) was calculated using Formula (2):

$$J = \frac{m}{\rho A \triangle t} \quad (2)$$

where m (kg) is the mass quality of infiltration water, A (m^2) is the effective membrane surface area, ρ is the density of water (1.0×10^3 kg m^{-3}), and Δt (h) is the filtration time. The BSA rejection rate R (%) of the membrane was calculated according to Formula (3):

$$R = \left(1 - \frac{C_p}{C_f}\right) \times 100\% \tag{3}$$

where C_f is the BSA concentration in the original solution, mg L^{-1}, and C_p is the BSA concentration in the solution after penetration, which was measured in terms of the absorbance at 278 nm using ultraviolet–visible (UV–vis) spectrophotometry.

The antifouling performance of the emulsified oil wastewater of the membrane was expressed by the flux recovery rate (FRR; %), as shown in the Formula (4):

$$FRR = \frac{J_{wc}}{J_{wv}} \times 100\% \tag{4}$$

where J_{wv} (LMH bar^{-1}) is the initial stable pure water flux and J_{wc} is the recovered water flux after filtering the emulsified oil wastewater.

The reversible fouling ratio (R_r), irreversible fouling ratio (R_{ir}), and total fouling ratio (R_t) were calculated using Equations (5)–(7): [59]

$$R_t = \left(\frac{J_{wv} - J_F}{J_{wv}}\right) \times 100\% \tag{5}$$

$$R_r = \left(\frac{J_{wc} - J_F}{J_{wv}}\right) \times 100\% \tag{6}$$

$$R_{ir} = \left(1 - \frac{J_{wc}}{J_{wv}}\right) \times 100\% \tag{7}$$

where J_F is the emulsified oil solution flux.

4. Conclusions

Membranes made from various TB/ZTB ratios were prepared using VIPS and utilized to separate emulsified oil wastewater. The relationships between membrane performance and various preparation parameters were investigated. The blended ZTB/TB MF membranes with zwitterionic properties demonstrated excellent hydrophilicity, high rejection rates, and a high antifouling performance when used for emulsified oil wastewater treatment. The hydrophilicity of the MF membrane gradually decreased upon increasing the ZTB content. The cross-sectional structure of the MF membrane exhibited a spongy bicontinuous structure resulting from the delayed phase separation mechanism during VIPS. Additionally, the blended MF membranes exhibited a significantly greater surface porosity and average surface pore diameter compared with the pristine TB MF membrane. Interactions between foulants and the membrane surface could be fine-tuned by regulating the surface charge and hydrophilicity in a synergistic manner, which can prevent irreversible fouling. This study demonstrates the potential for the development of high-performance MF membranes in the treatment of emulsified oily wastewater.

Author Contributions: Conceptualization, S.L. and H.T.; methodology, S.L. and H.T.; validation, S.L. and H.T.; formal analysis, M.W. and T.H.; investigation, T.H.; data curation, M.W. and T.H.; writing—original draft preparation, M.W. and T.H.; software, T.H.; writing—review and editing, M.S. (Meng Shan) and M.S. (Mei Sun); visualization, M.S. (Meng Shan) and M.S. (Mei Sun); funding acquisition, S.L. and H.T. All authors have read and agreed to the published version of the manuscript.

Funding: This research was funded by Anhui Natural Science Foundation (2108085ME188), the Anhui Polytechnic University Startup Foundation for Introduced Talents, China (No. 2021YQQ048), and the Key Program of Anhui Polytechnic University, China (No. Xjky2022115), National Innovative Entrepreneurship Training Program for Undergraduates (202210363059).

Institutional Review Board Statement: Not applicable.

Informed Consent Statement: Not applicable.

Data Availability Statement: Data are contained within the article.

Acknowledgments: The authors acknowledge Zijie Xu of Anhui Polytechnic University for his testing supporting.

Conflicts of Interest: The authors declare no conflict of interest.

References

1. Shi, P.; Zhang, R.; Pu, W.; Liu, R.; Fang, S. Coalescence and separation of surfactant-stabilized water-in-oil emulsion via membrane coalescer functionalized by demulsifier. *J. Clean. Prod.* **2022**, *330*, 129945. [CrossRef]
2. Xiang, B.; Shi, G.; Mu, P.; Li, J. Eco-friendly WBF/PAN nanofiber composite membrane for efficient separation various surfactant-stabilized oil-in-water emulsions. *Colloids Surf. A Physicochem. Eng. Asp.* **2022**, *645*, 128917. [CrossRef]
3. You, X.; Liao, Y.; Tian, M.; Chew, J.W.; Wang, R. Engineering highly effective nanofibrous membranes to demulsify surfactant-stabilized oil-in-water emulsions. *J. Membr. Sci.* **2020**, *611*, 118398. [CrossRef]
4. Deng, Y.; Dai, M.; Wu, Y.; Peng, C. Emulsion system, demulsification and membrane technology in oil–water emulsion separation: A comprehensive review. *Crit. Rev. Environ. Sci. Technol.* **2023**, *53*, 1254–1278. [CrossRef]
5. Chen, L.; Si, Y.; Zhu, H.; Jiang, T.; Guo, Z. A study on the fabrication of porous PVDF membranes by in-situ elimination and their applications in separating oil/water mixtures and nano-emulsions. *J. Membr. Sci.* **2016**, *520*, 760–768. [CrossRef]
6. Song, S.; Yang, H.; Zhou, C.; Cheng, J.; Jiang, Z.; Lu, Z.; Miao, J. Underwater superoleophobic mesh based on BiVO4 nanoparticles with sunlight-driven self-cleaning property for oil/water separation. *Chem. Eng. J.* **2017**, *320*, 342–351. [CrossRef]
7. Sun, H.; Tang, B.; Wu, P. Development of Hybrid Ultrafiltration Membranes with Improved Water Separation Properties Using Modified Superhydrophilic Metal–Organic Framework Nanoparticles. *ACS Appl. Mater. Interfaces* **2017**, *9*, 21473–21484. [CrossRef]
8. Liu, Y.; Su, Y.; Cao, J.; Guan, J.; Zhang, R.; He, M.; Fan, L.; Zhang, Q.; Jiang, Z. Antifouling, high-flux oil/water separation carbon nanotube membranes by polymer-mediated surface charging and hydrophilization. *J. Membr. Sci.* **2017**, *542*, 254–263. [CrossRef]
9. Mat Nawi, N.I.; Chean, H.M.; Shamsuddin, N.; Bilad, M.R.; Narkkun, T.; Faungnawakij, K.; Khan, A.L. Development of Hydrophilic PVDF Membrane Using Vapour Induced Phase Separation Method for Produced Water Treatment. *Membranes* **2020**, *10*, 121. [CrossRef] [PubMed]
10. Wang, M.; Xu, Z.; Guo, Y.; Hou, Y.; Li, P.; Niu, Q.J. Engineering a superwettable polyolefin membrane for highly efficient oil/water separation with excellent self-cleaning and photo-catalysis degradation property. *J. Membr. Sci.* **2020**, *611*, 118409. [CrossRef]
11. Liang, S.; Kang, Y.; Tiraferri, A.; Giannelis, E.P.; Huang, X.; Elimelech, M. Highly Hydrophilic Polyvinylidene Fluoride (PVDF) Ultrafiltration Membranes via Postfabrication Grafting of Surface-Tailored Silica Nanoparticles. *ACS Appl. Mater. Interfaces* **2013**, *5*, 6694–6703. [CrossRef]
12. Safarpour, M.; Hosseinpour, S.; Haddad Irani-nezhad, M.; Orooji, Y.; Khataee, A. Fabrication of Ti$_2$SnC-MAX Phase Blended PES Membranes with Improved Hydrophilicity and Antifouling Properties for Oil/Water Separation. *Molecules* **2022**, *27*, 8914. [CrossRef] [PubMed]
13. Song, C.; Rutledge, G.C. Electrospun Liquid-Infused Membranes for Emulsified Oil/Water Separation. *Langmuir* **2022**, *38*, 2301–2313. [CrossRef]
14. Li, P.; Ge, Q. Membrane Surface Engineering with Bifunctional Zwitterions for Efficient Oil–Water Separation. *ACS Appl. Mater. Interfaces* **2019**, *11*, 31328–31337. [CrossRef] [PubMed]
15. Wang, J.; Qiu, M.; He, C. A zwitterionic polymer/PES membrane for enhanced antifouling performance and promoting hemocompatibility. *J. Membr. Sci.* **2020**, *606*, 118119. [CrossRef]
16. Zang, L.; Zheng, S.; Wang, L.; Ma, J.; Sun, L. Zwitterionic nanogels modified nanofibrous membrane for efficient oil/water separation. *J. Membr. Sci.* **2020**, *612*, 118379. [CrossRef]
17. Ghaffar, A.; Zhu, X.; Chen, B. Biochar composite membrane for high performance pollutant management: Fabrication, structural characteristics and synergistic mechanisms. *Environ. Pollut.* **2018**, *233*, 1013–1023. [CrossRef] [PubMed]
18. Venault, A.; Wei, T.-C.; Shih, H.-L.; Yeh, C.-C.; Chinnathambi, A.; Alharbi, S.A.; Carretier, S.; Aimar, P.; Lai, J.-Y.; Chang, Y. Antifouling pseudo-zwitterionic poly(vinylidene fluoride) membranes with efficient mixed-charge surface grafting via glow dielectric barrier discharge plasma-induced copolymerization. *J. Membr. Sci.* **2016**, *516*, 13–25. [CrossRef]
19. Zhao, X.; Cheng, L.; Wang, R.; Jia, N.; Liu, L.; Gao, C. Bioinspired synthesis of polyzwitterion/titania functionalized carbon nanotube membrane with superwetting property for efficient oil-in-water emulsion separation. *J. Membr. Sci.* **2019**, *589*, 117257. [CrossRef]

20. Zhu, Y.; Wang, J.; Zhang, F.; Gao, S.; Wang, A.; Fang, W.; Jin, J. Zwitterionic Nanohydrogel Grafted PVDF Membranes with Comprehensive Antifouling Property and Superior Cycle Stability for Oil-in-Water Emulsion Separation. *Adv. Funct. Mater.* **2018**, *28*, 1804121. [CrossRef]
21. Maggay, I.V.; Suba, M.C.A.M.; Aini, H.N.; Wu, C.-J.; Tang, S.-H.; Aquino, R.B.; Chang, Y.; Venault, A. Thermostable antifouling zwitterionic vapor-induced phase separation membranes. *J. Membr. Sci.* **2021**, *627*, 119227. [CrossRef]
22. Folgado, E.; Ladmiral, V.; Semsarilar, M. Towards permanent hydrophilic PVDF membranes. Amphiphilic PVDF-b-PEG-b-PVDF triblock copolymer as membrane additive. *Eur. Polym. J.* **2020**, *131*, 109708. [CrossRef]
23. Venault, A.; Chiang, C.-H.; Chang, H.-Y.; Hung, W.-S.; Chang, Y. Graphene oxide/PVDF VIPS membranes for switchable, versatile and gravity-driven separation of oil and water. *J. Membr. Sci.* **2018**, *565*, 131–144. [CrossRef]
24. Nayak, M.C.; Isloor, A.M.; Moslehyani, A.; Ismail, N.; Ismail, A.F. Fabrication of novel PPSU/ZSM-5 ultrafiltration hollow fiber membranes for separation of proteins and hazardous reactive dyes. *J. Taiwan Inst. Chem. Eng.* **2018**, *82*, 342–350. [CrossRef]
25. Dehban, A.; Kargari, A.; Ashtiani, F.Z. Preparation and optimization of antifouling PPSU/PES/SiO$_2$ nanocomposite ultrafiltration membranes by VIPS-NIPS technique. *J. Ind. Eng. Chem.* **2020**, *88*, 292–311. [CrossRef]
26. Lin, H.-T.; Venault, A.; Chang, Y. Reducing the pathogenicity of wastewater with killer vapor-induced phase separation membranes. *J. Membr. Sci.* **2020**, *614*, 118543. [CrossRef]
27. Venault, A.; Chang, C.-Y.; Tsai, T.-C.; Chang, H.-Y.; Bouyer, D.; Lee, K.-R.; Chang, Y. Surface zwitterionization of PVDF VIPS membranes for oil and water separation. *J. Membr. Sci.* **2018**, *563*, 54–64. [CrossRef]
28. Peng, Y.; Fan, H.; Dong, Y.; Song, Y.; Han, H. Effects of exposure time on variations in the structure and hydrophobicity of polyvinylidene fluoride membranes prepared via vapor-induced phase separation. *Appl. Surf. Sci.* **2012**, *258*, 7872–7881. [CrossRef]
29. Abdulazeez, I.; Salhi, B.; Elsharif, A.M.; Ahmad, M.S.; Baig, N.; Abdelnaby, M.M. Hemin-Modified Multi-Walled Carbon Nanotube-Incorporated PVDF Membranes: Computational and Experimental Studies on Oil–Water Emulsion Separations. *Molecules* **2023**, *28*, 391. [CrossRef]
30. Zhang, M.; Wang, M.; Chen, J.; Dong, L.; Tian, Y.; Cui, Z.; Li, J.; He, B.; Yan, F. Demulsifier-Inspired Superhydrophilic/Underwater Superoleophobic Membrane Modified with Polyoxypropylene Polyoxyethylene Block Polymer for Enhanced Oil/Water Separation Properties. *Molecules* **2023**, *28*, 1282. [CrossRef]
31. Chen, W.; Long, N.; Xiao, T.; Yang, X. Tuning the Pore Structure of Poly(vinylidene fluoride) Membrane for Efficient Oil/Water Separation: A Novel Vapor-Induced Phase Separation Method Based on a Lower Critical Solution Temperature System. *Ind. Eng. Chem. Res.* **2020**, *59*, 14947–14959. [CrossRef]
32. Huang, T.; Yin, J.; Tang, H.; Zhang, Z.; Liu, D.; Liu, S.; Xu, Z.; Li, N. Improved permeability and antifouling performance of Tröger's base polymer-based ultrafiltration membrane via zwitterionization. *J. Membr. Sci.* **2022**, *646*, 120251. [CrossRef]
33. Venault, A.; Chang, Y.; Wang, D.-M.; Bouyer, D. A Review on Polymeric Membranes and Hydrogels Prepared by Vapor-Induced Phase Separation Process. *Polym. Rev.* **2013**, *53*, 568–626. [CrossRef]
34. Young, T.-H.; Chen, L.-W. Pore formation mechanism of membranes from phase inversion process. *Desalination* **1995**, *103*, 233–247. [CrossRef]
35. Ismail, N.; Venault, A.; Mikkola, J.-P.; Bouyer, D.; Drioli, E.; Tavajohi Hassan Kiadeh, N. Investigating the potential of membranes formed by the vapor induced phase separation process. *J. Membr. Sci.* **2020**, *597*, 117601. [CrossRef]
36. Zhao, Q.; Xie, R.; Luo, F.; Faraj, Y.; Liu, Z.; Ju, X.-J.; Wang, W.; Chu, L.-Y. Preparation of high strength poly(vinylidene fluoride) porous membranes with cellular structure via vapor-induced phase separation. *J. Membr. Sci.* **2018**, *549*, 151–164. [CrossRef]
37. Guillen, G.R.; Pan, Y.; Li, M.; Hoek, E.M.V. Preparation and Characterization of Membranes Formed by Nonsolvent Induced Phase Separation: A Review. *Ind. Eng. Chem. Res.* **2011**, *50*, 3798–3817. [CrossRef]
38. Li, H.-B.; Shi, W.-Y.; Zhang, Y.-F.; Liu, D.-Q.; Liu, X.-F. Effects of Additives on the Morphology and Performance of PPTA/PVDF in Situ Blend UF Membrane. *Polymers* **2014**, *6*, 1846–1861. [CrossRef]
39. Wang, J.; Liu, Y.; Liu, T.; Xu, X.; Hu, Y. Improving the perm-selectivity and anti-fouling property of UF membrane through the micro-phase separation of PSf-b-PEG block copolymers. *J. Membr. Sci.* **2020**, *599*, 117851. [CrossRef]
40. Xu, M.-H.; Xie, R.; Ju, X.-J.; Wang, W.; Liu, Z.; Chu, L.-Y. Antifouling membranes with bi-continuous porous structures and high fluxes prepared by vapor-induced phase separation. *J. Membr. Sci.* **2020**, *611*, 118256. [CrossRef]
41. Dehban, A.; Hosseini Saeedavi, F.; Kargari, A. A study on the mechanism of pore formation through VIPS-NIPS technique for membrane fabrication. *J. Ind. Eng. Chem.* **2022**, *108*, 54–71. [CrossRef]
42. Peng, Y.; Dong, Y.; Fan, H.; Chen, P.; Li, Z.; Jiang, Q. Preparation of polysulfone membranes via vapor-induced phase separation and simulation of direct-contact membrane distillation by measuring hydrophobic layer thickness. *Desalination* **2013**, *316*, 53–66. [CrossRef]
43. Yi, G.; Chen, S.; Quan, X.; Wei, G.; Fan, X.; Yu, H. Enhanced separation performance of carbon nanotube–polyvinyl alcohol composite membranes for emulsified oily wastewater treatment under electrical assistance. *Sep. Purif. Technol.* **2018**, *197*, 107–115. [CrossRef]
44. Dehban, A.; Kargari, A.; Zokaee Ashtiani, F. Preparation and characterization of an antifouling poly (phenyl sulfone) ultrafiltration membrane by vapor-induced phase separation technique. *Sep. Purif. Technol.* **2019**, *212*, 986–1000. [CrossRef]
45. Venault, A.; Chang, Y.; Wang, D.-M.; Lai, J.-Y. Surface anti-biofouling control of PEGylated poly(vinylidene fluoride) membranes via vapor-induced phase separation processing. *J. Membr. Sci.* **2012**, *423–424*, 53–64. [CrossRef]

46. Lu, D.; Zhang, T.; Gutierrez, L.; Ma, J.; Croué, J.-P. Influence of Surface Properties of Filtration-Layer Metal Oxide on Ceramic Membrane Fouling during Ultrafiltration of Oil/Water Emulsion. *Environ. Sci. Technol.* **2016**, *50*, 4668–4674. [CrossRef]
47. Liu, Z.; Xu, Z.; Liu, C.; Zhao, Y.; Xia, Q.; Fang, M.; Min, X.; Huang, Z.; Liu, Y.G.; Wu, X. Polydopamine Nanocluster Embedded Nanofibrous Membrane via Blow Spinning for Separation of Oil/Water Emulsions. *Molecules* **2021**, *26*, 3258. [CrossRef]
48. Tang, B.; Huo, Z.; Wu, P. Study on a novel polyester composite nanofiltration membrane by interfacial polymerization of triethanolamine (TEOA) and trimesoyl chloride (TMC): I. Preparation, characterization and nanofiltration properties test of membrane. *J. Membr. Sci.* **2008**, *320*, 198–205. [CrossRef]
49. Zhao, X.; Su, Y.; Liu, Y.; Li, Y.; Jiang, Z. Free-Standing Graphene Oxide-Palygorskite Nanohybrid Membrane for Oil/Water Separation. *ACS Appl. Mater. Interfaces* **2016**, *8*, 8247–8256. [CrossRef]
50. Tsai, J.T.; Su, Y.S.; Wang, D.M.; Kuo, J.L.; Lai, J.Y.; Deratani, A. Retainment of pore connectivity in membranes prepared with vapor-induced phase separation. *J. Membr. Sci.* **2010**, *362*, 360–373. [CrossRef]
51. Liu, Y.; Su, Y.; Zhao, X.; Li, Y.; Zhang, R.; Jiang, Z. Improved antifouling properties of polyethersulfone membrane by blending the amphiphilic surface modifier with crosslinked hydrophobic segments. *J. Membr. Sci.* **2015**, *486*, 195–206. [CrossRef]
52. Barambu, N.U.; Bilad, M.R.; Bustam, M.A.; Huda, N.; Jaafar, J.; Narkkun, T.; Faungnawakij, K. Development of Polysulfone Membrane via Vapor-Induced Phase Separation for Oil/Water Emulsion Filtration. *Polymers* **2020**, *12*, 2519. [CrossRef]
53. Yu, Y.; Han, Q.; Lin, H.; Zhang, S.; Yang, Q.; Liu, F. Fine regulation on hour-glass like spongy structure of polyphenylsulfone (PPSU)/sulfonated polysulfone (SPSf) MF membranes via a vapor-liquid induced phase separation (V-LIPS) technique. *J. Membr. Sci.* **2022**, *660*, 120872. [CrossRef]
54. Chang, H.-Y.; Venault, A. Adjusting the morphology of poly(vinylidene fluoride-co-hexafluoropropylene) membranes by the VIPS process for efficient oil-rich emulsion separation. *J. Membr. Sci.* **2019**, *581*, 178–194. [CrossRef]
55. Wang, Y.; Yang, H.; Yang, Y.; Zhu, L.; Zeng, Z.; Liu, S.; Li, Y.; Liang, Z. Poly(vinylidene fluoride) membranes with underwater superoleophobicity for highly efficient separation of oil-in-water emulsions in resisting fouling. *Sep. Purif. Technol.* **2022**, *285*, 120298. [CrossRef]
56. Ong, C.; Shi, Y.; Chang, J.; Alduraiei, F.; Wehbe, N.; Ahmed, Z.; Wang, P. Tannin-inspired robust fabrication of superwettability membranes for highly efficient separation of oil-in-water emulsions and immiscible oil/water mixtures. *Sep. Purif. Technol.* **2019**, *227*, 115657. [CrossRef]
57. Li, H.-N.; Yang, J.; Xu, Z.-K. Hollow fiber membranes with Janus surfaces for continuous deemulsification and separation of oil-in-water emulsions. *J. Membr. Sci.* **2020**, *602*, 117964. [CrossRef]
58. Lu, P.; Liang, S.; Qiu, L.; Gao, Y.; Wang, Q. Thin film nanocomposite forward osmosis membranes based on layered double hydroxide nanoparticles blended substrates. *J. Membr. Sci.* **2016**, *504*, 196–205. [CrossRef]
59. Zhang, C.; Huang, R.; Tang, H.; Zhang, Z.; Xu, Z.; Li, N. Enhanced antifouling and separation properties of Tröger's base polymer ultrafiltration membrane via ring-opening modification. *J. Membr. Sci.* **2020**, *597*, 117763. [CrossRef]

Disclaimer/Publisher's Note: The statements, opinions and data contained in all publications are solely those of the individual author(s) and contributor(s) and not of MDPI and/or the editor(s). MDPI and/or the editor(s) disclaim responsibility for any injury to people or property resulting from any ideas, methods, instructions or products referred to in the content.

MDPI AG
Grosspeteranlage 5
4052 Basel
Switzerland
Tel.: +41 61 683 77 34

Molecules Editorial Office
E-mail: molecules@mdpi.com
www.mdpi.com/journal/molecules

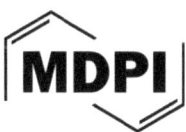

Disclaimer/Publisher's Note: The title and front matter of this reprint are at the discretion of the Guest Editor. The publisher is not responsible for their content or any associated concerns. The statements, opinions and data contained in all individual articles are solely those of the individual Editor and contributors and not of MDPI. MDPI disclaims responsibility for any injury to people or property resulting from any ideas, methods, instructions or products referred to in the content.

www.ingramcontent.com/pod-product-compliance
Lightning Source LLC
LaVergne TN
LVHW072346090526
838202LV00019B/2487